PROFESSIONAL PERSPECTIVES IN HEALTH CARE

Also by Carol Wilkinson

Nursing in Primary Care, *edited with Naomi Watson*
(Palgrave, 2001)

Professional Perspectives in Health Care

Edited by

Carol Wilkinson

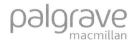

First published 2007 by
PALGRAVE MACMILLAN
Houndmills, Basingstoke, Hampshire RG21 6XS and
175 Fifth Avenue, New York, N.Y. 10010
Companies and representatives throughout the world

PALGRAVE MACMILLAN is the global academic imprint of the Palgrave Macmillan division of St. Martin's Press, LLC and of Palgrave Macmillan Ltd. Macmillan[®] is a registered trademark in the United States, United Kingdom and other countries. Palgrave is a registered trademark in the European Union and other countries.

ISBN 13: 978–1–4039–9058–7
ISBN 10: 1–4039–9058–1

This book is printed on paper suitable for recycling and made from fully managed and sustained forest sources. Logging, pulping and manufacturing processes are expected to conform to the environmental regulations of the country of origin.

A catalogue record for this book is available from the British Library.

10   9   8   7   6   5   4   3   2   1
16 15 14 13 12 11 10 09 08 07

Printed in China

To Nancy, Barry and David

Contents

List of Tables

List of Figures

Acknowledgements

The editor and contributors would like to thank the following: Lincolnshire South West Primary Care Trust, West Lincolnshire Primary Care Trust, Trent Research Development Support Unit, Milton Keynes NHS Trust, Lincolnshire Research Ethics Committee, East Midlands Mental Health Research Hub, Library Staff at the Universities of Lincoln, Sheffield, De Montfort and Nottingham, Heather DuMughn, Moira Gove, Steve Knight, the Parkin Family, Noreen Thorp, the Royal College of Nursing, Edinburgh.

A. Niroshan Siriwardena, the author of Chapter 1, would like to acknowledge that the final chapter section on knowledge translation draws on work that he completed as part of his doctoral thesis. He expresses particular thanks to Carol Wilkinson for her comments and suggestions, and to doctors on the South Trent MRCGP course on whom he tested the examples.

Notes on the Contributors

Lianne Aquilina trained originally as a dental nurse. Having completed a degree in Complementary Medicine, she is now a practising acupuncturist based in Stamford, Lincolnshire.

Katie Cook trained as a nurse and is currently Practice Placement Facilitator at the University of Hull. Her interests include the education and development of student nurses.

Jo Cooke is Health and Social Care Lead at Trent Research Support and Development Unit based in Sheffield.

Mark R. D. Johnson is Professor of Equality and Diversity in Health and Social Care at De Montfort University. He is Director of the Mary Seacole Research Centre.

Jo Middlemass trained originally as a nurse and health visitor. She has worked as Research Governance Lead for West Lincolnshire Primary Care Trust and is currently Senior Research Fellow at the University of Nottingham.

Anne Parkin is a practising medical herbalist based in Lincoln.

Gill Sarre is Health and Social Care Lead at Trent Research Support Development Unit based in Nottingham.

A. Niroshan Siriwardena is a general practitioner and Visiting Professor of Primary Care at the University of Lincoln. His research interests include primary care mental health, and innovation and education for professionals working in primary and pre-hospital care.

Judy Smith trained as a podiatrist and is currently working as Research and Development Facilitator for Lincolnshire South West Primary Care Trust. She is also a founder member of the East Nottinghamshire and Lincolnshire Designated Research Team.

Andrew Stableford is a practising medical herbalist with almost thirty years' experience, and a member of the National Institute of Medical Herbalists. He is also Senior Lecturer at the University of Lincoln where he is Programme Leader for Herbal Medicine degrees.

Nicola Waddie is Assistant Director of Nursing at the United Lincolnshire Hospitals Trust based in Lincolnshire. She has recently completed her PhD investigating the working lives of nurses. Her research interests include the study of pain. She is also Principal Lecturer at the University of Lincoln.

Carol Wilkinson is Principal Lecturer in Health Studies at the University of Lincoln. Her recent publications include *Fundamentals of Health at Work* and she is co-author of *Nursing in Primary Care* (also published by Palgrave Macmillan).

Introduction

This text presents a series of essays and empirical research projects undertaken within the field of health care. The work is discussed by a range of practising health professionals and academics who provide a rich and stimulating insight into the ways in which micro- and macro-health policies have and are currently affecting change within health services and health care delivery. The potential impact upon patients, health professionals, students and consumers of health care is discussed and analysed.

The range of material relates to practice, working relationships, opinions on complementary medicine and cultures across a selection of health care settings. The emphasis is on issues that influence health improvement: driving up standards, efficiency and effectiveness, and building research capacity to support and improve quality in health care for all users of the service and those involved in managing, supporting and delivering care.

Expression is also given to the interventions that exist for a more cohesive, dynamic and informed frame of reference for health care initiatives, and requirements for the future. The contributions are intended to give critical insight into developments that all health professionals, students and other interested parties will be able to relate to in their quest to find some fundamental answers to the health problems of the day.

The text is divided into two parts. Part I provides a context of the current concerns within health care, and Part II looks at a series of empirical research projects demonstrating various approaches to qualitative research and its use in health care. The intention is to demonstrate the effect of health policy upon different aspects of the service and to stimulate further debate.

Part I

The Effect of Policy Intervention upon Professional
Working Arrangements in Health Care

CHAPTER 1

Evidence-based Practice

A. NIROSHAN SIRIWARDENA

What is evidence-based practice?

It may come as something of a surprise to many of our patients that the advice we give and that they receive from us as practitioners is not based on the best available evidence – or indeed for that matter on any evidence at all. It may be even more of a revelation that there is a body of opinion that decries even the notion of evidence-based practice.

Evidence-based practice is the accessing, appraisal and application of appropriate best evidence applied with professional expertise and experience, having due consideration for patient preference and modified in light of local contextual factors, by health care practitioners to the management of patient, population and organizational problems presented in their professional practice. This is broader than previous definitions. For example, the often-quoted definition 'the conscientious, explicit, and judicious use of current best evidence in making decisions about the care of individual patients ... integrating individual clinical expertise with the best available external clinical evidence from systematic research' (Sackett et al. 1996) ignores the importance of accessing the literature appropriately (Rosenberg and Donald 1995), and the fact that as practitioners we are also making decisions about how we organize and deliver care for our practice populations based on research evidence. Rosenberg and Donald's (1995) definition 'systematically finding, appraising, and using contemporaneous research findings as the basis for clinical decisions', although acknowledging the issue of retrieval, ignores both clinical judgement and patient preference. Yet another definition, that by Greenhalgh (2001), 'the enhancement of a clinician's traditional skills in diagnosis, treatment and prevention and related areas through the systematic framing of relevant and answerable questions and the use of mathematical estimates of probability and risk' by emphasizing the quantitative overlooks the increasing relevance of qualitative research to individual care as well as to concerns of the population or system (Smith 1996) – see Figure 1.1.

The origins of evidence-based practice lie, arguably, in the explosion in biomedical literature in the past fifty years. This has been aided, in no small part, by the electronic revolution. Before this, a handful of anti-tuberculous

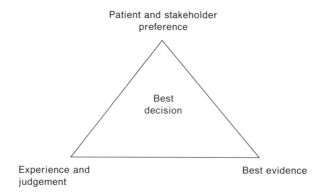

Figure 1.1 Relationship between patient preference, medical evidence and clinical experience

drugs and early antibiotics, together with drugs based on poisons such as foxglove, mercury and arsenic, were the mainstay of the therapeutic armamentarium of the practitioner. The massive increase in published evidence as well as increased access to evidence by practitioners and patients leads to inherent practical problems of retrieval, interpretation and application of the evidence, ethical dilemmas underlying the notion of evidence-based practice and conflicting effects on professional and expert power. There are a number of ethical dimensions to the use and abuse of evidence relating to beneficence (doing good), non-maleficence (doing no harm), distributive justice (equity) and autonomy (patients' rights to understand and determine their treatment).

This chapter will explore the broad notion of evidence-based practice in relation to today's health system by exploring the historical drivers and development of the idea, the ethical and professional issues and challenges that it raises, and its relevance to current practice. It will also discuss the use of evidence-based practice in detail, using a case study approach. Finally, there will be integration and synthesis of the path to evidence-based practice including evidence, beliefs about evidence and the implementation of evidence-based practice in its professional context using a new theoretical framework.

The history of evidence-based practice

Many of the original ideas on evidence-based practice were articulated in the seminal work of Archibald Cochrane. As a health services researcher he pioneered the notion that the health service should provide treatments based on evidence rather than anecdote (Cochrane 1972).

The evidence-based medicine movement subsequently developed rapidly in North America (for example, at McMaster University) and Australia, spreading swiftly to the United Kingdom, Europe and worldwide. From the first

Medline citation of 'evidence-based medicine' in 1992 to several thousand currently, and with over one million internet sites listed on Google, there is strong evidence for the phenomenal interest and importance of this area to researchers and health practitioners (Straus 2004). Clinical guidelines became an important instrument for the dissemination of evidence-based practice in North America and Europe (Siriwardena 1995) on the 1980s and 1990s. Evidence-based medicine rapidly incorporated evidence-based nursing (and other professional groups) to form evidence-based practice.

There are underlying assumptions to evidence-based practice including an innovation bias that good clinicians should use research that improves clinical practice and that scientific knowledge is required for effective change and efficient choices.

However, there has also been a backlash, with vociferous opponents of evidence-based medicine decrying the very values of the movement, some-times tongue in cheek (Clinicians for the Restoration of Autonomous Practice (CRAP) Writing Group 2002), leading to some proponents subtly reinventing and restating their case to address the criticisms (Sackett et al. 1996). Despite this, a number of centres of excellence have developed including the international Cochrane Collaboration, which was established in 1993, and the NHS Centre for Reviews and Dissemination at York, together with a number of other United Kingdom government initiatives promoting clinical effectiveness (NHS Executive 1996; NHS Management Executive 1993).

Since Cochrane there have been a number of opinion leaders and champions of the cause of evidence-based practice, notably David Sackett at Oxford and Trisha Greenhalgh in London, although many other influential figures in medicine, nursing and the allied health professions across the globe have contributed to developments in evidence-based practice.

The ethical basis of evidence-based practice

There are a number of fundamental ethical reasons why evidence-based practice has assumed such importance in health care. Firstly, one of the founding principles of many health services is the concept of justice, particularly distributive justice or equity. That there are considerable variations in health care delivery and that many of these might be unexplained by case-mix or any justifiable factor leads to the idea that injustice through unacceptable variations in health care is operating (for example, 'postcode' prescribing) and should be addressed.

Secondly, there is a natural logic to the idea that applying evidence appropriately will improve health outcomes thereby doing good (beneficence) as it will by applying treatments where benefits outweigh harms prevent negative consequences (non-maleficence). Thirdly, by taking into account patient preferences in decision-making, the principle of autonomy and informed choice is being upheld. A cost-effective application of limited resources in providing value for money also sits well with the notion of equity, freeing up resources for those interventions that are proven, whilst denying resources for practices that are dubious and wasteful of opportunities.

An alternative ethical analysis involves a consequentialist model, where consequentialism seeks to measure value based on the sequelae of an action. Problems with evidence-based practice include immeasurable or unmeasured outcomes of experimental studies such as harms, costs or long-term outcomes (most notably thalidomide). Also values of different stakeholders cannot always be reconciled and deciding between competing claims ultimately relies on judgement rather than science. Some studies, which have been carried out unethically, will contribute to the evidence base. Vested interests (for example, the pharmaceutical industry) will result in more evidence in certain areas and potentially greater health care resources being directed to those areas, such as drug therapy, in contrast with other areas that are more difficult to research or less attractive to funding bodies (for example psychological therapy or palliative care; see Kerridge et al. 1998).

Barriers and facilitators to evidence-based practice

Despite the potential of evidence-based practice for quality improvement and greater equity in health care and increasing awareness amongst health care workers of its importance (Hagdrup et al. 1998), there is evidence of considerable difficulties with the notion of evidence-based practice. The barriers are complex and may arise from practitioners due to negative attitudes, lack of confidence, poor knowledge (Khan et al. 2001), deficient skills and lack of time (McColl et al. 1998) for accessing and appraising evidence (Wilkinson et al. 2000). Practitioners on the one hand want expert groups or individuals to appraise evidence on their behalf because of lack of time, resources and expertise but at the same time remain suspicious of the quality of 'expert' reviews (McColl et al. 1998; Siriwardena et al. 2004), perhaps justifiably so, because expert reviewers tended to produce reviews of poorer quality than researchers who were not experts in the particular field (Oxman 1994). On a practical level, many practitioners consult colleagues and experts in preference to published evidence, sometimes because of lack of access to computers and literature or because of a lack of perceived relevance. Community staff, such as nurses and professions allied to medicine, have particular difficulties with accessing information technology (Falshaw et al. 2000) but nurses felt more confident than general practitioners in their skills in undertaking literature searches and appraisal (O'Donnell 2004).

Further problems occur in relating evidence to experience, applying evidence derived from secondary care to primary care, harmonizing evidence with local specialist guidance and in the weight given by colleagues to conflicting evidence, doubts about the permanence of evidence, individualizing care whilst maintaining the doctor patient relationship, and applying and communicating evidence in the context of the general practice consultation (Oswald and Bateman 2000; Temple 2002).

Practitioners also have real concerns about the quality and range of evidence available, the problem of changing behaviour as a result of evidence and the detrimental effect on professionalism from external pressure to implement evidence (Siriwardena et al. 2004). Some areas of health care, for example physical therapies, have particular challenges with designing valid experimental studies to prove effectiveness whereas other health care paradigms, such as some forms of complementary medicine, rejected traditional notions of scientific evidence altogether (Freeman and Sweeney 2001; Oswald and Bateman 1999). There are also real difficulties applying evidence from highly selected study populations in randomized controlled studies (Oswald and Bateman 1999), which often exclude women, the elderly and those with multiple conditions or comorbidities, and are therefore divorced from medical reality (Knottnerus and Dinant 1997).

Patient factors such as resistance or rejection of evidence (Freeman and Sweeney 2001) and factors relating to the evidence such as applicability, interpretation, validity or contradictory evidence (Hammersley 2001) are also important barriers to implementation, although it could be argued that by incorporating patient preference this fits in with an evidence-based approach.

Potential facilitators of evidence-based practice include protected time, increased resources (financial and staff) and training but also multiprofessional education and working, where professional staff, particularly non-medical perceive interprofessional boundaries as barriers to implementing evidence (O'Donnell 2004).

Evidence-based practice and professionalization

Hampton stridently declared in an editorial that 'clinical freedom is dead ... and no one need regret its passing.' It was 'at best a cloak for ignorance and at worst an excuse for quackery' (Hampton 1993). This statement, which highlights an apparent conflict between evidence-based practice and professional values, is partly explained by the concept of the indeterminacy–technicality ratio (Jamous and Pelloile 1970).

On the one hand, the implementation of evidence-based practice will enhance the professional status of the practitioner as a technical expert in the eyes of peers, other health care professionals and patients. However, at the same time, such knowledge when disseminated through publication becomes knowledge accessible to other professionals and patients and this may have the opposite effect of deprofessionalizing and emasculating the practitioner. This may occur by encouraging external control through 'top-down' or expert guidance, policy or protocol. By increasing fragmentation of the professional role into a subspecialist role through increasing technical and knowledge requirements, it enables other practitioners to develop the skills to care for patients in defined areas of technical expertise. This process has been termed deprofessionalization or proletarianization.

Indeterminacy or uncertainty is also a double-edged sword. The admission of complete uncertainty about the correct course of action in a situation will not usually enhance a practitioner's status in the eyes of professional colleagues or patients. If the knowledge of a patient or client is equal to that of the practitioner, then the professional becomes less valuable to the service user (Siriwardena 1995). But the art of the practitioner includes not only published evidence but also clinical experience, intuition and tacit knowledge (so-called 'sticky' knowledge because it sticks to the practitioner) which when applied to interpreting symptoms, solving complex problems and individualizing care, whether operating where there is clear evidence or in the grey zones of uncertainty (Naylor 1995), is part of the mystique and art of the healthcare practitioner.

To some extent even tacit knowledge can be written down in the form of narrative (Greenhalgh 1999) and analysed through qualitative research (Pope and Mays 1995).

Is current practice based on evidence?

The apocryphal tale is told of the eminent consultant on his ward round who states solemnly that at least half his treatments were based on good evidence – he just didn't know which half they were! A number of studies have been undertaken to assess whether and to what extent practice was based on evidence.

One study undertaken in a general medical ward at the Radcliffe Infirmary at Oxford contended that 82 per cent of inpatient interventions were evidence-based (Ellis et al. 1995). This was based on analysis relating the primary diagnosis of 109 patients managed during one month with evidence of randomized-controlled trial support of effectiveness of treatments used (53%) or unanimous agreement about supportive non-experimental evidence (29%). Another study of a suburban training practice in Leeds declared that 81 per cent of general practice interventions were evidence-based. This involved analysing 122 consultations over two days relating first recorded diagnosis to randomized-controlled trial (30%) or convincing non-experimental evidence (50%). Unfortunately, one fifth of the consultations were excluded because they involved referral or investigation, despite the importance of such interventions being based on evidence also. Both of these studies also failed to account for patients presenting with multiple diagnoses. Both studies used evidence from single randomized-controlled studies, which may give rise to opposite conclusions for the same intervention, rather than systematic reviews of evidence. A further study in forty psychiatric inpatients admitted during a month showed 65 per cent of interventions based on systematic reviews or randomized-controlled study evidence (Geddes et al. 1996).

However, the alternatives to evidence-based practice, where there is compelling evidence for a particular course of action, seem difficult to justify except when a fully informed patient declines. The alternatives including anecdotal medicine and 'expert' opinion (eminence-based practice) (Greenhalgh 2001) have little to commend them.

Discovering evidence-based practice

What do we mean by evidence?

Evidence in the context of evidence-based practice usually means published evidence. As well as scientific knowledge through experimentation, valid evidence can also be theoretical or practical. Expert, judicial and ethically derived evidence are also important categories of evidence. Despite the initial emphasis on quantitative evidence, the concept of evidence has broadened to include qualitative evidence including narrative. The advantage of narrative is that it is one way of externalizing and therefore exposing tacit knowledge and experience to analysis and deliberation (de Lusignan et al. 2002).

Formulating answerable questions: the patient or problem, intervention, comparisons, outcomes (PICO) model

The first step in accessing evidence is to formulate an answerable question in clear terms. Clinical questions arise from patients presenting to us with a clinical problem; non-clinical questions, for example relating to organization of services, also occur in day-to-day practice. The patient or organization's unmet need becomes a practitioner's educational need and the problem poses a potentially answerable question.

Practitioners often avoid asking this type of question. This may be because they think they know 'the answer' to 'the question' from earlier, even undergraduate, studies, even though this knowledge may have been acquired decades previously. They may also be put off asking questions because of a lack of awareness that this might be a gap in their knowledge (so-called 'unconscious incompetence'), lack of time, pressure of work, competing demands or other reasons. Even if a question comes to mind, this may not be addressed for similar reasons or it may not be formulated in an answerable way. Sometimes a question arises and is acted on, but the action involves asking a colleague who answers using outdated, incomplete or incorrect evidence or asking a question that has been incorrectly formulated and so does not apply to the patient or problem.

Table 1.1   Possible questions in a patient presenting with shoulder pain*

Patient/problem:	Age, occupation (sports/musician), duration, pathology (local/referred)
Intervention/test:	Physiotherapy (exercise/manipulation/ultrasound), chiropractic, osteopathy, analgesia, NSAID, nothing, positive vs. negative consultation from doctor, general practitioner, consultant rheumatologist, orthopaedic surgeon, soft tissue specialist or clinic, surgery, acupuncture, herbal, homeopathy
Comparison/alternative:	Placebo, sham, any of the other interventions
Outcome:	Pain, shoulder movements, quality of life, activities, patient preference or satisfaction for particular treatment

* This is not intended to be an exhaustive list.

For most clinical questions, it is important to be able to clarify the question in terms or the patient or problem (P), to understand the range of possible therapeutic interventions (I) available and what we are comparing any intervention with, that is to say the comparison (C) or alternative to that intervention, and finally to have a clear idea of the outcomes (O) that we are aiming for. See Table 1.1 for a good illustration of this.

The hierarchy of evidence reconsidered

The next step is to have a clear idea of what type of evidence to look for. Early formulations develop a simplistic notion of a hierarchy of evidence in which some forms of study design are considered intrinsically superior in quality to others. The quality of evidence in these hierarchies refers to our confidence in the estimate of effect or effect size of the intervention. For example, the widely cited Canadian Task Force on Prevention (Battista 1993), derived from work in the United States Agency (United States Department of Health and Human Services Agency for Health Care Policy and Research 1993), grades the quality of evidence according to the methodology of the study using the following scheme:

I   evidence from at least one properly randomized-controlled trial;
II-1   evidence from cohort and case control studies;
II-2   evidence from quasi-experimental studies or from exceptionally convincing uncontrolled experiments;
III   opinions of respected experts.

There are a number of problems with the validity of this notion. Firstly, it is clear that if you have more than one randomized-controlled study. Even when looking at similar patients, interventions, comparison groups and outcomes, they may produce effects of varying size. This problem can be addressed by making assessments of quality based on systematic reviews and using metaanalysis to determine effect size based on a number of comparable studies rather than a single study, particularly when these have been carried out with carefully developed, explicit and sound methods, for example using protocols developed according to the methodology developed by the Cochrane collaboration (Mulrow 1994).

Secondly, each study design is also susceptible to bias due to the way it is conducted. Problems in design, such as baseline imbalance, randomization or allocation concealment, can lead to over- or underestimation of effect sizes in experimental randomized controlled studies, giving rise to the possibility that a well-conducted non-randomized study may give a better estimate of effect size than a badly managed randomized-controlled study. Also randomized studies have been more likely to have rigid inclusion and exclusion criteria leading to differences in the study compared to a normal population (Britton et al. 1998), hence the importance of careful quality assessment of individual studies, rather than assuming that one method is superior to another.

Thirdly, experimental studies may be unnecessary (when effects are dramatic), inappropriate (outcomes are rare or distant) or dependent on active participation of subjects, impossible (difficult to recruit to, unethical, legally challenged, unfunded), unfeasible (because of risk of contamination or inadvertent spread of the intervention in control or limited by the volume of research that can be conducted) or inadequate because of problems of generalizability (Black 1996).

Finally, the clinical problem is not always about a therapeutic intervention and therefore a randomized-controlled trial may be an inappropriate method for answering such a question or effect size irrelevant as a measure of quality. For example, when a patient presents with a cough an appropriate and important question might relate to prognosis, for example 'How long will the cough last if left untreated?', a question that can be answered by a cohort study but not a randomized-controlled study. Many research questions relating to attitudes, beliefs and behaviour of practitioners and patients are best answered using qualitative research (Pope and Mays 1995).

These issues have been addressed by guideline developers refining the criteria for grading the quality of evidence depending on both method and quality of evidence and recommendations based on the balance between benefits and harms (Grades of Recommendation 2004).

Different types of study have different advantages and disadvantages. The main differences between the important study types are summarized in Table 1.2.

Accessing the evidence

Formulating answerable questions and understanding what type of evidence one is searching for is therefore the first step to accessing and retrieving evidence that might be capable of addressing these questions. A large number

Table 1.2 Types of study

	Advantages	Disadvantages
Case control	Small numbers, cheap, easy, quick Good for rare conditions Minimizes bias in case ascertainment Can study multiple exposures (causes) Calculates odds ratio (estimates relative risk when incidence is low)	Reliance on records or recall to determine exposure Not good for exposure to rare events Studies one outcome Selection of controls difficult Confounding Bias: control selection, recall bias, observer bias in assessing exposure
Cohort	Can study exposure to rare event and several outcomes Minimizes bias in measurement of exposure Easy to define controls Can measure incidence, absolute, relative and attributable risk Easy to generalize because studies whole populations	Large, expensive, time-consuming especially for rare outcomes Loss to follow-up ('drop-outs') Confounding Loss of enthusiasm by investigators Poor for diseases with long latent period unless retrospective Changes in diagnosis or ascertainment over time
Cross-sectional	Cheap, simple, quick, ethical Can study exposure and outcome Can determine prevalence	Determines association not causation Subject to unequal group sizes, confounding and recall bias
Randomized-controlled study	Gold standard Random allocation Reduces confounding Blinding and appropriate selection reduce bias	Exclusion, inclusion, generalizability Expensive, time-consuming Volunteer bias Failure of blinding
Systematic review	Pools data from smaller studies to increase power Can detect publication bias using funnel plots	Bias: publication, language Clustering around null of more precise studies in funnel plot suggests publication bias Heterogeneity, matching, pooling (populations, settings, time, interventions, outcomes), GIGO
Qualitative	Generate (vs. test) hypotheses Small numbers Validity vs. repeatability	Analysis difficult Requires triangulation Generalization may be difficult

Note: Mixing of diverse studies can make for a strange fruit salad: mixing apples and oranges may seem reasonable enough, but when sprouts, turnips or even an old sock are added, it can cast doubt on the meaning of any aggregate estimates from Bandolier on meta-analysis.

of electronic databases of medical literature are now available through an increasing number of portals. The large online databases, including Medline and EMBASE, have rendered obsolete the cumbersome Index Medicus, the impenetrable and voluminous paper catalogue of biomedical literature.

Some experts sensibly advise practitioners to restrict initial searches to a limited number of sources including PubMed, the Cochrane Library, and the TRIP (Turning Research into Practice) database from the Centre for Research Support at Cardiff (Clarke and Wentz 2000). The Cochrane Library consists of four databases, the Cochrane database of systematic reviews (CDSR), the database of abstracts of reviews of effectiveness (DARE), the Cochrane controlled trials register (CCTR), and Cochrane review methodology database (CRMD).

Theory
Hypothesis
Variables   Dependent (effect)
                             Independent (cause)
                             Intermediate (occurs in causal pathway e.g., urbanization →
                                 pollution, → asthma)
                             Confounding (can cause or prevent outcome of interest, is not
                                 intermediate and is not associated with independent variable)
                             (e.g., asthma → ↓ cancer; asthma → ↓ smoking → ↓ cancer
                             or HRT → ↓ MI, SC1 → ↑ HRT → ↓ MI)

Operationalization
Study type   Case-control, cross-sectional (observational), cohort
                             Randomized-controlled trial
                             Qualitative

Sample   Source, method, size
(representative)   Entry, exclusion, non-responders

Controls   Definition (i.e., no cases), source
(acceptable)   Matching, randomization, comparability

Intervention   Groups treated equally apart from intervention
                             Size of treatment effect (relative vs. absolute risk reduction, NNT)
                             Precision of treatment effect (confidence intervals)

Measurement   Quality: valid (sensitive, specific), repeatable, blinded
                             Completeness: compliance, missing data, dropouts, deaths

Problems   Bias (errors in design or execution)
                             Confounding (alternative explanations)
                             Repeatability (reproducible)
                             Internal validity (study showed what it purported to)
                             Generalizability or external validity (applicable to other settings)
                             Ethical

Relevance   Relevant to patients
                             Clinically important
                             Benefit vs. risks or harms
                             Cost-effectiveness

Figure 1.2   A critical appraisal checklist

Critical appraisal of evidence

Critical appraisal of evidence consists of three main elements. Firstly, it involves understanding and restating the aims and methods of the study in a clear and stylized manner. Secondly, it seeks to identify problems in the research aims or method in order to verify the internal validity (did the study actually show what it claims to?), external validity or generalizability (does the study apply to other settings?) and repeatability of the study by examining sources of bias (errors in design or execution of the study) or confounding (alternative explanations of the findings). Finally, it examines the relevance and applicability of the study to individual patients or practice. This is often done using a checklist; the example shown in Figure 1.2 has been developed from many previous examples (Fowkes and Fulton 1991) and enables a systematic approach. Figure 1.3 applies the checklist to a particular paper.

Applying evidence in practice

Many practitioners feel that their most important role is to apply the findings of research to their practice (McColl et al. 1998). When trying to understand and teach how to apply evidence to practice, there is considerable benefit to using examples from day-to-day work. The following examples take results from studies that are frequently used in practice to illustrate how this can be done.

Statistical significance and clinical importance

The precision of a study in comparing outcomes is often expressed as a p value or confidence interval, as in the following example:

Example 1

p values and confidence intervals

Hypertension in elderly in primary care (Coope and Warrender 1986)
A randomized trial of the treatment of hypertension in 884 patients aged 60 to 79 years at the onset showed a reduction of 18/11 mm Hg in blood pressure over a mean follow-up period of 4.4 years. The principal antihypertensive agents were atenolol and bendrofluazide (bendroflumethiazide). There was a reduction in the rate of fatal stroke in the treatment group to 30% of that in the control group (95% confidence interval 11–84%, p less than 0.025). The rate of all strokes (fatal and non-fatal) in the treatment group was 58% of that in the control group (95% confidence interval 35–96%, p less than 0.03).

To understand 'p values' we need to understand the concept of the 'null hypothesis' that states that there is no difference between the intervention and

Theory	'Doctor as a drug' (Balint).[†]
Hypothesis	'Positive' consultations improve patient outcome.
Variables	Independent (cause or exposure): consultation type positive/ negative + /- placebo. Dependent (effect or outcome): patient satisfaction, recovery from illness.
Operationalization	Recovery from illness -- self-administered postal questionnaire after 2/52. Patient satisfaction -- self-administered questionnaire after consultation.
Study type	Randomized study comparing four different interventions. Did the randomization lead to different groups i.e., 'chance imbalance'? There was no attempt to compare the different groups for differences such as age, sex, etc.
Sample	Patients receiving appointments with one doctor during 59 consecutive surgeries. This was a self-selected sample preferring to see one particular doctor. Patients were also selected by one doctor as having no 'definite' diagnosis. The information on completeness of follow-up was not clear.
Controls	The comparison group included alternative interventions.
Results	64% of patients recovered within two weeks of a positive consultation vs. 39% after a negative consultation.
Bias	Experimenter bias: subtle cues may have affected patient responses in the experimenter's desired direction. Dr Thomas had adopted a positive consulting style and become adept at this style presumably because he believed it was better. Selection bias: patients selected by doctor on basis of inability to make a diagnosis. Difficult to reproduce: it is difficult to reproduce inadequate clinical skills (negative consultations). It would be difficult to produce a valid patient sample including those with self-limiting (e.g., viral) illness only. Respondent bias: acquiescence (a tendency to produce the findings that the patient believes the doctor or experimenter wants) would tend to affect groups in the same direction.
Confounding (alternative explanations)	Usually, confounding is not possible in a randomized trial because the intervention is constant. However, patients may have selected a general practitioner for their particular consulting style and would be disappointed if the GP adopted another style. Hence unnatural consulting style (style to which the doctor was unaccustomed) may have been the explanation for a worse outcome).
Problems: Repeatability	Single experimenter/particular patient type but may be repeated in another setting.
Validity	Study design problems shown by sources of bias.
Generalizability	Single experimenter with a particular preferred style may not be applicable to doctors with an alternative preferred style.
Ethics	Lack of consent to participate. Dubious use of placebos.

Figure 1.3 A critical appraisal of practice consultation papers

Relevance   Doctors' consulting behaviour is an important area of research.
                           Interesting study with findings potentially relevant to everyday
                           general practice.
                           Important sources of bias (experimenter, selection) and
                           confounding (unnatural consulting style) throw doubt on the
                           findings.
                           May not be generalizable to other general practitioners with
                           alternative preferred consulting styles.
                           Ethical considerations would prevent this study being repeated.

Source: K.B. Thomas, 'General practice consultations: is there any point in being
positive?', *British Medical Journal* (1987) 294: 1200–2.

[†] M. Balint, *The Doctor, His Patient and the Illness* (London: Pitman Publishing, 1957).

Fig. 1.3 *Continued*

comparison groups. In this example comparing a treatment (antihypertensive)
with a placebo, the null hypothesis states that there is no difference between
antihypertensive treatment (atenolol or bendroflumethiazide) and placebo.
The researchers use statistical analysis to compare the effect of treatment and
comparison groups. The p value is the probability that the null hypothesis is
true. The smaller the p value, the less likely the null hypothesis becomes, i.e.
the more likely the groups being tested are different. By convention $p < 0.05$
(5%) is taken to be significant. It is important to realize that if there are more
than 20 variables in a study, then one is likely to be significant by chance and
therefore a lower p value is often sought after.

Another way of comparing intervention and comparison groups is the
confidence interval. The 95% confidence interval is the range within which, if
the study were to be repeated, the true result will lie 95% of the time.
Confidence intervals that cross zero mean that the null hypothesis is true.
Wide confidence intervals mean that the results of a study are less precise.

It is important to understand that statistical significance is not the same as
clinical importance. For example, it is possible to have a study in which there
is a significant improvement in an important outcome but in which the
difference in clinical outcome between the intervention and comparison
group is so small as to be irrelevant in the clinical situation.

Comparing outcomes

There are a number of different ways of expressing how good a treatment is
compared to a placebo or alternative treatment (Box 1). One can simply state
that treatment A is better than treatment B. However, this gives little
indication of the relative or absolute benefit of one treatment against a
comparison.

Box 1 Different ways of comparing outcomes

A is better than B
Relative risk vs. absolute risk
Numbers needed to treat or harm
Odds ratios
Investigations: sensitivity, specificity, etc., e.g. urine glucose
Economic: cost per QALY

Another way of comparing outcomes is to use relative risk, absolute and attributable risk and numbers needed to treat or harm. A frequent example in primary care clinical practice is the risk of hormone replacement therapy (Example 2).

Example 2 Understanding and explaining risk
   Effect of hormone replacement therapy (HRT) on breast cancer risk: oestrogen versus oestrogen plus progestin (Ross et al. 2000)
   If the relative risk (RR) after five years of HRT is 1.3, i.e. 30% greater risk per year;
   Assuming that the absolute risk (AR) of breast cancer without HRT is 3/1000 per year.
   Calculate from this data:[1]
   Absolute risk on HRT =
   Attributable risk of HRT =
   Number needed to harm (NNH) on HRT =
   How could you explain this to one of your patients?

There are a number of different ways of explaining this to your patients. For example, you could say that there is a 30 per cent increase in risk of breast cancer after five years' use of HRT. This might sound worryingly large to some patients. Alternatively you could say that it would take 1000 years for the average patient to develop breast cancer on HRT. This would make the possibility of cancer seem very remote. Using the concept of number needed to harm, one could explain that you would need to treat 100 patients for one year with HRT to cause an additional breast cancer. This seems the most truthful way of conveying what is a real but rare risk.

Another common example in clinical practice is the risk of deep vein thrombosis with the combined oral contraceptive pill. Example 3 uses a cohort study to illustrate the risk of deep vein thrombosis in the period just before and just after the 'pill scare' when there was widespread publicity about the risk of third generation (desogestrel or gestodene-containing) combined pills.

---

1 **Answers**: Absolute risk (AR) of breast cancer without HRT = 3/1000 per year, (AR) on HRT = 4/1000 per year, attributable risk = 1/100 per year, number needed to harm (NNH) = 1000 per year.

Example 3 Relative risk

Incidence of venous thromboembolism comparing third-generation oral contraceptives with oral contraceptives with levonorgestrel (Jick et al. 2000)

Study period	Progestogen	Women with thromboembolism	Women years at risk	Incidence per 100,000 person years	Relative risk ratio
January 1993 to	Levonorgestrel	17	85,000	? [20/100,000]	1.0
October 1995	Desogestrel or gestodene	50	125,000	? [40/100,000]	? [2.0]
January 1996 to	Levonorgestrel	25	100,000	? [25/100,000]	1.0
December 1999	Desogestrel or gestodene	10	25,000	? [40/100,000]	? [1.6]

Calculate incidence and relative risk ratios completing the table from this data
Why have the relative risk ratios changed between the two time periods?[2]
Using the data above, calculate relative risk increase (RR), attributable risk and number needed to harm (NNH) third vs. second-generation contraceptive pills and DVT[3]

Answers:
2   The relative risk ratios changed between the two time periods because of switching to alternative second generation pills especially amongst high-risk users.
3   RR $= 2 \times$ risk of DVT per year
Attributable risk $= 40/100,000 - 20/100,000 = 20/100,000$ per year
NNH $= 5000$ per year

Example 4 Odds ratios

Distribution of exposure to oral contraceptives in cases and controls and adjusted odds ratios of idiopathic venous thromboembolism (Jick et al. 2000)

Study period	Oral contraceptive	Cases (n = 100)	Odds	Controls (n = 600)	Odds	Odds ratio	Adjusted odds ratio
January 1993 to	Levonorgestrel	20	? [1/4]	150	? [1/3]	? [3/4]	1.0
October 1995	Desogestrel or gestodene	50	? [1/1]	240	? [2/3]	? [3/2]	? [2.0]
January 1996 to	Levonorgestrel	25	1/3	150	? [1/3]	1	1.0
December 1999	Desogestrel or gestodene	10	? [1/9]	30	? [1/19]	? [2 + 1/19]	? [2.1]

Calculate odds ratios from this data (1/9 = 0.1): [Answers in square brackets]
Why are the adjusted odds ratios the same between the two time periods?[4]

4   Unlike the cohort data in Example 3, Example 4 uses a case control method in which cases and controls are matched for other sik factors. this is the explanation for the odds rations being similar whereas the risk rations in the previous example differ after the pill scare.

The same authors used a case control method and odds ratios to illustrate the phenomenon (Example 4). Odds are simply another way of expressing a probability. In the case of a die, the *probability* of throwing a six is one in six (1/6) whereas the *odds* of throwing a six is one to five (1/5).

The data from Example 3 can be used to calculate relative risk, absolute risk and number needed to harm comparing second- and third-generation combined oral contraceptives (Example 5).

Example 5 Relative risk, absolute risk and number needed to harm
Calculate relative risk increase, attributable risk & number needed to harm (NNH) of third- vs. second-generation contraceptive pills and DVT from the data above.
Relative risk =
Absolute risk =
Attributable risk =
NNH =

How could you explain this to one of your patients?

What happened in the pill scare and why was the government advice reversed?[5]

Example 6 Number needed to treat
Hypertension in the elderly in primary care (Coope and Warrender 1986)
Approx. 900 adults aged 60–79, drug treatment of mild hypertension with bendro-fluazide or atenolol over five years (450 allocated to treatment and 450 controls). Cerebrovascular events (fatal and non-fatal): control group 45 intervention 22.5.

Calculate relative risk (RR), absolute risk reduction (ARR) and number needed to treat (NNT) from the data above.[6]

Example 7 Effect of prevalence
MRC trial of treatment of mild hypertension (MRC Working Party 1985)
Approx. 20,000 adults aged 35–64, drug treatment of mild hypertension with bendrofluazide or propranolol over five years.
  Cerebrovascular events (fatal and non-fatal): control group 100, intervention 50.

---

5   Example 5 answers: RR = 2 × risk of DVT per year, AR = 40/100,000 per year, Attributable risk = 40/100,000 − 20/100,000 = 20/100,000 per year, NNH = 5000 per yhear. In the pill scare women were advised that the risk of third generation pills was double that of older combined contracpetive pills leading to many of them coming off the pill and an increase in unwanted pregnancies. This advice was changed when it became understood that the attributable risk was so small.

6   RR   = 50% (½)
    ARR = 45/450 − 22.5/450 over 5 years
        = 10/100 − 5/100 over 5 years
        = 5/100 over 5 years
        = 1/100 over 1 years
    NNT = 20 over 5 years
        = 100 over 1 year

Calculate relative risk (RR), absolute risk reduction (ARR) and number needed to treat (NNT) from the data above.[7]

Why is there a difference in the NNT when the relative risk reduction is the same?

Who would you treat, young or elderly?

Examples 6 and 7 illustrate how relative risk reduction for prevention of stroke in mild hypertension with antihypertensive medication is the same for young or elderly patients but, because of the much higher prevalence of stroke in the elderly, the benefits in terms of strokes prevented is greater and this is reflected in a lower number needed to treat.

Example 8 Calculating sensitivity and specificity
Exercise tolerance tests
A 50-year-old male patient registers with you and tells you he recently had an exercise test at the hospital. His previous general practitioner told him the test was normal and advised him to stop his treatment for angina. What would you do? (Froelicher et al. 1998)

	Angiogram	
ETT	*CHD*	*Normal coronaries*
ETT + (n = 50)	40 (TP)	10 (FP)
ETT − (n = 50)	20 (FN)	30 (TN)

$4/9 = 0.44$

Define and calculate the following:[8]

Sensitivity =

Specificity =

Positive predictive value =

Negative predictive value =

Accuracy =

Likelihood ratio of a positive test =

Likelihood ratio of a negative test =

7 RR $= 50\% \ (\frac{1}{2})$
   ARR $= 100/10{,}000 - 50/10{,}000$ over 5 years
        $= 10/1000 - 5/1000$ over 5 years
        $= 5/1000$ over 5 years
        $= 1/1000$ over 1 years
   NNT $= 200$ over 5 years
        $= 1000$ over 1 year
8 Sensitivity: Ability to pick up true positives $= TP/TP + FN = 40/(40 + 20) = 66\%$
   Specificity: Ability to pick up true negatives $= TN/TN + FP = 30/(30 + 10) = 75\%$
   Positive predictive value = Probability of positive test having the condition $= TP/TP + FP = 40/(40 + 10) = 80\%$

To understand this problem better, one must have a grasp of the concept of likelihood ratios. Exercise testing has relatively low sensitivity and specificity. This results in a likelihood ratio that means if your clinical opinion was one of angina then a negative exercise test should not dissuade you from continuing to manage your patient on the basis of your clinical diagnosis.

Knowledge translation

Unfortunately, there is considerable evidence that the implementation systems to improve utilization of evidence and knowledge translation are poorly developed.

Models of implementation of evidence-based practice need to be based on the wider context of health policy and organizations, as well as on individual agents for change, the underlying evidence and associated outcomes of evidence-based health technologies and also the interventions required to implement change. To understand the complexity, range and effects of interventions designed to implement evidence-based practice, it is important to have a conceptual framework to draw on (Siriwardena 2003).

Implementation strategies may be classified according to the target of the intervention (e.g., patients, providers, or systems), the type of intervention (e.g., education, reminders, feedback), or the social theory (e.g., social influence, marketing) that underpins the intervention (Stone et al. 2002). One useful framework (Figure 1.4) explains how and why interventions affect their targets and also how one intervention type (for example a media campaign) can potentially affect more than one target (for example, both patients and practitioners).

However, this framework does not consider the outcome of the intervention or the evidence base for it. In implying cause and effect, a linear model such as this portrays the targets of the intervention as passive recipients when in fact patients, providers and systems are also agents of change in a complex interactive process.

The factors that determine which interventions are used and how they are applied are examples of organizational learning (Carroll and Edmondson 2002). These factors may be linked to previous practice, belief systems (what practitioners believed was most effective and appropriate in their

---

Negative predictive value = Probability of negative test excluding the condition = TN/ TN + FN = 30/(30 + 20) = 60%

Accuracy = Probability of test giving correct result = True positives + True negatives/ All = 40 + 30/100 = 70%

Likelihood ratio of a positive test = How much more likely that a positive test is found in a person with the condition than without = sensitivity/(1-specificity) = 2/3/(1/4) = 2.66

Likelihood ratio of a negative test = How much more likely that a negative test is found in a person without the condition than a person with it = 1-sensitivity/specificity = 1/3/(3/4) = 0.44

If you thought the chances were even 50% that the patient had angina, i.e., 1:1, then by doing the test the chances would only be reduced to 40% by finding a negative result.

Target	Intervention type
Patient(s)	Patient education (leaflets, posters, advice)
	Media and advertising
	Patient reminders
	Financial incentives to patients
Provider(s)	Practitioner education
	Practitioner prompts: reminders, recall
	Financial incentives to health workers
	Media and advertising
	Teamwork
	Feedback
System (practice, primary care organization, national health service)	Team based education (organizational learning)
	Practitioner prompts: reminders, recall
	Media and advertising
	Teamwork
	Feedback
	Policy (practice, national)
	Regulation
Theoretical basis	
Social theory underlying intervention types	Social influence
	Marketing and outreach
	Active learning
	Visual appeal
	Barriers and facilitators
	Teamwork
	Management support

Figure 1.4   Conceptual framework for interventions to improve adult vaccination rates (adapted from Stone et al. 2002)

previous experience), feedback (how practices compared with their peers and particularly how results compared with peers who might have been employing different strategies), relative costs (of using alternative arrangements) as well as specific learning about these issues from literature, media and team discussions.

Another useful model which does include evidence as a key component is the Promoting Action on Research Implementation in Health Services (PARIHS) framework (Rycroft-Malone et al. 2002). The three components of this model are evidence, context and facilitation. Evidence includes not only the strength of the science in relation to the research question being asked but also takes into account patient need and the acceptance of the evidence by professionals and patients. The context describes the setting in which the health technology is delivered. This includes the organizations, teams and individuals involved, together with their culture, which refers to the motivation and beliefs of the individuals and organizations and also includes health policy. Facilitation incorporates the various types of interventions, which may be internal or external to the organization, that are used to implement the health technology.

This model recognizes the importance of evidence and moreover how it might affect the beliefs of patients and practitioners. Also, by having these groupings of evidence, context and facilitation, we are able to see more clearly the possibilities for interaction within and between them. A drawback of this framework is that the centrality of the patient, both as the recipient and the motivator for some health care interventions is not adequately addressed. Another anomaly is that health policy is more often an intervention or facilitator rather than part of the context.

Both these models, whilst recognizing that the various components interact, provide little explanation of how they might do so. The third model, that more fully considers this interaction, is based on complexity theory. This theory has been explored in the primary care setting by Miller and others in the Unites States (Miller et al. 1998). The model sees general practice, its users and health professionals, together with its supporting organizations (or the 'context' in the previous model) as a complex adaptive system. Complex adaptive systems could be seen as ever-changing webs, containing many organisms and threads, each interacting uniquely with another and each affecting the whole structure, leading to change in the system, sometimes in an unpredictable manner. The potential changes in the web depend on its initial boundaries (organizational mission, priorities and history), the agents within it (patients, practitioners, health workers, pharmaceutical representatives, administrators, etc.) who are both targets and initiators of change, their pattern of interaction (relationships), the immediate surroundings (neighbouring or related complex adaptive systems existing in the same environment), together with wider influences (from the health organizations, national bodies, culture, finances and regulation) (Miller et al. 2001).

By combining these notions, a new model is derived (Figure 1.5), the three main elements of which are the context, interventions (or facilitators) and evidence. The context includes the change agents or various individuals and organizations involved in producing changes in performance (items shown within circles). This ranges from the patient, the provider (health care professional) working in a general practice team through to the various supporting organizations, such as the primary care trust and Department of Health. The outcome of interest and evidence are also shown (both as triangles). The overlap between providers and organizations is depicted by the overlap between their respective circles. This is because providers, such as general practitioners and nurses, as well as being individual agents also function within larger teams, general practices, community nursing teams, primary care trusts or at even higher organizational levels of the health service. The interactions between the components that form the context are shown as dashed arrows.

The final element, represented at the top of the diagram by a diamond, is the intervention or facilitator of change. The specific interventions are shown in boxes and, where they impact on the various change agents, are shown as solid arrows. The interventions are also classified as to their nature to the

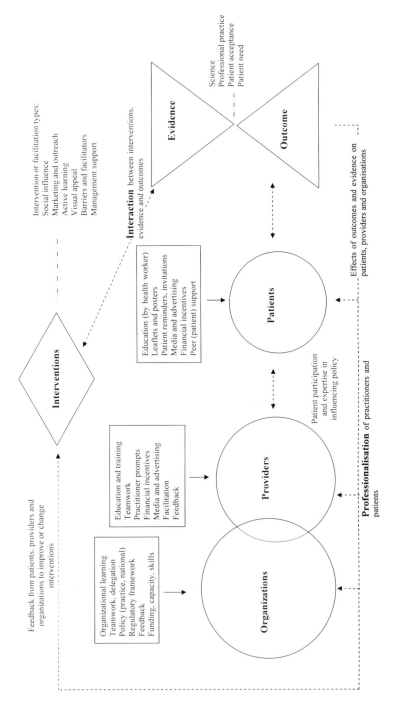

Figure 1.5 Diagrammatic representation of conceptual framework for interventions to improve prevention

right of the rhomboid. These intervention types and the specific interventions themselves are predominantly, and it will be argued most importantly, educational in their nature. They are educational in that they mostly involve learning, questioning (or iteration) and interaction. Interaction occurs between the agents, interventions and outcomes in an organic and complex way rather than in simple linear manner (Dopson et al. 2002). The importance of education lies in the fact that learning is fundamental to change in a highly professionalized organization such as primary care. Professionals, because of their background of learning, competence and expertise, are likely to be highly influenced by rationality and, although political influences may also be a significant factor in change, these can also be seen as part of the learning process. The model acknowledges that the various change agents, particularly providers and professionals but also patients, are able to influence the intervention types through feedback. Although practitioners within primary care organizations will learn from various sources, including their patients, the organization and professionals within it ultimately have the power to block change from occurring.

This theoretical model begins to explain why knowledge translation is such a difficult process and why the implementation of evidence depends on the evidence itself and what outcomes result, but also the agents of change, including practitioners, the organizations and patients that they serve and the interactions between them. However, it also lays the foundations for understanding how we can translate evidence into practice by using educational and change management strategies that address barriers to change, break down professional barriers and more closely link the producers and users of evidence (Landry et al. 2002).

References

Battista, R. N. (1993) Practice guidelines for preventive care: the Canadian experience. *British Journal of General Practitioners*, **43**: 301–3.

Black, N. (1996) Why we need observational studies to evaluate the effectiveness of health care. *British Medical Journal*, **312**: 1215–18.

Britton, A., McKee, M., Black, N., McPherson, K., Sanderson, C. and Bain, C. (1998) Choosing between randomised and non-randomised studies: a systematic review. *Health Technology Assessment*, **2**:

Carroll, J. S. and Edmondson, A. C. (2002) Leading organisational learning in health care. Qual. Saf Health Care, **11**: 51–6.

Clarke, J. and Wentz, R. (2000) Pragmatic approach is effective in evidence based health care. *British Medical Journal*, **321**: 566–7.

Clinicians for the Restoration of Autonomous Practice (CRAP) Writing Group (2002) EBM: unmasking the ugly truth. *British Medical Journal*, **325**: 1496–8.

Cochrane, A. (1972) Effectiveness and efficiency: random reflections on health services (London: Nuffield Provincial Hospital Trust).

Coope, J. & Warrender, T. S. (1986) Randomised trial of treatment of hypertension in elderly patients in primary care. *British Medical Journal* (Clin. Res. Ed), 293: 1145–51.

de Lusignan, S., Wells, S. and Singleton, A. (2002) Learning environments must be created that capitalise on teams' wealth of knowledge. *British Medical Journal*, 324: 674–74.

Dopson, S., Fitzgerald, L., Ferlie, E., Gabbay, J. and Locock, L. (2002) No magic targets! Changing clinical practice to become more evidence based. *Health Care Management Review*, 27: 35–47.

Ellis, J., Mulligan, I., Rowe, J. and Sackett, D. L. (1995) Inpatient general medicine is evidence based. A-Team, Nuffield Department of Clinical Medicine. *Lancet*, 346: 407–10.

Falshaw, M., Carter, Y. H. and Gray, R. W. (2000) Evidence should be accessible as well as relevant. *British Medical Journal*, 321: 567.

Fowkes, F. G. and Fulton, P. M. (1991) Critical appraisal of published research: introductory guidelines. *British Medical Journal*, 302: 1136–140.

Freeman, A. C. and Sweeney, K. (2001) Why general practitioners do not implement evidence: qualitative study. *British Medical Journal*, 323: 1100–102.

Froelicher, V. F., Lehmann, K. G., Thomas, R., Goldman, S., Morrison, D., Edson, R., Lavori, P., Myers, J., Dennis, C., Shabetai, R., Do, D. and Froning, J. (1998) The electrocardiographic exercise test in a population with reduced workup bias: diagnostic performance, computerized interpretation, and multivariable prediction. Veterans Affairs Cooperative Study in Health Services no. 016 (QUEXTA) Study Group. Quantitative Exercise Testing and Angiography. *Annals of Internal Medicine*, 128: 965–74.

Geddes, J. R., Game, D., Jenkins, N. E., Peterson, L. A., Pottinger, G. R. and Sackett, D. L. (1996) What proportion of primary psychiatric interventions are based on evidence from randomised controlled trials? *Qual. Health Care*, 5: 215–17.

Grades of Recommendation, A. D. a. E. G. W. G. (2004) Grading quality of evidence and strength of recommendations. *British Medical Journal*, 328: 1490–4.

Greenhalgh, T. (1999) Narrative based medicine: narrative based medicine in an evidence based world. *British Medical Journal*, 318: 323–5.

Greenhalgh, T. (2001) How to read a paper: the basics of evidence based medicine.

Hagdrup, N., Falshaw, M., Gray, R. W. and Carter, Y. H. (1998) All members of primary care team are aware of importance of evidence based medicine. *British Medical Journal*, 317: 282–282.

Hammersley, M. (2001) Some questions about evidence-based practice in education. www.leeds.ac.uk/educol/documents/00001819.htm, pp. 1–17. Paper presented at the symposium on 'Evidence-based practice in education' at the Annual Conference of the British Educational Research Association, University of Leeds, September 13–15, 2001. 3.

Hampton, J. R. (1993) The end of clinical freedom. *British Medical Journal*, 287: 1237–8.

Jamous, H. and Pelloile, B. (1970) Changes in the French university hospital system, in *Professions and Professionalisation* (ed. J. A. Jackson), Cambridge: Cambridge University Press, pp. 111–52.

Jick, H., Kaye, J. A., Vasilakis-Scaramozza, C. and Jick, S. S. (2000) Risk of venous thromboembolism among users of third generation oral contraceptives compared with users of oral contraceptives with levonorgestrel before and after 1995: cohort and case-control study. *British Medical Journal*, 321: 1190–5.

Kerridge, I., Lowe, M. and Henry, D. (1998) Ethics and evidence based medicine. *British Medical Journal*, 316: 1151–3.

Khan, K. S., Awonuga, A. O., Dwarakanath, L. S. and Taylor, R. (2001) Assessments in evidence-based medicine workshops: loose connection between perception of knowledge and its objective assessment. *Med. Teach.*, 23: 92–4.

Knottnerus, J. A. and Dinant, G. J. (1997) Medicine based evidence, a prerequisite for evidence based medicine. *British Medical Journal*, 315: 1109–10.

Landry, R., Amaro, N. and Ouimet, M. (2002) *Research Transfer in Natural Sciences and Engineering*. (Quebec: Laval University).

McColl, A., Smith, H., White, P. and Field, J. (1998) General practitioners' perceptions of the route to evidence based medicine: a questionnaire survey. *British Medical Journal*, 316: 361–5.

Miller, W. L., Crabtree, B. F., McDaniel, R. and Stange, K. C. (1998) Understanding change in primary care practice using complexity theory. *Journal of Family Practitioners*, 46: 369–76.

Miller, W. L., McDaniel, R. R., Jr., Crabtree, B. F. and Stange, K. C. (2001) Practice jazz: understanding variation in family practices using complexity science. *Journal of Family Practitioners*, 50: 872–8.

MRC Working Party (1985) MRC trial of treatment of mild hypertension: principal results. Medical Research Council Working Party. *British Medical Journal*, 291: 97–104.

Mulrow, C. D. (1994) Rationale for systematic reviews. *British Medical Journal*, 309: 597–9.

Naylor, C. D. (1995) Grey zones of clinical practice: some limits to evidence based medicine. *Lancet*, 345: 840–2.

NHS Executive (1996) Promoting clinical effectiveness: a framework for action in and through the NHS. (Leeds, Department of Health).

NHS Management Executive (1993) Improving clinical effectiveness. *EL* (93) 115. (Leeds, Department of Health).

O'Donnell, C. (2004) Attitudes and knowledge of primary care professionals towards evidence-based practice: a postal survey. *Journal of Evaluative Clinical Practice*, 10: 197–205.

Oswald, N. and Bateman, H. (1999) Applying research evidence to individuals in primary care: a study using non-rheumatic atrial fibrillation. *Journal of Family Practitioners*, 16: 414–19.

Oswald, N. and Bateman, H. (2000) Treating individuals according to evidence: why do primary care practitioners do what they do? *Journal of Evaluative Clinical Practice*, 6: 139–48.

Oxman, A. (1994) Checklists for review articles. *British Medical Journal*, 309: 648–51.

Pope, C. and Mays, N. (1995) Reaching the parts other methods cannot reach: an introduction to qualitative methods in health and health services research. *British Medical Journal*, 311: 42–5.

Rosenberg, W. and Donald, A. (1995) Evidence based medicine: an approach to clinical problem solving. *British Medical Journal*, 310: 1122–6.

Ross, R. K., Paganini-Hill, A., Wan, P. C. and Pike, M. C. (2000) Effect of hormone replacement therapy on breast cancer risk: estrogen versus estrogen plus progestin. *J. Natl. Cancer Inst.*, 92: 328–32.

Rycroft-Malone, J., Kitson, A., Harvey, G., McCormack, B., Seers, K., Titchen, A. & Estabrooks, C. (2002) Ingredients for change: revisiting a conceptual framework. *Quality and Safety in Health Care*, 11: 174–80.

Sackett, D. L., Rosenberg, W. M., Gray, J. A., Haynes, R. B. and Richardson, W. S. (1996) Evidence based medicine: what it is and what it isn't. *British Medical Journal*, **312**: 71–2.

Siriwardena, A. N. (1995) Guidelines in primary care: an investigation of general practitioners' attitudes and behaviour towards clinical guidelines, 1–98 (Nottingham University).

Siriwardena, A. N. (2003) *The Impact of Educational Interventions on Influenza and Pneumococcal Vaccination Rates in Primary Care* (De Montfort University, Leicester).

Siriwardena, A. N., Sandars, J. and Scott, K. (2004) *Attitudes of GP Trainers to Teaching Evidence Based Medicine* (Education for Primary Care).

Smith, B. H. (1996) Evidence-based medicine: rich sources of evidence are ignored. *British Medical Journal*, **313**: 169.

Stone, E. G., Morton, S. C., Hulscher, M. E., Maglione, M. A., Roth, E. A., Grimshaw, J. M., Mittman, B. S., Rubenstein, L. V., Rubenstein, L. Z. and Shekelle, P. G. (2002) Interventions that increase use of adult immunization and cancer screening services: a meta-analysis. *Ann. Intern. Med.*, **136**: 641–51.

Straus, S. (2004) What's the E for EBM? *British Medical Journal*, **328**: 535–6.

Temple, J. (2002) Why general practitioners do not implement evidence. Evidence seem to change frequently. *British Medical Journal*, **324**: 674.

United States Department of Health and Human Services Agency for Health Care Policy and Research (1993) Acute pain management: operative or medical procedures and trauma. (Clinical practice guideline No 1, ACHPR publication No 9200023), 107. (Rockville, MD, AHCPR).

Wilkinson, E. K., McColl, A., Exworthy, M., Roderick, P., Smith, H., Moore, M. and Gabbay, J. (2000) Reactions to the use of evidence-based performance indicators in primary care: a qualitative study. *Qual. Health Care*, **9**: 166–74.

CHAPTER 2

Patient Information and Society

CAROL WILKINSON

This chapter is intended to explore the increasing drive towards patient centredness within health care delivery. Specific reference is made to the increasing availability of health-related information within society, which has contributed to the empowerment of the patient as consumer of health care services. This aspect of empowerment has revised the debate about the authority of health professionals and whether issues concerning working in partnership with patients should become the order of the day or whether there are still undercurrents of authority being expressed in different ways by health professionals. It also attempts to determine whether or not the patient as consumer can rely upon the information that exists within the public domain to argue their case for better health care within society.

The context within which patients have been empowered

In 2001, the Labour government decided that they were not going to revise the *Patient Charter* developed by the previous government, but instead produce a booklet entitled *Your Guide to the NHS*. The emphasis of the document rested on the principles of maintaining quality and high standards of care, of partnership with patients as being integral to the needs of patients, and the provision of care and treatment on the basis of need rather than ability to pay.

It is apparent within the document that the government saw patients as integral to the service, with less of a requirement to underline their rights and obligations within the service. This approach differed from the previous government's in the sense that the patient, as consumer, has a voice which is integral to the development and maintenance of the health service.

The involvement of patients in the NHS has evolved from a number of standpoints. Firstly, there is the user involvement movement which has long established roots in mental health and social care, particularly where patients and their relatives assist in arriving at the decisions made about their care, and the development of services. Secondly, there is increasing dissatisfaction with aspects of the health service, in particular with visiting times, waiting times and, in some cases, with the actions of health professionals. This is endorsed by the mass media who invariably highlight the hotspots and tensions that exist in health care and the potential to detriment in health care consumer confidence, for example, in the case relating to the Bristol enquiry, and the Shipman case of the recent past. This has opened up questions of patient safety and health professionals' trustworthiness and competence. More recently, there have been issues concerning hospital cleanliness, highlighted by outbreaks of MRSA. The need for vigilance is also pointed up in television dramas such as *Casualty* and *Holby City* (BBC News, April 2003; BBC News, July 2003; BBC News, September 2005).

The third point relates to the increasing value placed on consumers and their needs, providing them with more choices in health care market. This has increased demand, driving up competition, which has drawn with it elements of efficiency, effectiveness and a desire to maintain the highest standards possible so consumers will continue to use and recommend the service to others (DoH 2003).

Finally, there is an increased use of technology in medicine and health care, providing patient access to health information, for example through television, radio and, more recently, the internet. Consumer access to knowledge regarding health has expanded considerably since the increase in technology use.

Telephone helplines that provide alternative access routes to medical advice are also a relatively recent development. For example, in some countries, there are helplines staffed by health professionals who are available for 24 hours a day to enable patients to seek advice about any aspect of health care. Callers can describe their symptoms and obtain information about their condition or request a second opinion regarding a prescription or side effects of treatment. One such helpline is NHS Direct; similar services exist in Spain and Italy. In Switzerland and Sweden they are also considered useful for advice on minor health problems (Coulter and Meager 2003).

The NHS Plan (DoH 2000) paved the way for increasing patient and public involvement in terms of extending their voice in the planning and development of the health service. In addition to this, the Health and Social Care Act 2001 placed a duty on strategic health authorities, primary care trusts and NHS Trusts to make arrangements to involve and consult patients and the public. Indeed, NHS organizations are required by law to consult on substantial variations and developments to services separately from the requirements of section 11 (DoH 2003).

The introduction of section 11 in the Act imposes a wider duty to involve and consult patients and the public. Such involvement has taken place on a number of levels including aspects of planning services, the formulation of proposals for change and the decision-making processes affecting the daily operation of delivery in patient care. The process of inclusion has incorporated the opinions of patients and the public, culminating in disclosure of their values, beliefs, ideas and experiences as users of the service. Allied to this a culture has evolved where patients and the public can discuss their concerns and share in the creation of solutions, as well as in effecting changes in attitude. This in turn has led to an increased responsiveness and strict accountability of health professionals who have attempted to make their plans for action visible to consumers for the benefit of health care delivery. To assist in this process, good information and intelligence have become necessary elements in meeting patient needs.

A good example of such activity is the voluntary sector. The Compact launched in 1998 provided a framework which set out the principles that formed the background of the relationship between the voluntary sector, the government and the community. The Compact created an approach for working in partnership through building effective relationships and developing codes of practice and local agreements. The emphasis upon working in partnership with patients as consumers is seen as a clear indication of their becoming empowered. But why is this important and how has the notion of empowerment evolved within health care?

Answering the latter question will involve exploring the notion of empowerment, whereas answering the former requires an examination of the evolution of the consumer movement in health care and the penetration of its values and requirements over a considerable period of time.

Defining the notion of empowerment

Empowerment as a concept has political, psychosocial and ethical components (Keiffer 1984). The idea of empowerment is rooted in the social action ideology of the 1960s and the self-help perspectives popularized globally over thirty years ago. From a health care perspective, the early works of Haug make this clear in observations of American and British society and of the challenges faced by professionals, particularly in education, law and health care at the time (Haug 1973; Haug 1975; Haug and Lavin 1984). Empowerment has been linked with strategies for the prevention of health problems and with community intervention within the evolution of health promotion (Tones 1991). It was Rappaport (1984) who introduced the concept in 1981 with a view to stimulating and guiding mental health policies.

Empowerment is a difficult concept to define and is sometimes easier understood by its absence as sensed in powerlessness, hopelessness, helplessness and alienation (Hegar and Huzenker 1988; Hurty 1984; Keiffer 1984; Shaw 1987; Wallerstein and Bernstein 1988). It is associated with coping skills, manual support systems, community organization, neighbourhood participation, personal efficacy and competence as well as self-sufficiency and self-esteem. In a broad sense, empowerment is a process by which people, organizations and communities gain some mastery over their own lives.

The notion of empowerment also implies a relationship with others in the form of a transaction. Often there is some involvement in meeting the needs of people through collaborative efforts. Wallerstein and Bernstein (1988) stated that empowerment involved much more than increasing individual esteem and self-efficacy or promoting positive health behaviours in individuals. It also involves environmental change because the process of empowerment has necessitated an alteration in policy, ideas, and thinking amongst specific groups or within an organization or profession. The ability to meet the needs of consumers will have precipitated such evolution.

Katz (1984) stated there are some internal and external connections between individual and community empowerment. For Katz, empowerment is a synergistic framework where there is an interrelation between people sharing resources and where collaboration is encouraged. The process entails mutually beneficial interactions that strengthen the mediating structures between individuals and the larger society. For example, this could include patients who require specific information about care and treatment whilst in hospital. The ward staff could assist by developing a patient booklet that provides the details requested, with some patient input in its development as a result of undertakings within a focus group meeting or in the first instance a simple survey of opinion of a particular aspect of the service.

Empowerment in health care

Other writers state there is a need to understand the complex social, political and economic aspects that shape people's lives. This makes the notion of empowerment a multidimensional concept as well (Keiffer 1984; Butterfield 1990). Empowerment is also a dynamic concept where power is both taken and given, in other words, power is shared. There is a need to consider not only how the powerless attempt to take power but also how the powerful release power. Many authors have discussed this very element of exchange. Elements that are useful in application to health care are referred to here:

(a) Feminist perspective

The feminist view of power can be encapsulated in the notion of empowerment. This is often conceptualized as a condition of being able to achieve some objective in cooperation with others. This contrasts with the masculine view of power which sees a limited supply that must be struggled for and defended against others (Hurty 1984; Watts 1990; Wheeler and Chinn 1989). The former position is useful when working with patients to achieve effective care, its maintenance and a successful outcome of treatment. Consequently, this perspective on empowerment may also be considered a democratic concept as the underlying process suggests a redistribution of power and the advancement of others, even social justice. However, despite this, the real issue may rest not so much in having actual power but in feeling more powerful.

The emphasis on power-sharing and cooperation has been the subject of discussion within the nursing literature and has been in some measure implemented in health care settings in the USA and Britain. The notion of shared governance emerges from the need for nurses to be responsible, accountable and demonstrate authority within their working lives and relationships with others in the health care setting (Porter O'Grady 1992). It is about shared decision-making, working collaboratively, making people feel valued, and generating ideas to maximize best patient care and to improve the quality of nursing.

This encouraging of a shift in culture within health care organizations was the subject of implementation in Leicester General Hospital, England. In 1998 they introduced the Trusts Nursing and Midwifery Strategy which included clinical supervision and a review of post-registration education, as well as leadership. The model used was the councillor type, reflecting contemporary nursing priorities, clinical practice, research, professional development and quality. The aspects of shared governance in practice led to the development of action plans and individual wards developing specific care standards, and patients and their relatives becoming involved in evaluating basic care standards. This led to an improvement in standards and overall satisfaction, and a reduction in complaints (Doherty and Hope 2000).

(b) Acculturation perspective

One of the early writers on empowerment viewed it in a developmental sense as a process of 'becoming'. It is described as a journey that the individual makes in achieving some form of empowered status. Keiffer (1984) considers this as a long-term process, an ordered and progressive development of participatory skills and political understanding. There are four stages identified in this process.

- The first stage is the 'era of entry' that parallels the developmental stage of infancy. In this stage, the participation of the individual is exploratory, unknown and uncertain, while authority structures and power are demystified. This is a process of initiation and familiarization.
- The second stage is an 'era of advancement', often characterized by a mentoring relationship as well as support from peers. In this process, opportunities for collaboration and mutually supportive problem-solving occur. A critical understanding of the situation is gained with the assistance of an external enabler. The individual develops mechanisms for action and accepts responsibility for choices. Additionally, rudimentary political skills are developed.

- The third stage is known as the 'era of incorporation', a phase where activities are more focused, confronting and contending with the permanence and painfulness of structural or institutional barriers to self-determination. In this phase, organizational, leadership and survival skills are developed.
- The final stage in Keiffer's analysis relates to an 'era of commitment' that parallels adulthood and is a period in which the individual integrates new personal knowledge and skills into the reality and structure of the everyday life world.

The implication within the description of this process is that it is a labour-intensive process; the journey is long and sometimes protracted. There is no indication that there will necessarily be successful advancement through each stage to achieve empowerment, hence Keiffer's emphasis on 'becoming'. Empowerment is therefore a goal to be striven for.

Empowerment, therefore, relates to a process of assisting individuals and groups to gain critical awareness of the root causes of their problems and a readiness to act on this awareness. This process is revolutionary in the sense that its focus may be on changing structures rather than integrating into existing structures.

The notion of empowerment is not without its critics. Conger and Kanungo (1988) developed a concept of empowerment from the perspective of motivational theory. Leadership theories, they argued, interpret empowerment too narrowly, as being concerned solely with the distribution and delegation of power. These definitions have limited scope, are regarded as ambiguous and even, in some measure, misunderstood. The idea of the instrumental exercise of power, the sharing of power leading automatically to empowerment, is problematic (Thomas and Velthouse 1990; Page 1992; Skelton 1994). This is because the actions that precipitate a drive towards empowerment are generated through an individual's behaviour, actions and relationships with others. It is the individual's standing, expertise and possibilities to act to acquire information which lead to that achievement (Foucault 1976; McNay 1994). For example, the requirement for information relating to care and treatment as well as success rates in such treatment is necessary to enable patients to make informed choices, regardless of ability to acquire or share power with health care professionals. It is the main concern of health care professionals to be able to assist in this process.

Policies including *The NHS Plan*, *Making a Difference* and *Modern Matrons* all espouse the notion of empowerment, particularly for patients and for nurses at all levels within the NHS (DoH 1998; DoH 2000; NHSME 2001). But why the renewed drive towards consumer empowerment in health care and why now?

There appear to be several reasons. One school of thought suggests the language of patient power is increasingly more acceptable as it generates the impression that consumers of health care have a real stake in health care delivery development. Commentators such as Edmonstone (2000) imply that on the political front at least, this notion emerged in the late 1980s and early 1990s. This was a time when right-wing governments and their management increasingly turned to left-of-centre notions such as empowerment in order to describe their initiatives in a liberating language, as a means of gaining commitment to them. It was also suggested that terms which once appeared to belong to the vocabularies and progressive ideologies of the radical left were re-articulated into competing right-of-centre frames of reference (Clarke and Newman 1997). The language once used by social movements to express conceptions that necessitated collective action, such as inequality and oppression, subsequently entered the political language of organizational and managerial transformation with an emphasis on individual freedom. It can be argued also that health professionals have another use for this weapon – to gain more resources for their sector of the service.

Another argument which has driven patient empowerment is simple economics. Within health care, as is the case in many organizations, growing economic competition has been the driving force towards achieving excellence which means that employees need to be able to:

- accommodate changing circumstances with new knowledge and skills acquired within the system;
- improve performance at varying levels within the organization;
- work across occupational boundaries and work in multi-occupational teams;
- work with change and a developing agenda to suit the changing economic situation;
- diagnose relevant problems and opportunities and take action to bring about results;
- discover and acquire the knowledge and skill needed to cope with unfamiliar circumstances.

If the above is intended to have value within the health care setting, there needs to be some form of improvement, involving the fostering of self-esteem, self-efficacy and ways of coping that would mitigate against ongoing difficulties within the organization. Problems such as poor recruitment and working relationships within the hierarchical management structures in health care are often seen as a source of stress. There needs to be some fusing or accommodation of patient and health care worker empowerment for mutual benefit.

A third element is that of patient centredness. This is a feature of new Labour health policy thinking. Patient centredness is the adjunct to aspects of empowerment. Patients, as consumers, critics and supporters of a health service and health care delivery, have certain rights and obligations in receipt of a service. They also have rights to expect particular standards of service and the potential to make informed choices. To extend this further, consumers of health care should have access to:

- knowledge of the product, with increasing information about such procedures, written with the consumer in mind, and available within the public domain. For example, magazines and books relating to eye care or hip replacement.
- knowledge of the hospital or clinic setting. For example, information on the internet, and/or a brochure explaining services, opening and closing times and contact details have become the norm for many health care establishments.
- knowledge of treatment success. This may be acquired through direct questioning of doctors and other health personnel connected to the service. Alternatively, the latest CHAI reports are available through internet access.
- knowledge of care from personal experience, relatives and friends, reports in local newspapers pertaining to events or issues relating to the local service.
- rights of complaint, for example, in the event of not being able to achieve satisfactory care and treatment, the means to apply mechanisms for forwarding reasonable complaints. Health care establishments now have personnel with specific responsibilities for dealing with complaints and ensuring consumers achieve satisfaction where possible.
- issues regarding satisfaction surveys used by trusts to note patient responses to care and treatment.

Professionals in the health service will undoubtedly reveal that patient centredness has always been integral to their role in the delivery of health care, through innate process or indoctrination, since the day they began training. Patients have always been in a position to change their general practitioner if they felt they were not obtaining the service they require. So what's new?

In fact, under the *Patient Charter* in the UK, consumers have become increasingly alert to their rights and choices within the health care sector. Also, consumer movements in the US during the 1960s and 1970s gradually influenced health and social care developments in Britain and Europe and revived the debate concerning the need for better quality health care. Increasing demand for health care, and opportunities that have arisen as a result of globalization have resulted in the consumer having greater choice of health care provision. This has largely come about through access to better information concerning service, care and treatment. Consumers of health care know they have more of a choice than ever, because of the increasing health offer, meaning not just conventional orthodox medicine but greater access to and knowledge of complementary medicine in its various forms. There is, too, continuous advancement in science and technology, and an emphasis on youth, including an increasing acceptance that body parts can be replaced and preserved for as long as possible, therefore establishing the view that consumers do not have to give up on meeting their health needs if one treatment does not work (Horton 2003; Saks 1994).

There is of course another aspect of the movement towards consumer empowerment in health care: that is, a perceived reduction in medical authority. Increasing awareness of rights, obligations and aspects of care and treatment in an educated public has heightened the potential for litigation which reinforces a lack of trust, and leads to a reduction in the belief of the value of medicine. Challenges to health care service delivery have spurred the need for evidence-based medicine, something which has become more apparent over the years (Hafferty et al. 1993; Horton 2003). Not only do health professionals need greater evidence that specific care and treatment is suitable for their patients but patients also need to be convinced before they take a tablet or sign a consent form for an investigation that there will be some benefit to them, or at least some knowledge of the risks involved so they can make an informed choice.

There is, too, the notion of self-care with the increasing availability of literature, over-the-counter medication and telephone helplines that can assist individuals to make the most of what they can purchase to maintain health and well-being. The use of the internet and the encouragement of self-diagnosis have been an emerging trend within health care.

The increase in need for patient information, including sources available to health professionals, has become a feature of demand in all aspects of health care. For example, studies undertaken demonstrate that attention is paid by patients to the side effects of medication as well as the risks and benefits of screening.

Information and the health service consumer

The provision of advice and information to patients and their relatives has seen considerable improvement over the years. It was once the norm that health professionals carefully attempted to control the amount and type of information that patients received, largely contributing to uncertainty and anxiety for patients. This is well documented in early studies of hospital care (Macintosh 1974; Waitzkin and Stoeckle 1976). The major thinking uncovered in such early work revealed that doctors justified their information control on the assumption that patients did not want to be told the reality of their condition (Fietel 1965; Freidson 1970). This was the norm for many studies undertaken by Macintosh in the early 1970s, where many patients did not actually want to know about their condition but just wanted to get well (Macintosh 1974). However, much of the research indicated that patients generally felt they did not get enough information from health professionals. For example, patients with terminal conditions, including cancer, were frequently anxious to know about the condition and often reacted well to being given sufficient information; being informed that they had a condition *at all* was the issue that mattered most, rather than merely accepting treatment. This breakthrough in patient research gave weight to the position that not only was there a need for knowledge, but also for a further opportunity to discover more about the condition and range of treatment options. Hence, in health care over the years it has become necessary to view the patient as an active participant in their care and treatment rather than a passive consumer (Wilkes 1977).

Patients and their relatives require information for all kinds of reasons, but usually in relation to investigations, diagnosis and treatment, as well as prognosis. They want to know what is going to happen to them and when. In addition, they want information about the environment in which they will receive treatment, whether it be a hospital or other clinical setting, as well as about the range of expertise of the health professionals and success rates of the intervention that they are to receive. Denial of information to patients and their relatives can be construed as a denial of responsible adult status (Freidson 1970), with the implication that the patient is not capable of intelligent choice and self-control. Patients are unable to evaluate or make sense of their experiences or project what will happen in the future without adequate information sources. This has been regarded as a form of alienation in which the patient's body is surrendered to the care of health professionals without maintaining their adult status. They lose control because of a lack of sufficient information to make informed choices, or even of knowledge of what to expect in the clinical environment. This can have consequences for the patient's ability to recover and increase the likelihood of anxiety concerning their treatment and care (Cox and Wilson 2003; Watts, Merrell, Murphy and Williams 2004; Flayle and Keeley 1998; Wilson 2001).

Although the issue of alienation can occur in the patient–health professional relationship, health professionals have the right to exercise clinical judgement in the interest of their patients. Examples include access to health records, informed consent and the right to refuse treatment, as well as confidentiality (Dimond 2004). Some rights are difficult to define, for example, the right to give consent based on information has been established in law. However, there are still problems in defining informed consent in practice. The right to privacy and to be treated with dignity is complex and will depend on the quality of the services that exist. General expectations of what are considered to be acceptable standards will change as services become more proficient (Hogg 1994).

General information, information giving, the receipt of and making use of information to enable informed choice are all linked to the issue of consumerism. The role of consumerism and its rise in health care has already been established. In the dialectic of power relations, the increasing monopolization of medical knowledge and medical practice has led to the development of countervailing forces in the form of patient consumerism. This movement has become increasingly dominant in society and the struggle with consumerism operates in the relationship between the medical profession and patients, although today, with increasing specialization in health care professions, this has expanded to encapsulate all relationships with all types of health care professionals.

The patient as consumer is entitled to make choices regarding their care and treatment by obtaining the best resources to make an informed choice. It is for the service provider to enter a relationship where they can provide the best insight into the 'product', in this case, care; this is gained through access to service expertise. However, within the consumer situation, there is the issue of relationships. Some relationships are long established such as, say, that with the family doctor, and therefore access to information about health care services and treatment will be based on mutual understanding of need. For others, and especially in episodes of acute illness in hospital, the relationship with the health professional will take some time to become established, as the patient will initially be reliant on their initial impressions and experience within the service. Of course, as a consumer, the individual may find the service and information not to their liking and so be obliged to seek an alternative. Choice is important, or at least the ability to choose within the health care arena.

Involvement of consumers within health care is a situation which has evolved over the years and there has been considerable debate regarding the extent of knowledge needed to enable them to participate with and challenge the health care system and health professionals (Pollitt 1988, 1989, 1990, 1991). Others, such as Youll and Perring (1991), have described various care situations where consumer involvement has been beneficial, for example, long-term residential care settings within psychiatric services where information and education has been provided, membership of a variety of patient forums and mutual assistance groups where information sharing has been the key to success in establishing and maintaining good relationships within services and the improvement of standards of care and treatment from both perspectives. It has involved a form of power-sharing but, as can be appreciated, this can only be partial because of structure, function and status.

Strong evidence that patient expertise could be harnessed to play a part in addressing the challenge of the shifting burden of disease came from Professor Kate Lorig and her colleagues at Stanford University in California. She began to develop and evaluate programmes for people with arthritic conditions and sidestepped the traditional model of professionals educating patients. By means of a more radical and innovative solution, using trained lay leaders as educators, she equipped people who had arthritis or other chronic disease with the skills to manage their own conditions. She found that, compared with other patients, 'expert patients' could improve their self-rated health status, cope better with fatigue and other generic features of chronic disease such as role limitation and reduce their disability dependence on hospital care. The Lorig approach to self-help in chronic disease management was used by patients' organizations such as the Long-term Medical Conditions Alliance in the UK. This is a real move towards empowerment of patients working in partnership with health professionals. There is value in the approach for the management of long-term conditions and for assisting the patient in making informed choices regarding their care and treatment (DoH 2001).

The notion of 'expert' challenges the authority of health professionals because the monopoly of knowledge within the health care professions is less apparent than in the past. However, the question must be posited concerning where precisely this leaves health professionals in protecting their expert position, particularly in relation to the boundaries of medical knowledge. After all, the control of access to patient information was at one time considered to be fundamental to the maintenance of a position of authority over patients and their relatives. This was justified on the grounds that it ensured that there was compliance over care and treatment regimes, making the management of the patient less problematic for health staff. There was also a protective element for staff in situations where treatment had not been effective and where prognosis was poor and therefore medical status was threatened, not only in the patient's eyes but in the professional's own as well.

The professional loss of medical has been brought about in many ways, not only through the process of consumer empowerment in health care but also through the rise in self-help and self-diagnosis. The increasing popularity in many countries of the use of electronic sources of information has seen an alteration in the form of dialogue that is developing between health consumers and health professionals.

The use of the internet has made information accumulation and transfer possible across the professional and consumer divide, not least in the field of health care. On one level, the balance of power is, therefore, shifting. However, on another level, consumers still need to establish relationships and develop trust with the health professionals they encounter (Tann et al. 2003).

Generally, consumers of health care are likely to improve their understanding by seeking information not only from health professionals but also from other sources such as newspapers, magazines, radio and television and, increasingly, for those with access to computer facilities, the internet. The use of internet chat rooms, for example, has been beneficial in enabling consumers to obtain further information and comfort from others with similar experiences, or simply to check facts. The internet has also been regarded as a check on the health professional's competence, particularly that of doctors. This has made doctors increasingly aware of the influence of the medical web pages that patients access. They are mindful of the information that may reach the potentially vulnerable, and increasingly one aspect of the health professional's role is that of improving the dialogue they have with their patients in demystifying medical jargon, explaining the usefulness and validity of the information either on websites or in studies that are described. They are also sources for locating reliable websites and search-engine facilities for patients. This has been particularly useful for patients with long-term conditions for which they can obtain advice on risks of medication and side effects, as well as useful recipes in the case of those with cardiac, coeliac or diabetic conditions.

Studies in the United States on the use of email communication between doctor and patient found this form of communication to have increasing potential for patient involvement in the supervision and documenting of their health conditions. This has been particularly the situation in the field of oncology. The website Oncolink was established in 1994 and has visits of some 37,000 per month worldwide; the popularity of such sites has arisen because of the access to support services they provide (Van Biervleit and Edwards-Shafer 2004).

In primary care in the UK, the majority of general practice settings and pharmacies were originally computerized to enable data entry for treatment regimes and test results and are predominantly used by health staff. However, the use of email and search facilities for communicating with patients is still in its infancy, although practice nurses and GPs are aware of the support and advice that they can provide through this route to patients who have access to such facilities (Tann et al. 2003).

In relation to information exchange, patients generally have varying expectations depending on their circumstances. Some desire straightforward answers while others seek some form of negotiation in the decision-making process. Health professionals today act as information guides rather than simply providing the occasional pamphlet. Besides websites, there is a range of information available for use. The patient will of course need access to computer facilities to benefit from the services available to them on the internet. There are now supermarkets, pharmacy outlets and health clinics, as well as internet cafés and local public libraries where such facilities are available for use by the public.

The quality of the information available to patients must also be considered. There are hundreds of websites in many different languages. The level of information on specific issues ranges from the rudimentary to the more complex in specific topic areas (Tann et al. 2003). Keeping the information relevant and up to date is also a task – this presents a problem on some websites where information may be up to two years old. This is an area where health professionals have an advantage in the generation and provision of information as well as maintaining face-to-face contact in the education of patients while providing advice within their own areas of clinical expertise. Therefore, an introduction to health informatics can be a valuable aspect of training for all health professionals.

The shift in the relationship between patients-as-consumers and health care professionals presents some benefits in the sense that the better-informed consumer may prove a positive for the health professional in terms of more interesting consultations, better dialogue and shared learning.

The latest studies, however, still take the view that the authority and competence of health professionals, especially doctors, are an area for potential challenge (Hewit-Taylor 2004; Elliott and Turrell 1996; Smith 2002). This remains a problem now and for the future, as there is concern about maintaining competence and sufficient expert knowledge in the face of constant challenges from consumers, and the health professional must attempt to hold their value within a changing society where there is perceived erosion of professional dominance in health care. This points also to the arguments relating to the value of information on the internet and from other sources which enables self-diagnosis if this is what the public wants. Health professionals have a unique role, not just because of the knowledge they possess, but also because of the tasks they perform. Patients are generally preoccupied with their condition and desire to recover. They want to know about their treatment options, risks in medication, surgery, or any long-term effects that they are likely to experience, and where to locate their nearest centre of excellence; these are their main drivers for seeking information, but they are no substitute for care. As enablers, health professionals can assist in this process rather than seeing patients as a challenge to their authority or domain of health expertise.

References

Butterfield, P. (1990) Thinking upstream: nurturing a conceptual understanding of the social context of health behaviour. *Advanced Nursing Science*, **12** (2): 1–8.

Clarke, J. and Newman, J. (1997) *The Managerial State: Politics and Ideology in the Re-making of Social Welfare* (London: Sage).

Conger, J. and Kanungo, R. (1988) The empowerment process: Integrating theory and practice. *Academy of Management Review*, **13**: 471–82.

Coulter, A. and Meager, H. (2003) *The European Patient of the Future.* (Buckingham: Open University Press).

Cox, K. and Wilson, E. (2003) Follow-up for people with cancer: nurse-led services and telephone interventions. *Journal of Advanced Nursing*, **43** (1): 51–61.

Department of Health (1999) *Making a Difference* (London: Department of Health).

Department of Health (2000) *The NHS Plan* (London: Department of Health).

Department of Health (2002) *The Expert Patient: A New Approach to Chronic Disease Management in the 21st Century* (London: Department of Health).

Department of Health (2003) *Strengthening accountability: involving patients and the public: policy guidance, Section 11 of the Health and Social Care Act 2001* (London: Department of Health).

Dimond, B. (2004) *Legal Aspects of Nursing* (London: Pearson Higher Education).

Doherty, C. and Hope, W. (2000) Shared governance: nurses making a difference. *Journal of Nursing Management*, **8** (2): 77–81.

Edmonstone, J. (2000) Empowerment in the National Health Service: does shared governance offer a way forward? *Journal of Nursing Management* **8**: 259–64.

Elliott, M. and Turrell, A. (1996) Understanding the conflicts of patient empowerment. *Nursing Standard*, **10** (45): 43–7.

Fietel, H. (1965) The function of attitudes towards death. In Group for the Advancement of Psychiatry (eds), *Death and Dying: Attitudes of Patients and Doctors* (New York: GAP), ch. 5, pp. 632–41.

Flayle, J. F. and Keeley, P. (1998) Non-compliance and professional power. *Journal of Advanced Nursing*, **27**: 304–11.

Foucault, M. (1978) *The Archaeology of Knowledge* (London: Tavistock).

Freidson, E. (1970) Professional Dominance (New York: Atherton).

Haug, M. R (1973) Deprofessionalization: an alternative hypothesisfor the future. *Sociological Monograph*, **20**: 195–211.

Haug, M.R. (1975) The deprofessionalization of everyone. *Sociological Focus*, **8** (3): 197–213.

Haug, M. R. and Lavin, B. (1984) *Consumerism in Medicine: Challenging Physician Authority* (Beverly Hills, CA: Sage Publications).

Hegar, R. and Hunzeker, J. (1988) Moving toward empowerment based practice in public Child Welfare. *Social Work*, **33** (6): 499–502.

Hewit-Taylor, J. (2004) Challenging the balance of power: patient empowerment. *Nursing Standard*, **18** (22): 33–7.

Hogg, C. (1994) *Beyond the Patients' Charter: Working with Others* (London: Health Rights Publishing).

Horton, R. (2003) *Second Opinion: Doctors, Diseases and Decisions* (London: Granta Books).

Hurty, K. (1984) Power in a New Key: the hidden resources of empowerment. *Phillipine Journal of Nursing* **54** (2): 56–61.

Katz, R. (1984) Empowerment and synergy: expanding the community's healing resources. *Prevention in Human Services* **3**: 201–26.

Keiffer, C. (1984) Citizen empowerment: a developmental perspective. *Prevention in Human Services* **3**: 7–36.

Macintosh, J. (1974) Processes of communication, information seeking and control associated with cancer. *Social Science and Medicine* **8**: 167–87.

McNay, J. (1994) *Foucault: A Critical Introduction* (London: Polity).

Page, R. (1992) Empowerment, oppression and beyond: a coherent strategy? A reply to Ward and Mullender. *Critical Social Policy* **12** (2): 89–92.

Rappaport, J. (1984) Studies in empowerment: introduction to the issue. *Prevention in Human Sciences* **3**: 1–7.

Robbins, H., Hundley, V. and Osman, L. M. (2003) Minor illness education for parents of young children. *Journal of Advanced Nursing* **4**(3): 238–47.

Saks, M. (1994) The wheel turns? Professionalization and alternative medicine in Britain. *Journal of Interprofessional Care* **13** (2): 129–38.

Shaw, R. (1987) *Powerlessness in a Nursing Home Population: Classification of Nursing Diagnoses* (Toronto: Mosby).

Skelton, R. (1994) Nursing and empowerment: concepts and strategies. *Journal of Advanced Nursing* **19**: 415–23.

Smith, R. (2002) The discomfort of patient power. *British Medical Journal* **324**: 497–8.

Tann, J., Platts, A., Welch, S. and Allen, J. (2003) Patient power: medical perspectives and patient use of the internet. *Prometheus* **21** (2): 145–60.

Thomas, K. and Velthouse, B. (1990) Cognitive elements of empowerment: an 'interpretive' model of intrinsic task motivation. *Academy of Management Review* **15**: 666–81.

Tones, K. (1991) Health promotion and empowerment and the psychology of control. *Journal of the Institute of Health Education* **29** (1): 17–26.

Waitzkin, H. and Stoeckle, J. D. (1976) Information control and the micropolitics of health care: summary of an ongoing research project. *Social Science and Medicine* **10**: 263–76.

Wallerstein, N. and Bernstein, E. (1988) Empowerment education: Friere's ideas adapted to health education. *Health Education Quarterly* **15**(4): 379–94.

Watts, R. (1990) Democratization of health care: challenge for nursing. *Advances in Nursing Science* **12**(2): 37–46.

Watts, T., Merrell, J., Murphy, F. and Williams, A. (2004) Breast health information needs of women from minority ethnic groups. *Journal of Advanced Nursing* **47**(5): 526–35.

Wheeler, C. and Chinn, P. (1989) *Peace and Power: A Handbook of Feminist Process*, 2nd edn (New York: National League for Nursing).

Wilkes, E. (1977) Effects of the knowledge of diagnosis in terminal illness. *Nursing Times*, **73**(11): 1506–7.

Wilson, H. V. (2001) Power and partnership: a Critical analysis of the surveillance discourses of child health nurses. *Journal of Advanced Nursing* **36**(2): 294–301.

Youll, P. and Perring, C. (1991) *Voice and Choice: User Participation in Service Development and Evaluation* (The Hague: European Group for Public Administration Study Group on Quality and Productivity).

www.bbcnews.co.uk/bristol, BBC News (2003) Memorial to Bristol Heart Babies, 22 April 2003.

www.bbcnews.co.uk/scotland/mrsa, BBC News (2005) MRSA Scare in Hospital Baby Unit, 27 September 2005.

www.bbcnews.co.uk/england/manchester/shipman, BBC News (2003) Shipman Enquiry Criticises Police, 14 July 2003.

CHAPTER 3

Clinical Governance

JUDY SMITH

Whilst researching the correct and appropriate words to provide a definition of clinical governance, it all came flooding back – the initial concerns that occurred at the time the term was first introduced into National Health vocabulary. What was clinical governance, why did we need it, what were we supposed to do to make sure we complied with the requirements? This chapter will discuss clinical governance; it will consider how it has evolved and how it now works within primary care. It will look at some of the difficulties around delivering the clinical governance agenda and how our initial concerns have changed; finally it will consider what clinical governance is like in some other countries.

The specific words 'clinical governance' became particularly important for the National Health Service in 1997 when the Department of Health said that quality measures had to be introduced. *The New NHS* (DoH 1998) gave more information and things became clearer still in 1999 when the Health Bill gave NHS trusts a legal responsibility to put a quality framework in place. To ensure that clinical governance was given priority by chief executives, at a time when a lot was happening within the NHS, they were made accountable, with a statutory duty to provide 'a framework through which NHS organisations are accountable for continually improving the quality of their services and safeguarding high standards of care by creating an environment in which excellence of clinical care will flourish' (DoH 1998). This, then, was the definition of clinical governance from the Department of Health.

If many people within the NHS originally appeared unclear about exactly what clinical governance was and why we needed it, this might have been because trusts were already working towards ensuring a quality service. The need to formalize and perhaps perceivably bureaucratize what already was occurring certainly meant that some clinicians treated clinical governance with caution. People were already carrying out audit as well as developing and using evidence-based guidelines, so some wondered why there was a need to take things further. Others recognized that the new requirements aimed to put a system in place that would raise the standards of health care and identify and improve poor performance; trusts needed to be able to demonstrate to others that this work was being undertaken. It was not enough just to comply with this strategy; it was essential that the process could be evidenced. No longer was it sufficient to monitor services; we needed to demonstrate that, when appropriate, changes were being made to improve them.

Accountability as a driver of clinical governance was not a new concept – way back in 1990, Irvine discussed the accountability of health professionals and commented that governments wanted value for money and responsive services. The Labour government of 1999 was now putting the responsibility for efficient services – the accountability – firmly in the hands of the Chief Executives.

The NHS reforms that occurred as a result of the NHS review (DoH 1989) had led to service contracts, including negotiated quality standards and targets, in agreements between purchasers and providers (Leathard 2000). Fundholding GPs had the opportunity to decide where to purchase hospital care and it may be that this process had not been as effective in driving up standards as had been hoped. Or perhaps the standards and targets were focused on meeting required numbers or 'bed days' without fully considering the actual quality of care delivered. In many cases, the standards were only driving forward improvements in secondary care, as generally primary care was purchased from secondary care rather than the other way around.

As the 1990s commenced, tension grew between clinicians and managers as managers tried to streamline for efficiency and clinicians perceived that quality of care was being reduced. The internal market developed, yet the government did not robustly evaluate the results of its reforms. Consequently, later in the decade it seemed that outcomes were not always positive as what was later known as a 'postcode lottery' became apparent, when some trusts and GPs could afford certain treatments and care while others could not. In fact, the reforms may themselves have led to increased managerial costs due to the contracting and management process which reduced funds available for direct patient care. Ultimately research by the Audit Commission (1996) demonstrated that only innovative and well-organized practices were able to use fundholding to improve the quality of care for their patients and generally it was felt that the introduction of competition into the NHS was not yet working as had been hoped.

Another driver for clinical governance may well have been an indirect result of 'patient power' as public confidence in health care was dwindling. The Patients' Charter, a Conservative Party initiative in 1991, had led to greater expectations for patients and public and, as people realized that they were not getting what they wanted, so they began to grumble. In fact the production of the Charter was aimed at generating accountability to service users; naturally they wanted the best care in the best place and if they could not get their appointments when and where they wanted, they began to complain. Some staff found this quite threatening and there was a perception that all the 'power' had shifted to the patient; consequently morale in some areas became very poor.

It is interesting on reflection to realize that we saw complaints as a negative process whereas now we see them as opportunities to learn and improve – although we would still prefer not to have them! Perhaps one of the reasons we initially struggled with the concept of clinical governance was because we felt threatened by it. Perhaps, because there was no specific and clear definition, it was difficult to understand exactly what it meant, so we were confused. Was it going to remove all professional decision-making? Would we lose our professional autonomy?

Why were we now having these doubts when as far back as 1960 Donabedian had raised the issues of quality of health care? He continued to publish his views and in 1980 brought one aspect of clinical governance quality to the forefront of health care by highlighting the need to demonstrate our effectiveness, for example, by measuring against pre-set standards. We needed good quality evidence to measure against; we needed to have measurable outcomes, we needed quality research, clinical audit and bench-marking. Now the government wanted to be assured that the NHS was delivering a quality and safe service. Clearly despite all the work that had previously been carried out, there was a need to make such quality care a legal requirement.

In 1993 clinical audit, a tool already well established for nursing staff, became more relevant to the rest of the NHS as the health reforms brought it within everyone's remit. As local trusts developed, so they embraced audit and many set up specific audit departments and training for their staff so that peers could audit each other. Initially it seemed that as long as we were seen to be auditing then all would be well; in some cases it was mere lip service to quality improvements. However, before long the emphasis became learning from audit rather than using it as a tool for management: making changes, closing the loop, repeating the audit cycle to demonstrate that change had been effective. Doing the right thing for the right person in the right way in the right place with the right clinician ...

As things progressed, it became clear that clinical governance was going to apply throughout the NHS – not even consultants would be exempt (Tyndall 1998). Healthcare standards were introduced although, as Gaster (1995) argues, standards are not a substitute for policy but can be important symbols and tools for policy. Gradually various initiatives were introduced such as 'Chimp', the name of which was swiftly changed to CHI – the Commission for Health Improvement. This was a statutory body which undertook inspection of all NHS trusts to assess local arrangements for clinical governance. Then in 1999 we had NICE (the National Institute for Clinical Excellence) – originally set up to provide guidance on effectiveness and quality. Health Action Zones (HAZs), Health Improvement Programmes (HImps), league tables, benchmarking, essence of care and National Service Frameworks have all played, and some continue to play, their part in providing a structure to assist effective clinical governance processes and outcomes.

Where we are now

Muir Gray put it quite nicely (1997), commenting that we have moved through the 1970s and 1980s from doing things right (cheaper/better) to doing the right things (more good than harm) in the 1990s and now in the 2000s we have to do the right things right. So we need to do more good than harm and do it cheaper and better! We also need to do things in a co-ordinated way.

Just as in the early 1990s, many trusts had their own specific audit department, so later in that decade and continuing into the 21st century, most have chosen to set up a clinical governance department. Occasionally these departments have become mini-industries, embracing clinical effectiveness, risk management and audit sections. Consequently some clinicians seemed to think that they did not need to worry about clinical governance; after all there was a department who took that responsibility. In some cases it took a while for people to realize that clinical governance was everyone's business and that we all had to take responsibility to ensure we provided effective, responsive and safe care for our patients, that clinical governance should be seen as underpinning everything that is happening within a PCT. It has always been there, implicitly, for clinicians but since the onus has been firmly put into the hands of the Chief Executives, the ethos has spread through PCTs like ink through blotting paper – gradually the message is seeping through. The culture is changing; we question more and, moreover, we link financial issues to clinical governance. Clinical governance is and in fact needs to be much more than any one department's business. The Royal College of Nursing (2003) provided a useful description when claiming that clinical governance integrates all the activities that impact on patient care in one framework, and it is an umbrella term for everything that helps to maintain and improve high standards of care.

So it encompasses standard-based and cyclical audit, it uses benchmarking, it exploits National Service Frameworks (NSFs) to encourage cross-boundary working. It requires evidence-based guidelines to be developed and implemented; it encourages quality and applicable research; it needs professional competency and ongoing training with continual professional development for all staff. It includes dealing with poor performance, self-regulation, clinical leadership and it necessitates a positive organizational culture.

As Strategic Health Authorities shift the balance of power, so accountability has moved closer to the primary care trusts, practices, dentists, opthamologists, pharmacists and every clinician. More than that, each individual member of the NHS staff has a part to play in ensuring that clinical governance requirements are met. The new GMS contracts are integral to its further development comprising standards for appraisal, training, education and continual personal development that are now tied to the purses of practitioners. It is rolling out to other health professionals as the dental PMS and new pharmacy contracts come into force. NSFs are encouraging partnership working amongst disease-focused practitioners. Such working has been encouraged in order to streamline the patient's journey (Secretary of State 1997) and whilst this is still happening only gradually, there is a feeling 'on the ground' that this way of working is growing; there is also a perception that clinicians are becoming less possessive of their own field of work and are starting to see the benefits for patients of skill mix.

The more latterly integrated Healthcare Commission Standards which aim to reduce the amount of 'checking up' for PCTs also provide a useful stimulus to maintain and improve clinical governance. It is too early to assess whether the standards make clinical governance more straightforward or if they reduce the bureaucracy associated with having multiple agencies checking standards; whilst the number of criteria may be reduced, the detail by which the criteria appear to be judged seems to be as complicated as ever.

How it works in primary care

Primary care is where a patient first attends; for example it might be a dental practice or a health centre, with various clinicians such as a therapist, an allied health professional, a nurse or a General Practitioner. Each Primary Care Trust, individual practice or service usually has a lead for clinical governance.

A qualitative study was conducted by Meal et al. (2004) to investigate the views of general practice clinical governance leads on their role in relation to the delivery of clinical governance. These were generally positive and showed an ongoing commitment to quality despite some initial reluctance to take on the role. After a year, attitudes had evolved – roles were developing beyond practice into link roles with others and with primary care organizations. The research recommended protected time to help GPs make the most of clinical governance.

If time for clinical governance was an issue for GPs, then it was just such a problem for the rest of the primary care team. Take the example of research governance; following incidents like that at Alderhay, the requirements to meet research governance have become massively bureaucratic and consequently have put people off research. Perhaps it has even discouraged people from applying for local and ethical approval, bringing greater risks to the researcher, subjects and relevant organizations. People might choose to call their research by another name – audit/evaluation/service development, etc. – rather than contend with the relevant paperwork and form-filling. Fortunately the Department of Health realized what was happening and has tried to reduce the relevant paperwork. Nevertheless, it can still act as a deterrent. If we are to have evidence-based care, we clearly need research to take place, so a balance needs to be achieved between governance requirements and practicalities. Good researchers understand the reasons behind the paperwork and, when bidding for funding, allow for the extra time that this requires.

Nurses and therapists have become used to clinical governance – they have been trained to practise reflectively – to consider what they did, whether it worked or could be improved. They have also learned how to manage unusual or difficult situations via clinical supervision which allows clinicians to discuss any issues which may have arisen in a safe and secure environment. They may wish to discuss issues such as a problem with a particular patient or illness; their supervisor can steer the clinician towards uncovering the solution to their problem themselves, suggest opportunities for continuing their professional development and support the clinician through the learning process. Supervision might use reflection as a tool; reflective practice encourages clinicians to think about how their clinical work has gone – the outcomes, whether good or less satisfactory. This practice means that they can learn from their experiences and then continue with successful care, changing things that can be improved. For example they might consider how, if near misses have happened, to reduce risks in future.

All PCTs and practitioners have an obligation to report untoward and 'near miss' incidents; this information can then be shared with others, either locally or nationally, to allow learning from this experience. The sharing of such information is vital; however, not all practitioners feel secure about this process, believing that if they self-report incidents they may be disciplined. There is still a perceived 'blame' culture within the NHS and this is something that needs addressing, else how are we to learn from and identify common trends? This blame culture also seems to prevent people from 'whistle blowing', the practice in which colleagues bring inappropriate or dangerous practice to management's attention. There appears to be a resistance to 'turning in' one's colleagues, some sort of misguided protection of a professional by a fellow professional.

If incidents are reported, so too are potential risks; clinical risk management is where potential risks are considered and risk forms completed, which identify risks and consider possible solutions. The risks and the financial costs to reducing them are considered, and a decision is made as to whether the risk will be accepted or whether suggested actions should be implemented to reduce the risk.

Clinical governance was given an additional incentive with the introduction of new regulations on instrument sterility. This was the result of learning from the experiences of Creutzfeldt-Jakob disease, when instruments with ferrules were found to have live viral deposits post autoclaving. The regulations have led to a debate about whether to use central sterilizing depots, to continue with benchtop autoclaves or to use disposable instruments. Where sterilization is carried out locally, a stringent protocol needs to be followed. This has meant that continual training is needed to ensure that staff know how to do things correctly.

Training and continuing professional development is fundamental to clinical governance. Some might consider that we need to train not just the staff but also those in schools and higher education establishments as well as others in professional training. An example is the drive to reduce hospital-gained infections; the media have encouraged patients to ask all who come to deliver them care, food and so on if that person has washed their hands. This drive has meant that more people are beginning to understand what causes the problem and how to decrease the risk. So public health departments and educators, as well as the whole of our society, have a pivotal role to play in clinical governance.

Yet one could argue that the NHS workforce could be the most effective cog in the governance wheel. This is evident outside overtly clinical issues; for example, the current trend of increasing greater skill mix with the skilled not registered workforce can reduce cost to the NHS whilst still delivering quality of care. Those financial savings can then be put to other uses and clinicians can use their particular skills more appropriately and concentrate on clinical work. Thus back to Muir Gray and 'more good than harm and cheaper and better!'

Appropriate continual professional development is now firmly linked to payment by results within the Skills and Knowledge Framework as part of the Agenda for Change. For any member of staff to progress through the next pay 'gateway', they need to be able to demonstrate that they are meeting required competencies. Hopefully this will be a very effective tool in the governance armoury, as nothing motivates like money! The new GMS contract also encourages payment by results for independent practitioners – for example within the Quality Outcome Framework, where practices receive funding for each point awarded. Consequently, there is an impetus for practices to participate in appraisal, research, patient surveys and audit and so forth.

Audit itself continues to play its role. Audit has matured and is now targeted to those areas where there is a perceived need so that appropriate changes are made and re-audit is carried out to ensure that these changes are effective. Thus we measure/monitor/evaluate and look at inputs/through-puts/outputs/outcomes as we map the patients' journeys. Then we remodel/re-audit/re-evaluate and the process again moves forward, all in the name of clinical governance.

So does all this activity have a positive effect? Are there fewer complaints, fewer untoward incidents? Are patients safer and happier?

Patients and public involvement in clinical governance

Patients and the public are crucial to clinical governance, but how do we engage with them in a meaningful manner? Practices are encouraged to conduct annual patient satisfaction surveys and respond accordingly, and PCTs usually appoint a patient and public engagement officer as part of a move towards a patient-led NHS. We allow for diversity, as all people need to feel safe accessing NHS services and to be able to become involved in shaping the way that services are delivered. Kendall (2001) highlighted that recent policies were leading to a more patient-centred service; however, patient experience in 2000 was typically not perceived as good. Patients were struggling to get what they wanted, where they wanted and with whom they wanted. More recently, the Choice Initiative has been introduced and patients will drive clinical governance as they choose to be treated at places or sites more convenient to them and more quickly, according to their preference. They may choose a different provider; for example, foot surgery may be with a podiatric surgeon in day surgery under local anaesthetic rather than with an orthopaedic surgeon, who is then free to concentrate on other surgery like replacement knees, hips and so on.

The patient/professional relationship is central to perceptions of level of care (Kendall 2001). As telemedicine becomes more widespread in the delivery of health care, how will we measure its value, how will we govern that? Will patients gain the satisfaction that occurs in good one-to-one relationships? Or if care is given by specialist disease-focused teams, will that mean that patients will need to be seen by one team for diabetes, one team for their arthritis and yet another team for cardio- vascular disease, instead of receiving all their care within their GP surgery? Or will the changes occurring in 2005 mean that we end up with a 'health village' model – only time will tell.

Potential for improvement

One major flaw with current clinical governance as it is happening in PCTs is its failure to link health economics with outcomes. It would be useful if research could be undertaken to identify how this could best work. Financial costs need to be considered alongside benefits of care and delivery of service. These need to consider more than 'actual' costs and obvious benefits; they should reflect quality of life outcomes and costs/ benefits to society as a whole. Whilst PCTs and all health communities have an obligation to break even financially, this may sometimes make clinical decisions feel unethical; clinicians and patients alike could benefit from support and training so that they can see the bigger picture and thus understand the reasons behind difficult decisions. We are yet to see the effect that streamlining of assessment has on PCTs and whether it reduces the bureaucratic workload. Such a reduction will be a positive step towards reducing an administrative and financial burden.

Housing estates will need to be considered more carefully if buildings are to support appropriate clinical care; they need to have suitable air conditioning, floor coverings, wall coverings and so on to reduce the risk of cross-infection and to facilitate adequate cleanliness. As NHS organizations close buildings and sell off land to assist with financial restraints, they must not ignore the fact that existing and new buildings need to be appropriate.

Robust information technology is needed to support clinical governance, and research is taking place to show how this can best work. This will be useful to help implement evidence-based practice, using the National Electronic Library for Health, computerized GP data-base systems with prompts and the many other support systems. The new nationwide IT system, once it is finally in place, will enable better data analysis so that areas for improvement can be identified. This could include prescribing patterns which should help reduce inappropriate prescribing; it might identify practices and PCTs with better outcomes, enabling their work to be scrutinized so that improvements for others can be achieved.

The change to NHS data systems, where the whole of the United Kingdom will be linked, enabling patients' medical records to be accessed wherever they are needed, will be useful in reducing risks. It will mean that someone's allergies are identified so that appropriate and safe prescriptions and treatment can be given. It will also allow identification of patients who need closer scrutiny, and so enable health behaviour changes to be encouraged. Better use of IT will mean that services can be developed and changed to provide more timely and effective care. It might help identify where skill mix could be effectively used in order to meet the needs of patients within the financial constraints of the NHS budget. The change to NHS data systems, where the whole of the UK will be linked, will be useful in risk reduction as appropriate and safe prescriptions and treatment can be given.

As previously mentioned, the opportunities arising through the Agenda for Change and the Knowledge and Skills framework could prove very beneficial in driving forward clinical governance. To support this, we need to ensure that educational needs are identified and provided for through appraisal or needs analysis. Then we need adequate mentoring and supervisory capability; this should be there for all staff, not just clinicians. Barriers to clinical governance have been evident; in particular a lack of time had been identified (Johnston et al. 2000). Some GP practices have a hierarchical structure which may not lend itself well to joint decision making (Haycock-Stuart and Houston 2005). Team members may have different objectives and incentives. For example a practice nurse may want to attend a particular training session but their practice manager may not have funds to provide appropriate clinical cover. Use of protected time for GPs has reduced that obstacle for them, but has it done so for the rest of the practice team?

The time for continuing professional development needs to be protected and practices should be accountable for the way it is used. Patients belonging to the practice could ask staff how they use their time and suggest areas where they think the practice teams could improve. It is of interest that Haycock-Stuart and Houston's (2005) study found that primary health care team members value education within protected time, clinicians especially so, but administrative staff to a lesser extent. This could be because they do not see clinical governance as so relevant to them and maybe this is one of the key learning points – that clinical governance is everybody's business.

Government itself is not exempt from room for improvement; greater consideration still needs to be given to both professional registration and regulation. It is questionable if self-regulation is sufficiently transparent to satisfy the public that wants to see that health care is being provided by properly trained and educated staff and that medical errors are dealt with appropriately. There is still a feeling that an 'old boys' network exists with a reluctance to inform on colleagues who may be underperforming. This does not create a feeling of security. PCTs have been able to instil clinical governance policies and procedures in their directly employed staff more easily than in GPs; here there is still a tension between autonomy and accountability. PCTs have responsibility yet GPs are independent contractors. The PCT can offer help, advice and support but cannot insist that things are done in a particular way. They can send out NICE guidelines and bring guidance to GPs' attention; GPs do not always agree with guidelines and can choose not to use them and may be proved correct in their judgement, as for example in the case of the Cox inhibitor guidelines.

It could be that the move away from service provision will enable PCTs to deal with these issues in a more direct way, as potential conflicts of interest will be reduced, yet it is difficult to direct independent contractors who are, after all, running their own small businesses.

We still do not perform as well as we should in recognizing and replicating good practice; while there have been networks like CHAIN, these have struggled for survival. Why should we believe a reliable network and communication mechanism exists to transfer knowledge between NHS organizations when there may not be a totally effective network within the individual organizations themselves? Why is this and why do individuals in a health community not know about other projects and roles within that community? Communication surveys are carried out regularly and there is some improvement; people try to publicize new roles and services, yet it is questionable if staff read newsletters and emails as their time for reading is limited. Emails themselves are a wonderful thing for enabling communication; however, since we are nearly all connected, they can have their downside as mail boxes fill up at alarming rates.

Other areas which could be improved include geographical discrepancies which can produce postcode lotteries for some specific treatments, particularly prescriptions. The difficulties surrounding league tables have been well documented and the general public is realizing that they can be taken at face value; they see that more mortality is likely to occur where there are higher risk procedures or where higher risk patients are being treated.

We should not underestimate our patients; as we involve and empower them, they are managing their care themselves. Where in the learning process for self-care do we fit clinical governance? Should we be measuring these improvements or deteriorations and, if so, how do we do this? There is no doubt that the public has the greatest role to play in clinical governance. Today's patients have been encouraged to become 'expert' patients and to know what the most effective treatments are; they are well read and want the best, despite realizing that there is no bottomless pot of money. Staff are not always in a position to make autonomous decisions in support of patients' preferences and may not be able to respond to their demands. Coote (1993) has identified the potential for increased demand where practitioners have to perform a balancing act between patients' wishes and available services. Perhaps the patient who more actively researches information ends up getting the best care – he who shouts loudest? This could result in excellent quality of care for a few but poorer quality for the masses.

The drive to move patients from secondary to primary care, in effect to prevent the need for hospital admission at all, has undoubted financial benefits, yet this is not proving a positive benefit for the public or for primary care. Patients and staff see hospital wards close, yet do not see improvements in primary care. Certainly a vertical patient costs less to look after than a horizontal one, but why has the money not followed the patient and been transferred to this area?

Another challenge in the move to bring patients out of expensive secondary care into less costly primary care is the increase in workload for general practitioners. The work is then shifted from GP to nurse, and from nurse to health care support worker, so that the patient may be cared for by competent rather than expert staff – if expertise is acquired through practice. In practices team support acts as a safety net.

Partnership working is one of the opportunities for really improving clinical governance; we need to be working not just with other health and social care organizations but also with academic and educational institutions and councils. Using the same support structures will save money and we can also learn from each other – that is, assuming we can set up effective communication processes!

Learning may be derived from problems, such as those that occurred with research governance; following incidents at Alderhay and Bristol, and in some ways exacerbated by directives from the European Community, clinical governance became massively bureaucratic. It is now improving but researchers are still frustrated by the level of governance as it is not always risk related. So in some cases there has been a disregard for ethical issues; academic institutions may encourage researchers to design their studies so as to avoid having to subject them to ethical and governance processes; this can lead to it being less useful and can diminish patient and public involvement. So when Government considers legislation, policies or procedures, it should ponder whether they will actually have the desired effect or whether they will self-destruct.

If clinical governance is to be truly effective, there is a need to identify strong leadership, so that clinical teams can be supported through the ongoing changes within the NHS. There have been so many structural changes that many people have become disillusioned and demotivated. Others see the reasoning behind the changes and have been able to seize the opportunities that have consequently arisen. Nevertheless, when jobs are at risk that affects staff morale in general. The agenda change has, along with its potential benefits, brought massive disruption as so many staff have been removed from their existing roles in order to support the process. Perhaps what we really need is a period of stability so that staff can grow in confidence and regain their innovative flair which seems to diminish with successive changes.

Most recently, Nigel Crisp (DoH 2005) in *A Patient-led NHS* talks about 'recognising that some services are indispensable while others can be replaced'. While this is undoubtedly true, it may indicate that parts of some services will disappear. This may be an acknowledgement that we cannot do all things for all people and will surely encourage the use of evidence-based practice.

Payment by results will add to the evidence-based impetus as money will follow effective care; already, critical appraisal training is gaining popularity not just with researchers but also with managers and clinical staff. We should now be offering this to the public, perhaps teaching this skill in schools and colleges, as papers and magazines report and reflect new research. This will allow public and patients to discuss treatment options and effectiveness in an informed manner, thus removing some of the difficulties for clinicians. Patients have learned to question decisions; now they need support to become intelligently involved in choices in their health care.

Clinical governance – some international differences

Clinical governance is not just a UK initiative; it has been and still is happening elsewhere. We can learn from these models, for example in New Zealand where they identified 'cultural safety' as an issue when the health of Maoris was put at risk by uninformed nursing and midwifery practice (Ramsden 1992). Now all people's views need to be seen as legitimate rather than ignorant and all nursing students are taught appropriately. Richardson and Carryer (2005) studied the teaching of cultural safety to explore the experience of both Maoris and Pakeha nursing students. They describe this teaching as unique to New Zealand. It is a good example of learning through experience and using bad practice to influence appropriate change. Now we need to learn from these experiences and consider the issues in the UK's diverse population. Although health organizations consider cultural safety for their patients and raise diversity awareness with their staff, specific cultural safety is not routinely a part of nursing or other health professional training.

Boulton et al. (2004) discussed the Maori health strategy that was a part of the New Zealand Public Health and Disability Act (2000). Research suggests this has been successful in encouraging greater Maori participation in governance issues. The UK challenge is to have representation from all communities participating in health decisions and governance.

It seems that there is a lot to learn from the experience of the New Zealand model and perhaps something has already been learnt. Malcolm and Mays (1999) discussed the independent practitioners in New Zealand's development of an integrated clinical and financial accountability that they identified as useful for health care groups in primary care in the UK. They considered that this was a better way of dealing with clinical governance than the more isolated approach being taken within the NHS. The independent practitioner associations in New Zealand were established in 1992, when GPs there felt threatened by health reforms. They took responsibility for non-general medical service budgets for things such as laboratory and pharmaceutical services, giving them the opportunity to affect the quality of clinical decisions. It also allowed them to make savings and use this money for, among other things, developing new services. This was way ahead of the NHS where many PCTs have only recently started to build quality standards into contracts. Since then a District Health Board system has been implemented; one reason for this is to democratize health care governance. Consequently, boards are no longer appointed by government but are elected.

Australia has seen an increase in attention given to clinical governance (Callaly et al. 2005) as a unifying concept aimed at providing structure and systems to ensure and improve the quality of clinical services through an integrated and organization-wide approach. They suggest that some practitioners may find this hard as they might feel their clinical autonomy is being threatened. This reflects the views of some UK practitioners.

Research by Coulter and Rozansky (2004) demonstrated that shared decision-making is delivered in a more paternalistic way in the United Kingdom compared with New Zealand, Australia, Canada and the United States of America. This was supported by findings from the Healthcare Commission (2005) in Accident and Emergency departments where 20 per cent of patients did not feel that they had sufficient information to be fully involved in their own care. These few examples seem to show that the UK is learning but could learn still more from other countries' experiences; it is not just decision-making that needs to be shared.

In conclusion, there is still a perception that clinical governance is not as robust as it might be in some PCTs. In 2002, NICE felt it appropriate to publish a book on clinical audit, saying that 'the time has come for everyone in the NHS to take clinical audit very seriously.' This made me wonder what had been happening previously. NICE said that clinical audit was at the heart of clinical governance. I think that those words could have been better chosen – it is a part of it but not the heart of it. The heart of clinical governance must be the culture of the organization. Clinical governance legally starts with Chief Executives; however, we have argued that the responsibility goes much further than that. It started out simply as a framework to draw all its components together in a more formal process.

Now we use research to support clinical effectiveness, we keep practice current and we check to ensure that it is working as it ought. 'Prove it, learn it, use it, audit it, update it.' So we produce evidence-based guidelines, we put procedures and policies in place. We look at financial risk and corporate governance; we integrate clinical and cost accountability and we adopt a risk-based approach, focusing on patient care and safety. Yet we still need to get patients well and truly involved in their care and support and that may mean allowing practitioners to deviate from guidelines. If we want quality indicators, then perhaps the best question is: does the treatment work for the patient? Do they feel better? Perhaps we spend too much time looking at medical outcomes and insufficient time talking to patients about how they feel.

It is strange really that at the time of writing, a case is being made for the advancement of clinical governance, yet we are still dismissive of this to some degree, suspecting that getting other organizations to accept that they are partners in health might be tricky. It may help focus on the real possibilities if one considers countries where poverty is rife, for example in Africa where more than 50,000 people die every day. We would not dream of suggesting that the solution there is clinical governance framework; we can all see that their need is much more far-reaching than that. There is no need for double-checking prescriptions when tablets are themselves a luxury. As demonstrated by the Make Poverty History and Live8 campaigns, millions of people recognize that there are things that other countries besides Africa could do to influence change. So we need to grasp the concept of public health and public accountability, of clinical governance being everybody's business. We must learn from experience, not just local experience but national and pan-national experience; not just from health but from all societal experience.

Way back in 1980, Donabedian discussed the benefits of the unifying model of quality – benefits/risks/costs – best balance. For clinical governance to be really effective, a cultural shift needs to take place throughout the NHS and beyond; it cannot be done in isolation. It is not just up to the NHS trusts and its social services partners; it is the responsibility of education, academic institutes, government and its civil servants, local authorities and councils.

The shifting the balance of power continues to instil clinical governance more deeply into the culture of the NHS – it is devolving to the 'ground floor' so that clinicians are more often influencing service design and change and thinking about how best to spend their limited resources. Ownership gives responsibility. The NHS is 'owned' by the whole of UK society and therefore the true responsibility lies with each and every person within the UK. Clinical governance is the foundation on which good clinical practice is built. To be truly effective, responsibility for it must be taken by the whole of our society.

References

Audit Commission (1996) *What the Doctor Ordered: A Study of GP Fundholders in England and Wales* (London: HMSO).

Boulton, A., Simonsen, K., Walker, T., Cumming, J. and Cunningham, C. (2004) Indigenous participation in the 'new' New Zealand health structure. *Journal of Health Service Research Policy* 9 (2): 35–40.

Callaly, T., Arya, D. and Minas, H. (2005) Quality, risk management and governance in mental health: an overview. *Australasia Psychiatry* 13 (1): 16–20.

Coote, A. (1993) Understanding quality. *Journal of Interprofessional Care* 7 (2): 141–50.

Coulter, A. and Rozansky, D. (2004) Full engagement in health. *British Medical Journal* 329: 1197–8.

Currie, L., Morrell, C. and Scrivener, R. (2004) Clinical Governance: quality at centre of services. *British Journal of Midwifery* 12 (5): 330–4.

Department of Health (1989) *Working for Patients: The Health Service, Caring for the 1990s* (London: HMSO).

Department of Health (1991) *The Patients' Charter* (London: Department of Health).

Department of Health (1998) *The New NHS, Modern and Dependable: A National Framework for Assessing Performance* (London: HMSO).

Department of Health (2005) *A Patient-led NHS* (London: Department of Health).

Donabedian, A. (1966) Evaluating the quality of medical care. *Millbank Memorial Fund Quarterly* 3 (2): 166–207.

Donabedian, A. (1980) The definition of quality: a conceptual exploration. In Donabedian, A. and Arbour, A. (eds) *Explorations in Quality Assessment and Monitoring*, vol. 1: *The Definition of Quality and Approaches to Its Assessment* (Michigan: Health Administration Press).

Donabedian, A. (1988) The quality of care: how can it be assessed? *Journal of American Medical Association* 260 (12): 1743–8.

Gaster, C. (1995) *Quality in Public Services* (Buckingham: Open University Press).

Haycock-Stuart, E. and Houston, N. (2005) Evaluation study of a resource for developing education, audit and teamwork in primary care. *Primary Health Care Research and Development* 6: 251–68.

Healthcare Commission Feb 2005

Health Funding Authority of New Zealand (1998) *The Next Five Years in Practice* (Wellington: Health Funding Authority).

Irvine, D. (1990) *Managing for Quality in General Practice* (London: Kings Fund).

Johnston, G., Crombie, I., Davies, H., Alder, E. and Millard, A. (2000) Reviewing audit: barriers and facilitating factors for effective clinical audit. *Quality in Health Care* 9: 23–36.

Kendall, L. (2001) *The Future Patient* (London: IPPR).

Leathard, A. (2000) *Health Care Provision Past, Present and into the 21st Century* (Cheltenham: Stanley Thornes).

Malcolm, L. and Mays, N. (1999) New Zealand's independent practitioner associations: a working model of clinical governance in primary care? *British Medical Journal* 319: 1340–2.

Meal, A., Wynn, A., Pringle, M., Carter, R. and Hippisley-Cox, J. (2004) Forging links: evolving attitudes of clinical governance leads in general practice. *Quality in Primary Care* 12 (1): 59–64.

Muir Gray, J. A. (1997) *Evidence-Based Healthcare* (London: Churchill Livingstone).

National Institute for Clinical Excellence. (2002) *Principles for Best Practice: I Clinical Audit* (Oxford: Radcliffe Medical Press).

Patten, S., Mitton, C. and Donaldson, C. (2005) From the trenches: views from decision makers on health services priority setting. *Health Service Management Research* 18 (2): 100–8.

Ramsden, I. (1992) *Kawa Whakaruruhau: Guidelines for Nursing and Midwifery Education* (Wellington: Nursing Council of New Zealand).

Richardson, F. and Carryer, J. (2005) Teaching cultural safety in a New Zealand nursing education program. *Journal of Nurse Educator* **44** (5): 210–18.

Royal College of Nursing (2003) *Clinical Governance: A Resource Guide* (London: RCN).

Secretary of State for Health (1997) *The New NHS: Modern – Dependable* (London: HMSO).

Sowden, D. (2005) Clinical governance and the interface with education and the assessment of learning. *Developing an Effective Workforce Conference* (Nottingham: Trent SHA).

Tyndall, R. (1998) Clinical governance: shift workers. *Health Service Journal* **108** (5631): 27–9.

CHAPTER 4

Interprofessional Working

NICOLA WADDIE

This chapter explores the way in which interprofessional working has arisen and the way in which its development influences, in particular, nursing practice.

Interprofessional working is a complex paradigm with the potential to impact at organizational, professional and personal levels of working. The notion of collaboration between health authorities and local authorities became a major policy objective in the early 1970s, as both health and local government were reorganized in recognition that health and social policies were essentially intertwined (Chapman et al. 1995). However, interprofessional working is a relatively new concept in health and social care, rising out of the development of The Third Way, a philosophy aiming to prevent the domination of health policies by changing political attitudes and priorities (Giddens 1998). Instead, interprofessional working aims to replace competition with partnerships and, in doing so, facilitate working that crosses professional and organizational boundaries (Salmon and Jones 2001). Barrett et al. (2005) suggest that the efficacy of different professionals working together indicates the quality of the service received. Thus, interprofessional working not only aims to support the objectives of the NHS plan (DoH 2000) but also to reduce, if not eliminate, professional rivalries that potentially inhibit the delivery of excellence in health care. It is significant to note, despite its recent emergence, that this construct is an integral aspect of government policy, for use as a tool to bring about significant changes in the way in which the National Health Service (NHS) is structured and the way in which it will function in future (DoH 1997, 1998, 2000). Pietroni (1994: 81) states: 'All areas of activity – hospitals, general practice, community nursing and personal social services – are being completely re-organized, and several fundamental changes will ensure that professional working patterns will alter substantially.'

Despite the newness of this innovation, the rapid uptake of the philosophy has potentially far-reaching implications for the professionals working across the whole range of health and social care settings. The legal ramifications of the proposed developments would require that revolutionary transformations be made within organizational infrastructures to ensure the support of such collaborative initiatives at an operational level. The constructive engagement of individuals at all levels across the NHS will be necessary if such transformations are to occur. This narrative will focus, in particular, on the implications of such events for nursing practice and explore the impact they may have on future nursing developments.

This chapter also explores the definitions of the wide range of terms associated with interprofessional working as well as its antecedents and thus demonstrates the differences between interprofessional working and other collaborative initiatives, including those such as multidisciplinary or multi-professional working. These issues will be considered in light of the current political agenda reflecting planned or actual changes in health and social care policies. The role of the UK government in supporting the expansion of nursing clinical practice will be evaluated.

The chapter will also discuss proposals put forward to ensure that the introduction of interprofessional working is successful, reviewing potential benefits and disadvantages of progression along this route. The key role of education within the introduction of interprofessional working will be explored.

The rhetoric of interprofessional working

There exists a range of vocabulary associated with health and social care professionals that intimates that joint working and collaboration is abundant in the NHS. This extensive vocabulary represents something of a 'terminological quagmire' (Leathard 1994: 5) and makes clear that collaborative working has a much longer history than the relatively new terminology of interprofessional working. The multitude of definitions and objectives of interprofessional working within government documentation for the NHS similarly indicates a lack of clarity (Finch 2000). Significant quantities of the existing literature focus on the potential problems of facilitating successful working relationships between practitioners from a variety of professional groups (Molyneux 2001). Nonetheless Molyneux advocates the importance of evaluating the positive, rather than the negative, characteristics of such ways of working. However, the extent to which interprofessional working is a reality within the clinical situation is not by any means clear, even where the vernacular suggests it is. Despite the prevalence of Leathard's terminological quagmire, the rhetoric has, to date, remained external to the practical internal operations; furthermore, Kenny (2002a) suggests that, predominantly, such concepts have had no impact at ward level. Therefore, Kenny argues, interprofessional working has no impact on the operational activity of the nursing profession. However, he also argues that the drive to implement such change, in fact, is acting as a facilitator of transformation within the health service and will continue to do so. It is for that reason imperative that there is an understanding of such constructs, as well as of their potential impact at ward level, to allow nurses to participate fully in this initiative. If there is no successful dissemination of information throughout nursing, including at the operational 'coalface', then nurses will be disadvantaged.

If interprofessional working is to enhance a holistic method of providing care, then engagement of all health and social care professionals is essential. Furthermore, Molyneux (2001: 33) found in her research that success is dependent on the appointment of 'motivated, committed and experienced staff' willing to develop and sustain flexible approaches to working practice. Dennis-Jones (2005) puts more emphasis on individual attitude, suggesting there is a requirement for personal commitment to a common goal, as well as effective communication and support from the institution. The potential, discussed later in this chapter, for a redistribution of power structures within the NHS to result from the adoption of interprofessional working practices, means that these developments are particularly significant for nursing. As such, an engagement in the transformation will allow nurses to influence change and development in the National Health Service in ways they have never been able to before, as power redistribution is on a more equitable basis and, thus, less concentrated in the hands of medics and managers. A failure to disseminate this philosophy and adjuvant information will, therefore, restrict, if not deny, nurses the potential for involvement at the centre of such innovative opportunities.

What interprofessional working is not

Multidisciplinary and multiprofessional working

Multidisciplinary or multiprofessional working is perhaps the most colloquially recognized language for describing a team approach to health and social care. It represents a number of professionals participating in the process of both delivering and also determining the type and extent of care required. Multidisciplinary or multiprofessional working is, therefore, aptly described as a team approach involving a number of professional services, the precise nature of which will vary with the requirements and the requisite resources essential to meet the needs of each individual patient (Couchman 1995). The number of professional groups potentially involved is extensive and, whilst the list below is far from exhaustive, it does help to indicate the complexities involved. Health care professional groups may include doctors, nurses, pharmacists, psychologists, occupational therapists and physiotherapists. This does not, however, include recognition of the role of social care professionals in meeting the needs of the individual but it is important to understand the key roles fulfilled by these individuals, or groups, who may also be involved in this approach as and when apposite.

This approach to health care delivery allows for a number of professional bodies to be involved in the process of providing patient care. This may be through practical involvement in the course of participation in direct care, or indirectly through influencing clinical decision-makers, or by ensuring the adequate provision of resources necessary to allow clinical care to be provided. The potential impact of evidence-based practice in the process is significant. There needs to be a concurrent recognition of the requirement to balance carefully resources and needs. This method of care recognizes the importance of the contribution of each of the professional groups, acknowledging that one profession alone cannot provide the expertise required to ensure efficient and effective care is delivered. Efficacy is dependent on more than a single profession.

Multi-agency/interagency

Multi-agency/interagency working is another concept differing in principle from interprofessional working. This concept incorporates both NHS and local government services. Working in this way has developed as a result of wide policy issues that ultimately control NHS and local government priorities and, significantly, resource allocation. The NHS and Community Care Act (1990) set objectives that promised seamless interagency working, uniting both NHS and local government bodies to provide collaborative care. *The New NHS, Modern, Dependable* (DoH 1997), set out to address some of the complex organizational problems by assimilating new frameworks for standards of care and quality, which endeavoured to make certain that coordinated and responsive care was available. 'It widely recognised that effective community care services depend on successful integration and coordination between health and social care' (Vernon 2000: 282–7).

Recognition of the inextricable links between health and social care needs is fundamental to the success of multi-agency working. Within this style of work, however, each professional group continues to be independent of the others although, as cited above, there is increased recognition of the need for several professionals to work together to provide quality of care. Furthermore, Malby (1995: 127) argues that it is not possible to isolate the individual professional contributions, as 'the reality is that high quality care is seldom achieved by people from a single-discipline.' To look for single discipline solutions to the problems of health and social care, given the complexity of current societal situations, hardly seems to be an appropriate response from rational professional disciplines. The solutions are more complex and require a fuller integration of services and of the professionals providing them.

Collaborative working

Collaborative working is a nebulous concept. This is imprecise terminology and refers to teamwork in the broadest sense. It can be used to describe any or all of the processes of working across professional boundaries or working within professional groups. It quite simply means working with somebody else.

Uniprofessional and intraprofessional working

Other terms encountered in the literature are uniprofessional and intraprofessional, where individuals work only with others from the same professional group. This may be used to describe ways, for example, in which nurses from differing backgrounds work together. Boon et al. (2000) demonstrate this approach as just one aspect of their exploration of how to manage effectively a community-based patient with a large, malodorous and leaking fungating wound, that was malignant in origin. The primary care team worked closely with stoma care nurses to achieve a successful solution, which significantly, was also eventually an acceptable method of care to the patient, as well as to the health care teams involved.

Intraprofessional working is also a term used to describe joint working within one professional group, but may allow for working across other divides and boundaries, such as primary and secondary care collaborative working, or primary and secondary care working in collaboration with tertiary care.

Each of the terms above has a different meaning, aiming to meet differing objectives. In one sense, the volume of terminology relating to joint working indicates that neither the inherent philosophy nor the operational out-working of any of these concepts has achieved its desired end. This plethora of vocabulary also indicates the complex nature of contemporary health care. There is a wide range of professional groups involved in meeting the diverse demands of modern health and social care needs. Significantly, this makes it evident that no single professional group can expect to be able to provide the necessary expertise for all areas of the care for any one client. There is no capacity for single-professional domination of the current health and social care paradigms. It is therefore important to note that the historical domination of the NHS by medical practitioners does not provide a useful way forward for health care delivery.

None of these definitions has provided a generic meaning of health and social care team-working collaboratives. On the other hand, the diversity of the language suggests that this is a reflection of the different approaches to different working initiatives and, as such, may be appropriate to success in achieving local objectives for local teams. This locality attitude and potential for success should not be dismissed when seeking a broader and more collective approach. Nevertheless, however admirable local examples of excellence in practice may be, these approaches have not led to broad or generic structural changes in the ways in which health and social care professionals have worked together within both the National Health Service and local government provision of care. Indeed, it would seem unreasonable to expect them to do so. Such pockets of excellence may lead the way, through the provision of examples for others to emulate, but will lack the persuasive influence and power to exert wide-reaching reform across the whole NHS.

Much of this terminology, therefore, has been provided by the antecedents of interprofessional working. Øvretveit et al. (1997) consider that professionals have been trained to uphold a professional-centric view of the world that encourages individuals to uphold the 'myth of the omnipotence of the individual practitioner' (Øvretveit et al. 1997: 1). Beattie (1995), writing about tribal boundaries in health care, suggests these were derived not only from the cultural, class and societal divisions of Victorian Britain, but are perpetuated by the impact of training that socializes professional members to form a common identity and value for their own and others' professions. The New Labour government, elected in 1997, stated its intention to strive towards the breakdown of these professional boundaries, considering this the optimum method of producing improvements in effective service delivery. New Labour hoped that by working in new ways they would have fiscal rewards as well as benefits for client groups. However, within a policy context, the belief that interprofessional working will result in efficient working and economic benefit is as yet not proven (Kenny 2002b). This may be considered, in part, to be the result of the lack of evidence on which to base such judgements.

So what is interprofessional working?

The term 'interprofessional working', although comparatively new, is an important patient-based concept of care. As such, it is readily acceptable to both the health and social care professionals where the importance of the patient or client as a central issue underpins both philosophies of care and educational principles. Interprofessional working arose out of academic deliberations (Giddens 1998) in an attempt to facilitate an integrated care system within the NHS, thus improving the delivery of services across the broadest spectrum of both health care and social care. The increasingly more complex systems of both health and social services, allied to a proliferation in the expenditure required to provide the services needed to meet the burgeoning demand from an ageing population, necessitates a governmental approach to facilitate a rationalization of resources and reduce duplication of both effort and cost. The resultant theory of interprofessional working differs from the surfeit of other expressions of joint working that, as has been shown, allows one professional group within health and social care to associate, or indeed to distance itself, from other professional groupings. Interprofessional relationships allow for any number of professional groups or agencies to work together, in partnership, to ensure a seamless service and the provision of the package of care that best suit the individual client. The essential nature of such collaborations is that patients benefit and such benefit must result directly as a consequence of the efforts made.

Despite a lack of clarity within the literature regarding terminology allied to collaborations between health and social services, as well as an associated paucity of definitions of interprofessional working, certain key aspects are consistently indicated. Predominantly, these refer to the need for such a collaboration to result in improvements in health and social care which unequivocally advantage the client groups. This is a key principle in the establishment and maintenance of interprofessional working, as it is from this academic basis that the concept evolved. Fundamentally, those engaging in the process, or endeavouring to see such an alliance established within their own area of practice, consider health care can be improved through the instigation of interprofessional working. Central government also supports the concept and this may be seen as a driving force for the implementation of such changes (Leathard 2003). Government support and drive will be required to ensure that this system of working is effective across the whole remit of health and social care. It will be a requisite to prevent the development of pockets of excellence and areas of mediocrity, creating an NHS that is neither equitable nor acceptable.

It has, notwithstanding its recent emergence, been high on the political agenda, advocated as the way forward for modern health care to be delivered yet, despite this priority status, progress has been relatively slow (Roberts and Priest 1997). Roberts and Priest further suggest that for such major changes to be made, several challenges need to be met. They also advocate the development of research into the field of interprofessional working to support the pace of change and highlight areas for future action. Such a research base will also facilitate further changes and developments to advise and guide other potential projects and innovations.

Øvretveit et al. (1997) describe interprofessional working as occurring both within teams that have already been established (as occurs in multi-professional working) but also extending beyond these teams to include other professionals outside the established teams. However, Jones (1992) proposes that multiprofessional teams are often not teams at all, but a random group of people who do not adhere to the same principles, policy or ideology. In such circumstances mutual understanding and support do not occur. Therefore, for such team initiatives to be successful, to be planned and effective and not the result of ad hoc circumstances, Øvretveit et al. (1997) propose it is important to understand the nature and functioning of teams and that fundamental to this process is the central issue of communication. The primary difference between multiprofessional and interprofessional teams relates to the priorities of the individual members. Within multiprofessional teams, the individual team members still have a greater alliance to their own professional group, leading to an approach to care which is fragmented and potentially failing to provide a quality of service. Miller et al. (2001) purport that the less team cohesion, the less the professional commits to the work project, therefore the less obligation to the subsequent success of the team and the more they will associate within their own professional boundaries. Within multiprofessional working, meetings may occur only when identified clients or patients need a specific, and usually complex, situation to be resolved and those members of the team required to assist in resolving the problems may not be at each, or indeed any, meeting, reflecting a lack of allegiance to a team approach. In sharp contrast to this, interprofessional working brings together a group of professionals aiming to meet the needs of a population or community and not simply to respond to a single crisis. Øvretveit (1997) considers interprofessional working requires integration and not networking to ensure effective and successful outcomes.

Interprofessional working, therefore, is about partnership and interaction with other professionals as well as with the patient or client groups (Kenny 2002b). It focuses on the need to both learn and understand about the role and responsibilities of other professionals, in order to support and enhance collaborative working. A key aspect of this understanding is to recognize and articulate the identity of one's own profession as well. The whole process is dependent on communication for its success. It is more than paying lip service to the roles of other groups or individuals; it requires a comprehensive knowledge and understanding of the work of other professional groups and, thus, an acknowledgement of the roles and contributions of the other group or person. The predominant aim of these processes, taking precedence over the development of mutual appreciation for each other arising from such an initiative, is to make certain that patient care is effectively delivered, ensuring the optimum outcome for the patient and those social groupings such as family and friends that surround them. This requires a commitment to communication and the development of the team providing care depends on the nature of the communication process. The process of communication is a direct result of the extent to which the participant groups retain and work within their professional cultures or the extent to which they develop a team culture (Miller et al. 2001). The more integrated the team, the stronger the team culture that develops that, in turn, is a corollary of the input of the professionals involved. Interprofessional working is dependent on the commitment of the professionals participating in the process. The evolution of a truly integrated team creates and sustains a series of structures and processes that allow for mutual understanding of all the roles involved and create a situation in which successful communication can take place, ultimately to the benefit of the recipient of the care planned and then effectively delivered.

For this manner of communication and understanding to take place, there must be a commitment from all participants to learn from one another and, as a consequence of this expectation to learn together, an associated willingness to share and teach one another. There is a need for a 'safe' working environment based on mutual respect and a desire to promote the health and well-being of the patient or client for this to flourish.

Interprofessional working is not only about individuals working together in response to local needs, or client needs, but also about their needs to be a part of a wider organizational culture spanning both health and social care providers, as well as groups beyond this remit, as appropriate. Individuals working together to provide care which is client-focused and therefore responsive to the needs of individual clients may provide examples of excellence in practice that may be copied by other groups. However, such collaboration may lead to exhaustion and burn-out for the professionals involved, as they strive to continue to provide a service in a wider, contemporary health care system that recognizes such a fundamental basis of practice only in its rhetoric and not in its performance. For interprofessional working to be successful across health and social services, it requires, as discussed earlier, more than isolated examples of good practice.

However, even where examples of successful interprofessional working exist, it does not mean that all participants are equal partners. Traditional backgrounds and professional jealousies integrated into the hierarchical structure of the National Health Service have the potential to ensure that bigotry and prejudice can adversely influence patient or client care. Whilst this may not be the case, it is equally not a line of reasoning that can be easily ignored. Cultural differences and professional socialization processes have sustained professional elitism, thus maintaining arbitrary boundaries between professional groups (Roberts and Priest 1997). As discussed earlier, Beattie (1995) claims these have a long-standing history but, perhaps most significantly, are sustained in the contemporary health care setting through the secondary socialization processes involved in the development of professional training programmes. As a result of educational strategies, these professional and elitist beliefs have remained predominantly unchallenged and therefore, unchanged, for decades (Pietroni 1994). There are a number of facets that make up professional groups and the rewards of conformity, or the sanctions for not conforming, work to ensure that members of the groups understand and abide by the rules. These rules are taught as an integral aspect of professional training and this process takes place early within the training period. Furthermore, there is a strengthening and consolidation of these rules by professional regulatory bodies. Therefore, the professional groups are not set up to accept the notion of interprofessional working. Furthermore, Pietroni (1994) suggests some may even be trained to oppose interprofessional working, as interprofessional working will erode the occupational monopoly of the group. Pietroni does consider that one potential solution could be found through focusing on communication skills, recognizing that this must be simultaneously supported by the organizations or institutions involved, in addition to the professional regulatory bodies. Tackling the education and training process is an important step in developing interprofessional working. 'What has been missing in all these tumultuous changes is a proper reappraisal of the educational and training needs for the future health and social care workers. The move towards interprofessional care that such a review is is long overdue' (Pietroni 1994: 87).

Nevertheless, despite potential educational barriers to interprofessional working, it must be remembered that all professional groups have a valuable and distinct contribution to make to the provision of health and social care. As such, it is important to note that no one group is more significant than any other, in every situation. The emphasis on or lead by any group at any point of the care delivery pathway should reflect the needs of the client, or the population group, at that time. All groups involved have to accept the responsibility and the associated accountability that is inherent in any progression from professional insularity to interprofessional working. This process will result in a state of flux. Change is integral to the process as it responds to constantly evolving and developing scenarios.

The dynamic nature of working in such a way in itself may provide significant challenges for which professional groups need adequate preparation and, when in this situation, appropriate support mechanisms need to be in place. Consideration of these issues is needed if working in such environs is to be professionally beneficial, as well as ensuring the provision of the best care for any individual patient or client, at any point in time. Throughout these deliberations, the centrality of the patient or client is the single most important factor.

It is important, therefore, for nurses to ensure the integration of nursing values into the collaborations, to allow for recognition of changes and developments in nursing. It is also important that the role of nursing, notably within health care, is recognized. Nurses, in the guise of practitioners or consultants, are now able to take on a number of responsibilities traditionally considered the domain of general practitioners (Price and Williams 2003) and this progression of nursing development should be recognized through interprofessional working along with a number of other potential and revolutionary changes to professional roles. The opportunities this offers to nurses are significant, so a failure to engage in the process may be to the detriment of the nursing profession and, more importantly, to the patient or client groups.

Doctors and nurses have always worked together, haven't they?

Doctors are frequently seen as the closest working partner with nurses in the provision of health care. In fact, close working relationships between doctors and nurses do not have a long history and date only from the time of Florence Nightingale with the evolution of modern nursing (Baly 1988). Before that time, history shows that doctors tended to the needs of the patient themselves, performing even the most fundamental of care tasks (Astley 1990). Advances in medical knowledge, and the early developments which consequently were established, required doctors to look for assistants;

nurses were to provide the answer. Blue and Fitzgerald support the argument for the emergence and continuance of these divergent relationships, between the doctors and the nurses: 'Although there is a symbiotic relationship between doctors and nurses, at least in terms of their wish to care for and cure humankind of illness, their respective philosophies and history are different' (Blue and Fitzgerald 2002: 314).

The discursive formation that is nursing is made up of a complex system of concepts and rules that have evolved throughout its history and that form the basis of power within nursing. These forces determine the power that nurses hold as well as the powers to which nurses are answerable and the complicated history that is an integral aspect of nursing has been shaped by political, social and economic events that have distributed and redistributed power. External forces both endow nursing with power and, simultaneously, work to restrict nursing power. However, the power ascribed to nursing is not a state of authority or domination; rather, it is the strategic situation in which nurses work, where they are subjected to pressure from external forces and arguably such power is dependent on areas of resistance to maintain its own existence (Smart 1985). The work that nurses perform, in which they act as conduits or controlling gates for the passage of information between individual clients and other health care professionals, confirms this as a key perspective. Nursing has a pivotal role in health care delivery across a spectrum of environments and thus needs to ensure it is integrated and its values reflected in collaborative projects such as interprofessional working.

Doctors were dominant in health care in the Victorian society as the male doctor held both professional and societal supremacy over nurses. It continues to be so as doctors, over time, have persistently applied pressure to a variety of social structures, and recruited government support to enhance their domination, securing their position as principal players in health care scenarios (Blane 1997). These liaisons have resulted, in part, in the establishment of a legal monopoly and formalization of the professional status of doctors, representing the consequence of a protracted and continual effort by doctors on their own behalf.

Thus, the dominance of the doctor in the medical profession continues, despite the number of nurses working within health care far outstripping that of doctors and keeping nursing in a subordinate role. The issues involved are clearly more complex than mere numerical supremacy. Mackay (1995) argues that nurses and doctors carry out routine performances, in which both nurses and doctors assume the doctor has the leading role. Despite the increasing number of roles that are taken on by nursing staff which were previously the domain of doctors, nurses remain in a subordinate position and doctors retain dominance in the relationship. These performances are surrounded by rituals and traditional practices that need to be reviewed and challenged if interprofessional working is to be successful beyond the realms of superficial rhetoric. The two parties need to understand the interrelationships and their carefully orchestrated interactions to allow the system to be challenged effectively.

Over time, nurses have striven towards the establishment and maintenance of a recognized professional status. Professionalism allows for the identification of those characteristics that distinguish a group and simultaneously separate them from any other group. This desire to professionalize, Saks (1998) proposes, can and, in fact, often does involve the subordination of a less powerful group as professions establish and maintain a power base. The corollary of this achievement is the subjugation of another and separate group of staff, intentionally or otherwise. Just as doctors dominate nurses, nurses in turn seek domination of health care assistants, and in doing so allow themselves to maintain their position in the professional pecking order. The distance between the levels within this professional pecking order is created and maintained through the development of specialist skills and specialist knowledge. Both of these allow boundaries to be established which in turn provide a continual reminder of the differences between the professional groups and, thus, sustain the segregation.

Despite the efforts of nurses, professional status did not bring the advantages it had previously brought to doctors. Nurses did not gain significantly, for whilst they successfully established a chain of command within the profession with all that this entails, the work they perform continues to be dictated from outside the professional grouping, namely from doctors (Blane 1997). The majority of nurses still work to a timetable established by and for the doctors, within which they have little scope for negotiation (Morgan et al. 1985).

The restrictions on their professional status may also result, to some extent, from a lack of a clear, recognized body of knowledge belonging to nursing and only nursing. The difficulty is compounded as wide ranges of individuals, from registered nurses to health care assistants, also perform nursing work in differing ways and with differing levels of accountability. In addition, pay levels are lower than for other professional groups, revealing the cost implications to the National Health Service of ensuring equity of pay: 'As a largely female workforce confronting a predominantly male medical profession and administrative civil service, nurses may be met by assumptions of superiority and the belief that women do not need to be paid a "family wage" ' (Blane 1997: 218).

Joseph (1994) argues that nursing is a good example of the subordination of women to patriarchy. In addition, he argues, nurses are socialized into a female role that equates nursing with motherhood and domesticity. Nursing and caring are inextricably linked with the female gender and the work of women continues to be held 'in low esteem' (Joseph 1994: 12). By contrast, Joseph proposes nursing should be seen as a full profession and efforts should be made to show how the nature of professional ideologies could be used to show professionalism in nursing. In order to achieve this, some of the populist views and stereotypes of nurses need to be discarded to allow dialogue that is more meaningful.

The significance of the professional developments of doctors and nurses rests in allowing recognition of current work situations. To understand the present situation, an appreciation of how it developed and was then sustained is essential. The demarcation and boundaries between any of the health care professional groups, as exemplified by doctors and nurses, play a role in allowing, or inhibiting, the development of interprofessional working. Whilst some health and social care staff, irrespective of their professional background, will be able to report excellent examples in their own practice where professional groups work successfully together to achieve optimum benefit for their client group, this will not be the experience of all. The differences between any of the health care professional groups permit or inhibit the development of interprofessional working. The vastly divergent educational backgrounds and the differences resulting from professional socialization will provide barriers to interprofessional collaboration. Although the different philosophies of professional groups represent potential barriers by sustaining professional identities, for interprofessional working to be successful it is imperative that the advantages of such initiatives are highlighted clearly and understood by all involved in such innovative changes.

Advantages of interprofessional working

Interprofessional tensions can threaten the delivery of quality health care in a hospital setting ... Repeated calls have been made for improved collaboration, communication, congruence and equity within health care teams as ways of improving quality of care and protecting patient safety.

(Lingard et al. 2004: 403)

Leathard (1994) postulates that interprofessional working allows for the separate and distinct professional skills available throughout both health and social care to be brought together in response to the growing complexity of contemporary health and social care. In addition, the expansion of knowledge can facilitate increased specialization and with it, a reduction in duplication of effort and a simultaneous reduction of wasted resources, not least the time of professional groups. A fully integrated service can also be used advantageously to manage resources efficiently.

The Department of Health wants to reduce the number of health care professionals in contact with patients or clients. Using interprofessional working to achieve these ends, such as reductions in team size, is possible only where the professionals have knowledge of each other's function within contemporary health and social care settings (Miller et al. 2001). It is not appropriate to allow historical perceptions of the professional groups to dominate, as these will in all probability reduce the potential for interprofessional working and enhance the dividing barriers. Mackay (1993) believed these generalized perceptions lead to a failure of understanding between disciplines. There is an expectation that patients and clients will benefit from the smaller team approach, where there are fewer opportunities for poor communication to cloud issues, cause confusion and engender professional tribalism, if not actually lead to outright conflict. Øvretveit (1997) writes how recipients of care often question the standard of communication between professionals resulting in questions being repeated and, an expectation that they will provide the same, or similar, answers to a number of different professionals. Furthermore, the professional boundaries fail to be meaningful in light of the patient or client position that regularly and frequently transcends all such arbitrary boundaries (McKenna 1992).

In addition to easing channels of communication, the escalating number of 'patient pathways', guidelines and algorithms to inform care decisions can be seen as directly benefiting the patient or client. These developments are reliant on the use of evidence-based interventions and facilitate the implementation of good practice that is of obvious benefit to the recipient. However, the process also relies on a number of professional groups to develop pathways. This, in itself, can be a complex and time-consuming initiative, with little evidentiary documentation to support the concept that, once established, the pathways will ultimately reduce workload (de Luc 2000; Johnson, 2000). However, through interprofessional working there can be a facilitation of the development of care pathways that benefits from the reciprocal awareness of professional strengths and weaknesses. Following this sequence of events, interprofessional working may be beneficial, as this development allows a widening of mutual understanding and appreciation of another's role.

Nurses who do not speak out and express their opinions are not useful allies to patients (Mackay 1995); furthermore, when nurses are given a subservient role, as discussed above, it reduces confidence in their own opinions and ability. Whilst not all nurses accept the role of subordination, Mackay (1995) reports it continues to be common in hospital environments. Interprofessional working echoes the holistic approach to care adopted by nursing. Such a philosophy underpinning a care system makes it attractive to nurses, but nurses have retained their subordinate status and, in doing so, are not able to advocate successfully for their patients. If interprofessional working is to reap benefits for the patients, then it is important that nurses think carefully about the performances they give and the roles they play in their work lives. Nurses who fail to review their roles will contribute to barriers inhibiting interprofessional working. It is now a requirement of the Nursing and Midwifery Council (2004) that nurses have the ability to 'demonstrate knowledge of effective interprofessional working practices which respect and utilise the contribution of members of the health and social care team.'

Resource allocation and the need to make the best use of finances and human resources, whilst keeping pace with an ever-expanding array of medical advances, is a key concept in contemporary health care. The promise of interprofessional working to bring together service planning and development, as well as assist in the formation of shared and agreed goals, is an advantage of the system for health and social care employees, for government bodies and, most importantly, for the recipients of the services. Where teams are established and the members of the teams demonstrate a commitment to working together and they communicate effectively, then maximum use can be made of physical resources as well as staff utilization, specialization and progression. Significantly, Leathard (1994) argues that involvement of the patient in the process is a fundamental part of any such course of action, especially where resource allocation is considered. However, not all aspects of interprofessional working are advantageous and it is important to consider why the collaboration may not be successful.

When does interprofessional working not work?

Although the concept of interprofessional working is supported by a generally held belief that collaboration is good, Leathard (1994) proposes that there is only modest verification to demonstrate it is effective: 'However, there is little evidence to substantiate the view that collaboration leads to an increase in the quality of care which has furthered the well-being of patients and services users' (Leathard,1994: 7). Therefore, whilst it remains a significant issue within the policy agenda, it is based on a largely unfounded assumption that better integration of services will result in improved outcomes for service users and patients (Davey et al. 2005). Perhaps it is this underlying assumption that contributes to a lack of success. The failure of interprofessional working is often as much to do with strategic and operational inhibiting factors as it is with the willingness of professional groups to harness together their working practices. Demarcations within the health service were recognized in the NHS plan and proposals put forward to show this as an area where effort was required to break down these traditional barriers (DoH 2000). However, barriers extend beyond any professional demarcations, they can be shown as existing in the range of service fragmentation that is aligned to the establishment of borders between purchasers and providers, primary and secondary care, resulting in financial boundaries, all leading to constraints in the development of interprofessional working practice (Roberts and Priest 1997). Financial limitations and concerns regarding the need to meet financial targets also have a role to play, as invoices have replaced more traditional 'give and take' and, in terms of personnel, releasing a staff member to help elsewhere also results in a cost pressure.

Although central government advocates interprofessional working, Roberts and Priest (1997) purport there have been no resource or policy initiatives to support such reform, particularly on a scale potentially embracing the whole NHS. Kenny (2002a), however, considers Department of Health publications have established a common vocabulary that will facilitate changes in professional practices, although the language has yet to impact at ward level. Despite the common linguistic structure, a failure to provide the appropriate reform of all other structures across health and social care will result in collaboration being a response to local needs and, potentiality, in a service more fragmented than at present (Roberts and Priest 1997), thereby defeating the original purpose of the development of interprofessional working.

The cultural differences between professions, reflecting their common sense of identity and shared social role, as well as the absence of a clear language to facilitate communication (Malby 1995), can also lead to the failure of interprofessional collaboration. The divergence of professional knowledge and perspectives can lead to a culture of fear and defensive behaviours. As has been discussed, a part of the definition of a profession is to have a distinct body of knowledge and set of skills. The differing styles of professional groups, their separate languages and values, make this perhaps the most difficult area to challenge. To overcome these biases will require innovative thinking to establish interprofessional trust, and this will take time. For interprofessional working to achieve its potential, traditional power bases have to be lost and hierarchies be worn away. However, Kenny (2002a) proposes that the reality of such power struggles may be a redrawing of the boundaries with the long-established, traditional historical power bases eventually maintained but under a new guise.

Alternatively, it is possible that nursing does not want to pursue the proposed utopia of interprofessional working. Despite the overabundance of anecdotal accounts in nursing literature claiming that, unlike nurses, doctors are distanced from their patients, Fletcher (2000) claims that nurses in fact fall foul of the same misconception. As nurses extend their clinical competencies, Fletcher believes they follow the route other professionals have taken and generate a professional mystique which detaches them from patients and the caring therapeutic relationship advocated by Watson (1985). Although an ethic of caring can be combined with professionalism, nurses may want to pursue a humanistic approach without concern for the expansion of professional responsibilities and may, furthermore, consider patients are better served by such an approach, rather than through the, as yet, poorly researched construct of interprofessional working.

If interprofessional working has the potential to fail in the provision of effective and financially robust health care delivery systems, then a method of breaking down barriers needs to be found. As will be shown, several authors have suggested what needs to take place within educational settings. There needs, in effect, to be a prevention of the formation of barriers, rather than an attempt to break these down at a later stage of the professional development of the individuals involved.

Education as a tool to facilitate interprofessional working

Professional training programmes have traditionally provided a separate educational base for each different profession, leading to each developing an unique approach to the delivery of health care (Masterson 2002). Now a plethora of interprofessional programmes are available for a diverse selection of providers. Education, of course, does not start and end with pre-registration training, and interprofessional education can be integral to both pre- and post-registration programmes. Interprofessional education is viewed as a central element in the process of restructuring health and welfare provision (Salmon and Jones 2001). Meaningful shared learning has the potential to prepare students for the complexities of real-life situations in interprofessional work environments (O'Neill et al. 2000). In addition, it can provide an environment which is supportive of professionals and encourages initiative and innovation (Roberts and Priest 1997). Hence, training and education have been reported on the one hand as being the source of problems in establishing interprofessional working, as they reiterate professional boundaries that promote professional identity and commonality, but on the other as tools that may also be the potential salvation of this complex concept.

Health and social care professionals are key to the well-being of the members of the population (Sullivan 2000) and, therefore, the ways in which these professional groups use their education and capabilities are fundamental within contemporary society. The education of these professionals and their proposed employment are significant aspects of the political agenda and thus important factors when considering interprofessional working. There has been increasing focus on interprofessional education in recent years (Tunstall-Pedoe et al. 2003). Tunstall-Pedoe et al. postulate that when students arrive to commence training, they already hold stereotyped views of each other, and already have strong affiliations with their own professional group. These individuals may be resistant to interprofessional working, considering some see shared learning as irrelevant and a threat to their perceived professional identity (Basford 1999). Hind et al. (2003:21) support the argument of Tunstall-Pedoe et al., proposing: 'Effective interprofessional working, which is widely considered as essential to high-quality health care, is influenced by the attitudes of health care professionals towards their own and other professional groups' (Tunstall-Pedoe et al. 2003). If, however, students arrive already sure of what each other does, then clearly either interprofessional education must work to eliminate these preconceptions or education must commence earlier. Furthermore, Hind et al. (2003) consider the greatest benefit of interprofessional education in facilitating interprofessional working is for this to occur as early in training programmes as possible in order to maximize students' positive attitudes both towards their own and other professional groups.

It is important, however, to note that interprofessional working and interprofessional education are not attempts to blur the edges of professional groups, thereby creating a generic worker, essentially a 'jack of all trades' and 'master of none'. Rather, central to the purpose of such an endeavour is to improve health care delivery through the development of collaborative working (Lax and Galvin 2002). The objective is to ensure that individual professionals are both competent in their own skills and their areas of proficiency, but are equally confident in the skills and abilities of other professional groups within health and social care. With a developed understanding of the roles played by all professionals, collegiate working can improve the health of communities. Interprofessional education, therefore, seeks to generate professionals who have no regard for the traditional hierarchies, but seek to provide an effective and efficient service for the community. The concept sits well within the clinical governance framework that requires individuals to be fit for purpose and competent to perform the tasks and activities required of them. Interprofessional education challenges professionals to modify their reference framework and develop a greater understanding of what it means to be professional (Kenny 2002b).

Whilst traditional education programmes have had a single-profession focus, nevertheless there is some shared learning taking place, most notably around the biomedical or behavioural sciences. Miller et al. (1999), however, in a study of actual or potential courses, found few that placed an emphasis on joint working or sharing of best practice information. Therefore, these courses do not achieve the desired outcomes of preventing insularity and encouraging professionals to engage in meaningful interactions that cross professional boundaries. Consequently, there is only minimal improvement in the efficacy of the service delivered by these professionals.

Roberts and Priest (1997) describe some of the problems of enacting interprofessional education, citing cultural differences between the professions and the methods employed in their education. They judge that these have delayed interprofessional working, allowing fear resulting from uncertainty to sustain intransigence. Long histories of professional elitism and variances in the vocabulary maintain such inflexibility as they compound communication barriers. Problems resulting from the different approaches taken by the regulatory bodies of health and social care professionals with regard to models of behaviour, standards of accreditation and professional regulation are all based on traditional philosophies. Furthermore, as with interprofessional working, there is, to date, little evidence that interprofessional education provides the desired outcome. Conversely, there is no substantive body of evidence to suggest it is not effective.

Despite the potential for fiscal rewards that some have argued (Hughes and Lewis 1998) are the initiative objectives, interprofessional working has the potential to radically reform the NHS. These negative issues need to be overcome to allow true interprofessional education to lead the way to interprofessional working. The process of necessity will be protracted. However, Masterson argues: 'the health workforce of the future is likely to develop in ways that are increasingly out of line with traditional health professional roles ... Training and education should support and develop joint working between health and social care' (Masterson 2002: 334–5). To be advantageous, interprofessional education needs to provide opportunities for professionals from across the spectrum of health and social care, both to learn together and, significantly, from and about each other at the same time. This approach is promoted in the policy literature discussed earlier. Such programmes of education aim to provide professionals with the ability to use their skills, and those of others, to maximum effect. Thus these programmes further enhance professional roles rather than diminish them.

The NHS Plan (DoH 2000) intends to utilize interprofessional working as an essential way forward to prevent unnecessary deaths and improve the quality of patient care, not just on an individual basis but through communities and populations as the infrastructures of the whole NHS change, allowing reform. Interprofessional working, based on interprofessional education, aims to remove arbitrary boundaries and thereby allow each member of staff, irrespective of background, to make the best possible contribution to health and social care. Similarly, the government recognizes shortfalls in recruitment and care delivery as a result of the absence of interprofessional working: 'For too long we have planned and trained staff in a uni-professional way without a clear and comprehensive look at the future. This means that some of our best plans for service improvement are thwarted because we can't recruit and deploy the best staff to provide the service we want' (DoH 2000a: 11).

Interprofessional training and education are crucial to the promotion of teamwork and collaborative partnerships between professionals, agencies and service users. Therefore, interactive learning between students of differing professions is clearly distinct from common learning or shared teaching, as outlined above. Interprofessional working is not a debate that it is possible to ignore in light of the increasing pressure for health and social care professionals to work and learn together, enabling them to meet the challenging and complicated needs of a modern, complex society. All professionals need to work together to engender professional respect and develop a meaningful perception of the contribution that each of the others makes. 'It is time that our understanding of team collaboration moved beyond the rhetoric ... towards a more authentic depiction of the skills required to function in the competitive setting of the interprofessional health care team' (Lingard et al. 2004: 407). Professional integration, therefore, needs to replace professional isolation to benefit the recipients of the care delivered, by ensuring this is well planned, communicated effectively and is appropriate to the needs of the community.

References

Astley, A. (1990) A history of pain. *Nursing*, 4 (17): 33–5.

Baly, M. E. (1988) *Florence Nightingale and the Legacy of Nursing* (Kent: Croom Helm).

Barrett, G., Sellman, D. and Thomas, J (2005) *Interprofessional Working in Health and Social Care: Professional Perspectives* (Basingstoke: Palgrave Macmillan).

Basford, I. (1999) Shared learning: a phenomena for celebration and a challenge to health educators. *Nurse Education Today*, **19**: 345–6.

Beattie, A. (1995) War and peace among the health tribes. In K. Soothill, L. Mackay and C. Webb (eds), *Interprofessional Relations in Health Care* (London: Edward Arnold).

Blane, D. (1997) Health professions. In G. Scambler (ed.), *Sociology as Applied to Medicine*, 4th edn (London: W. B. Saunders).

Blue, I. and Fitzgerald, M. (2002) Interprofessional relations: case studies of working relationships between registered nurses and general practitioners in rural Australia. *Journal of Clinical Nursing* **11**: 314–21.

Boon, H., Brophy, J and Lee, J. (2000) The community care of a patient with a fungating wound. *British Journal of Nursing* **9** (6): 35–8.

Chapman, T., Hugman, R. and Williams, A. (1995) Effectiveness of interprofessional relationships: a case illustration of joint working. In K. Soothill, L. Mackay and C. Webb (1995) *Interprofessional Relations in Health Care* (London: Arnold).

Couchman, W. (1995) Joint education for mental health teams. *Nursing Standard* **10** (7): 32–4.

Davey, B., Levin, E., Iliffe, S. and Kharicha, K. (2005) Integrating health and social care: implications for joint working and community care outcomes for older people. *Journal of Interprofessional Care* **19** (1): 22–34.

De Luc, K. (2000) Care pathways: an evaluation of their effectiveness. *Journal of Advanced Nursing* **32** (2): 485–96.

Dennis-Jones, C. (2005) Breaking down the barriers. *Therapy Weekly* 5 October accessed on line 24 May 2006.

Department of Health (1990) *The NHS and Community Care Act.* (London: HMSO).

Department of Health (1997) *The new NHS: Modern, Dependable.* (London: DoH).

Department of Health (1998) *A First Class Service: Quality in the New NHS* (London: DoH).

Department of Health (2000a) *The NHS Plan: A Plan for Investment, A Plan for Reform* (London: DoH).

Department of Health (2002b) *A Health Service of All the Talents: Developing the NHS Workforce* (London: DoH).

Finch, J. (2000) Interprofessional education and teamworking: a view from the education providers. *British Medical Journal* **321**: 1138–40.

Fletcher, M. (2000) Doctors have become more caring than nurses. *British Medical Journal* **320** (7241): 1083.

Giddens, A. (1998) *The Third Way: the Renewal of Democracy* (Cambridge: Cambridge University Press).

Hind, M., Norman, I., Cooper, S., Gill, E., Hilton, R., Judd, P. and Jones, S. (2003) Interprofessional perceptions of healthcare students. *Journal of Interprofessional Care* **17** (1): 21–34.

Hughes, G. and Lewis, G. (eds) (1998) *Unsettling Welfare: The Reconstruction of Social Policy* (London: Routledge).

Johnson, S. (2000) Factors influencing the success of ICP projects. *Professional Nurse* **15** (12): 776–9.

Jones, R. V. H. (1992) Teamwork in primary health care: how much do we know about it? *Journal of Interprofessional Care* **6**: 25–9.

Joseph, M. (1994) *Sociology for Nursing and Health Care* (Cambridge: Polity).

Kenny, G (2002a) The importance of nursing values in interprofessional collaboration. *British Journal of Nursing* **11**(1): 65–8.

Kenny, G. (2002b) Interprofessional working: opportunities and challenges. *Nursing Standard* **17** (6): 33–5.

Lax, W. and Galvin, K. (2002) Reflections on a community action research project: interprofessional issues and methodological problems. *Journal of Clinical Nursing* **11**: 376–86.

Leathard, A. (1994) *Going Interprofessional: Working Together for Health and Welfare* (London: Routledge).

Leathard, A. (2003) *Interprofessional Collaboration: From Policy to Practice in Health and Social Care* (Oxford: Blackwell).

Lingard, L., Espin, S., Evans, C. & Hawryluck, L. (2004) The rules of the game: interprofessional collaboration on the intensive care unit team. *Critical Care* **8** (6): 403–8.

Mackay, L. (1993) *Conflicts in Care: Medicine and Nursing* (London: Chapman and Hall).

Mackay, L. (1995) 'The patient as pawn in interprofessional relationships.' In K. Soothill, L. Mackay and C. Webb (1995) 'Interprofessional Relations in Health Care.' London. Arnold.

Malby, B. (1995) (ed.) *Clinical Audit for Nurses and Therapists* (London: Scutari Press).

Masterson, A. (2002) Cross-boundary working: a macro-political analysis of the impact on professional roles. *Journal of Clinical Nursing* **11**: 331–9.

McKenna, H. (1992) Quality quarantine: a call for less professional isolation. *Quality in Health Care* **1**: 215–16.

Miller, C., Ross, N. and Freeman, M. (1999) *The Role of Collaborative/Shared Learning in Pre- and Post-Registration Education in Nursing, Midwifery and Health Visiting* (London: English National Board).

Miller, C., Freeman, M. and Ross, N. (2001) *Interprofessional Practice in Health and Social Care: Challenging the Shared Learning Agenda* (London: Arnold).

Molyneux, J. (2001) Interprofessional teamworking: what makes teams work well? *Journal of Interprofessional Care* **15** (1): 29–35.

Morgan, M., Calnan, M. and Manning, N. (1985) *Sociological Approaches to Health and Medicine* (Beckenham: Croom Helm).

O'Neill, B., Wyness, A., McKinnon, S. and Granger, P. (2000). Partnership, collaboration and course design: An emerging model of interprofessional education. *www.cstudies.ubc.ca/facdev/services/registry/pcacdaemoie.html*

Øvretveit, J. (1997) How to describe interprofessional working. In Øvretveit, J., Mathias, P. and Thompson, T. (eds) *Interprofessional Working for Health and Social Care* (Basingstoke: Palgrave Macmillan).

Øvretveit, J., Mathias, P. and Thompson, T. (eds) (1997) *Interprofessional Working for Health and Social Care* (Basingstoke: Palgrave Macmillan).

Pietroni, P. (1994) Interprofessional teamwork: Its history and development in hospitals, general practice and community care. In: A. Leathard (ed.) *Going Interprofessional: Working Together for Health and Welfare* (London: Routledge).

Price, A. and Williams, A. (2003) Primary care nurse practitioners and the interface with secondary care: a qualitative study of referral practice. *Journal of Interprofessional Care* **17** (3): 239–50.

Roberts, P. and Priest, H. (1997) Achieving interprofessional working in mental health. *Nursing Standard* **12** (2): 39–41.

Salmon, D. and Jones, M. (2001) Shaping the interprofessional agenda: a study examining qualified nurses' perceptions of working with others. *Nurse Education Today* **21** (1): 18–25.

Saks, M. (1998) Professionalism and health care. In: D. Field and S. Taylor (eds) *Sociological Perspectives on Health and Health Care* (Oxford: Blackwell Publishing).

Smart, B. (1985) *Michel Foucault* (London: Routledge).

Sullivan, W. M. (2000) Medicine under threat: professionalism and professional identity. *Canadian Medical Association Journal* **162** (5): 673–6.

Tunstall-Pedoe, S., Rink, E. and Hilton, S. (2003) Student attitudes to undergraduate interprofessional education. *Journal of Interprofessional Care* **17** (2): 161–72.

Vernon, S. (2000) Assessment of older people: politics and practice in primary care. *Journal of Advanced Nursing* **31** (2): 282–7.

Watson, J. (1985) *Nursing: Human Science and Human Care. A Theory of Nursing.* (Connecticut: Appleton-Century-Crofts).

CHAPTER 5

A Professional Approach to Ethnic Diversity

MARK R. D. JOHNSON

The practice of health care is, and as far as can be established always has been, essentially multicultural and reliant on a diverse workforce. Even before the Chief Medical Officer for Britain announced in 2004 that he was setting the NHS a ten-point action plan to promote race equality, including action on recruitment and development opportunities (Godfrey 2004), the NHS had been reliant on migrant professionals and had taken a variety of steps to emphasize their value to the service. Indeed, it is now well recognized that the Minister of Health most responsible for accelerating this process was Enoch Powell (during the 1960s), despite his being better known among students of 'race relations' for his speeches attacking immigration (see obituary: http://politics.guardian.co.uk/politicsobituaries/story/0,1441,563473,00.html). In recent years, however, there has been a spate of government publications and policies aimed at underlining the vital connection between a diverse workforce and the development of a high quality health service able to meet the needs of all citizens.

In every situation, in every country across the world, the processes of globalization – of growing international migration and interlinkage of economies and societies – are meaning that professional staff in health and social care need to take account of ethnic diversity in their work. It is no longer possible, if indeed it was ever advisable, to treat everyone 'the same' and to assume that we are all members of the same human race and have the same needs and wants. It has been estimated that one in every eight people in Europe is not living in the country of their birth and similar figures could be true for most other continents and countries: in some cities, more than one in four of the population are 'strangers' or migrants. This has many consequences, not least in terms of the languages spoken at home, and familiarity with local health and social care services. Even when a migrant speaks the language of their adopted home fluently, they may be less familiar with the local organization of services, such as the procedures required to register with a doctor or where to obtain vaccinations for children. When they seek care, there may also be difficulties arising from cultural differences or misunderstandings relating to local and traditional customs. This can cause many problems, not least of which may be a risk to public health, as well as inequality in health care and outcomes. It is the responsibility of the health care professional to ensure that all those who need their help are treated equitably and sensitively, which means taking account of these issues. This must include the responsibility of the migrant worker to understand not only the culture (and language) of the country in which they are working, but also the cultures and specific needs of other migrants and settlers in that state, in order to be able to offer them the same level of service and respect that they themselves might expect. In return, however, it is important to recognize that the migrant health worker also is worthy of respect for their specialist knowledge of their own country and culture, and deserves recognition and protection from discrimination or harassment.

Legally and ethically, the health professional must, increasingly, be aware of and be prepared to meet, ethnic and cultural diversity. Monoculturalism, and racist or xenophobic attitudes, while historically present, are no longer acceptable within any profession. Britain has had significant inputs from a variety of ethnic and geographical backgrounds, and continues to receive migrant workers and refugees, many of whom present the health care professional with new challenges. The same is true in every other state in Europe and across the world. In Europe, the practitioner works against the background of the Treaty of Amsterdam, while internationally, there are the International Conventions on Human Rights and the Rights of the Child, and the Geneva Convention on Refugees and Asylum. Practitioners in New Zealand will be familiar with the Treaty of Waitangi (http://www.newhealth.govt.nz/ toolkits/tow.htm) which protects the rights of the indigenous Maori people, while in the United States of America it is a condition of federal funding (for example through the Medicare system) that services do not discriminate on the grounds of race or gender, and increasingly, laws are including obligations to address, or even use positive action to redress, historic inequalities. However, there are also competing pressures, as (at least in relation to the United Kingdom) there have been calls to reduce the reliance of the NHS on 'imported' medical and nursing professionals, in order to protect the health of the countries from which these have been recruited (see 'The great African doctor drain' (*Guardian* newspaper, G2 supplement, 18 November 2005; Hinsliff, G. (2004); 'NHS crackdown on headhunting African nurses' (*Observer* newspaper, 22 August 2004, p. 9).

Whereas for the migrant health professional, it is clear that there may be benefits from working in Europe or America compared to their possible career and salary in a 'third world' country, there is ample evidence that historically they have not received the same levels of opportunity and reward as 'native' staff. Indeed, this situation has continued (Vydelingum 2004) and is not confined to the UK (Dreachslin et al. 2000). Over forty years ago, nurses recruited from the Caribbean (under the initiative launched by Enoch

Powell) were diverted into less prestigious posts, or their registerable qualifications were ignored and they were directed into support grades (as state-enrolled, rather than state registered, nurses), from which promotion was much more difficult. No precise figures are available to say how many nurses were recruited from overseas in the 1960s and 1970s, but in 1971, overseas nurses formed nine per cent of the total hospital workforce, half of which came from the Caribbean (Thomas and Morton-Williams 1972). Nurses accepted from overseas for training were very rapidly put into working roles, and frequently they found themselves in psychiatric or other less popular specialist roles, rather than the general nursing and training posts they had anticipated. Few had any help in settling in, and none of those surveyed experienced a formal orientation programme. Indeed, for many their place in Britain was conditional on their work permit and it is clear that many were forced into lower-grade posts than might have been expected on the basis of their previous qualifications. Others were (mis)guided into the less prestigious, lower-paid state-enrolled nurse grades with little or no prospect of career advancement. Even in other hospital employment, they were segmented into the least attractive and most insecure elements of catering, domestic and portering work, and hardly ever accepted into the better-rated ambulance work (CRE 1983). Those who tried to upgrade their status faced a series of barriers and few were successful. In addition, many faced racial abuse from their patients and even from their colleagues (Lee-Cunin 1989; see also Bowler 1993) as well as being largely confined to night shifts, particularly in mental handicap, psychiatric and geriatric care wards, which are recognized as 'dead-ends' for subsequent promotion. Not surprisingly, one result has been a determination that their children should not repeat their own experience, even at the expense of having to work longer and harder themselves to support their children. As two of Lee-Cunin's respondents commented:

> *George*: I will stay in nursing, to keep my children away from it. I want them to be a doctor or lawyer. I have made my bed, so I have to lie in it.   (Lee-Cunin 1989: 9)

and

> *Elaine*: I wouldn't get a job now [following the 1988 regrading exercise]. No one would take me. I have to stay in nursing. Soon they will have no young black nurses in my hospital. They are not taking them, and anyway my kids are not going to get into that profession.   (Lee-Cunin 1989: 11)

More recent figures show that there have been significant changes in the health services, and there are indeed a few high-profile or highly graded staff of minority ethnic origin. Current monitoring of entrants to nursing, while showing that six per cent come from a 'minority' background, also shows that they are much more likely to describe themselves as being of black African origin (Gerrish et al. 1996). However, a survey by the MSF Trade Union (now

Amicus) in 1997 found that at least 100 NHS employers (health authorities, colleges or NHS Trust hospitals, ambulance services and community health trusts) were employing no black staff of Caribbean origin. Places such as Brent, Ealing and Lambeth, that have significant black populations, had proportions of black employees which were noticeably below the levels that might have reasonably been expected. Only a very few (such as Croydon Mayday NHS Trust) employed more black staff than might have been predicted on the basis of their catchment areas. There has been a dramatic fall in recruitment, so that while in 1995 8.7 per cent of nursing grade staff aged 55–64 were black (African-Caribbean origin), less than one in a hundred staff aged under 25 were so in those organizations for which data were available. This cannot be attributed to the lack of educational qualifications or labour-market engagement of this group: a high proportion are either in further educational study, or unemployed and seeking work (Owen 1994). The 1991 census shows a distinct move into clerical or secretarial work and self-employment (a trend continued in the census of 2001). Anecdotal and incidental evidence from other sources suggests that in some cases at least the move to self-employment arises from the development of nursing homes, following a 'West Indian' tendency to develop 'skill-based' entrepreneurial activity (Johnson 1988).

Amongst the migrant women in the 1996 Policy Studies Institute (PSI) survey of the Black and Minority Ethnic (BME) population, those of Caribbean origin were twice as likely (around six per cent) compared to whites to be nurses, and in general this was the most highly qualified of all migrant groups. Of older women, more than one in eight of all Caribbean female migrants were (or had been) nurses, but below the age of 44, the figure fell to less than one in twenty. The same survey also noted that 25 of the 32 Caribbean female employees in the hospital sector (out of 175 working Caribbean women in the survey), denied that there were 'equal opportunities' where they worked. These two facts, as was also suggested by Beishon's et al.'s study (1995) of the nursing profession, may be linked. Consequently, it is not surprising that NHS policy has increasingly insisted on the need for affirmative or at least protective action to assure staff of BME origins, and potential recruits to the service from these communities, that they will be valued and seen as an essential resource. Indeed, it is not only in the UK that this is true, but the recruitment of over 13,000 nurses and 4,000 doctors (in 2002) was a key statistic underlying a World Health Organisation workshop on International Migration, at which the global dimensions of the issue were explored, and British governmental action (such as an agreement of under-standing with the South African government) was seen as leading interna-tional developments in good practice (IoM 2005). Those agreements and discussions, however, appear to continue independently of the situation of 'overseas workers' within the recruiting countries, since however poorly migrant workers are treated, they may feel better rewarded here than in their underfunded countries of origin.

Positive action

It is clear from the history of racialized inequality in the NHS (and indeed in other sectors of employment) that change will only be slow unless some form of positive or 'affirmative' action is taken to compensate for many years of discrimination and exclusion. This has been a controversial issue, and for a long time was resisted as it was believed that 'positive discrimination' was illegal and might be damaging to recipients. However, recent and forthcoming legislation, relating to a range of dimensions of discrimination, age, gender, religion and belief, sexual orientation and disability, provides a timely opportunity for organizations to undertake positive action (Home Office 2005). It has to be admitted that there has been a good deal of uncertainty around positive action, but it is now recognized that it is legal and, in certain circumstances, encouraged by the Department of Health because it can assist in meeting certain priorities, including the ability of the NHS to meet the needs of minority communities and to address the imbalances which still exist between the profile of staff and the communities they serve. Further, it is recognized that widening the field of recruitment in this way can bring real benefits to organizations by broadening the input of experience, knowledge and ideas among their staff. A workforce that, at all levels, broadly reflects the community served will be better placed to understand its needs and provide an effective service.

Service pressures also underline the need for change. The NHS is keen to maximize the potential workforce that it can recruit from, since it is already failing to fill all its vacancies from UK recruitment – and (as shown above; see also Allan et al. 2004) international recruitment has not been without its own problems. It has, for example, been estimated that each year the NHS loses nine per cent of its entire workforce, which means that it has to find around 10,000 employees annually simply to provide the same level of service. The situation is likely to worsen since the workforce is ageing. Of nurses, 73,000 are aged between 50 and 55 and are due to retire over the next five to ten years. Almost half of all GPs intend to retire before they are 60. The situation is worse in the deprived areas of the country (including not only inner-city metropolitan districts but also such areas as the 'valleys' of south Wales) where 'the backbone of the GP workforce ... has come from the ranks of those qualifying in South Asian medical schools' (Gavin and Esmail 2002: 77), the majority of whom are expected to reach retirement age within the next five years. Significantly, the profile of the national BME population is bucking this trend and represents a younger workforce than its white counterparts. This therefore presents employers and recruiters with a challenge – and an opportunity – but one which will require some action to overcome the existing barriers or perceptions of inequality that affect current levels of application from these sources.[1]

It is worth repeating that positive discrimination is illegal in that it leads to employing or promoting persons because they are from a particular target group (for example, women, men, or ethnic groups). In the case of positive action, the bottom line is that the strongest candidate is appointed, regardless of background, but that members of hitherto underrepresented groups are given additional incentive or access to apply for consideration. This is now supported by key equal opportunities legislation, such as the Sex Discrimination Act (1975) and the Race Relations Act (1976), which allowed employers to target specific groups (including women or particular ethnic groups) in a legally acceptable way. In such cases there would need to be evidence of past discriminatory policies and practices against a specific group and/or under-representation of a specific group, within the workforce as a whole or at particular levels within it, during the previous twelve months.

If such evidence exists, the following actions are explicitly permitted by this legislation:

- provision of facilities to meet the special needs of people from particular groups in relation to their training, education or welfare;
- targeted job training for people from groups that are underrepresented in a particular area of work, or encouragement of them to apply for such work.

Such an approach is reinforced by more recent legislation, prohibiting discrimination in employment on the grounds of sexual orientation and religion or belief. This permits specific measures where it reasonably appears that the action 'prevents or compensates for disadvantages linked to sexual orientation' or 'for disadvantages linked to religion or belief'. However, there are no specific suggestions as to what might constitute positive action in the Disability Discrimination Act (1995) although there is a requirement for employers and service providers to make 'reasonable adjustments' to accommodate the needs of disabled people. The resultant removal of unnecessary barriers to access to jobs and services helps to redress the balance between disabled and non-disabled people.

Positive action is also implicitly sanctioned under law as public authorities are now explicitly required to show their response to the positive duty to actively promote good race relations (Race Relations (Amendment) Act 2000) and gender equality (Equality Bill, 2005) as well as equality of opportunity for disabled people (Disability Discrimination Bill 2005). Taken together, these provide ample support in legislation for specific types of positive action, in order to promote equality of opportunity in certain areas. None of these are based on targets or leave out of the equation individual ability: they are essentially enabling activities that help to redress the balance but do not provide an unfair advantage to previously disadvantaged groups at the expense of the majority.

Therefore, NHS Employers have come up with a working definition of positive action as follows:

> Positive action is a range of lawful actions which seek to address an imbalance in employment opportunities among targeted groups which have previously

experienced disadvantage, or which have been subject to discriminatory policies and practices, or which are under-represented in the workforce. (DoH 2005) its the positive action website detail in end refs

A selection of these legitimate actions could include:

- work experience placements
- job preparation training
- personal development support
- mentoring schemes
- assistance towards qualifications
- targeted recruitment
- recruitment stalls at community events
- targeted management development/leadership programmes
- community awareness programmes
- BME Leadership Programme
- apprenticeship schemes
- changes to policy, practice or working environment
- staff training and awareness raising

Some of these types of positive action are aimed at individuals or offered to groups of potential recruits, such as work experience placements, whereby paid or unpaid employment is offered to a potential employee for a limited period to provide experience of a working environment or specific type of work. Those who have completed the placement period should, it is felt, be in a better position to make a successful application and can point to having had some experience in doing the job. Linked to this approach might be the creation of apprenticeship schemes, or lower-level entry programmes that provide training to allow people on them to aspire to higher-level posts: examples include nurse cadetship schemes employing staff as health care support workers with release for coursework. Such placements and schemes also provide a link between the trust and minority groups and have been found to encourage individuals on the programme to apply for full-time posts in the trust or elsewhere. For staff already in post but lacking confidence or experience to apply for promotion, mentoring schemes (Thomas 2001) are also frequently advised and have been found to be successful, sometimes in conjunction with other forms of training (including assertiveness training and courses in specific management skills) (Szczepura et al. 2000).

There are a number of other 'positive action' approaches that do not require such direct interference with the lives of individuals, or the provision of specific training, but that hold the potential for significant change at low cost and, at the same time, may affect the whole perception of the organization, both internally and by communities. In particular, the use of targeted recruitment strategies can be very effective. Instead of the 'normal' placement of advertisements in conventional media (that has a relatively low impact in many cases, and may not be viewed by members of minority ethnic groups), the recruiting body makes more direct links with specific community groups by setting up job shops at local community events such as the growing number of 'Indian' Melas, carnival parades or just at 'health days' in temples and community centres. These might form part of a wider community awareness programme that could include more direct health promotion activity or outreach to increase the use of specific services (such as immunization or screening). Such activities, however, are generally most effective if they can draw on the organization's bilingual staff, thereby showcasing existing 'minority' staff.

General staff training around awareness of equality and diversity issues is *not* considered to be positive action. However, targeted training to carry out specific management tasks relating to equality and diversity *can* be classed as positive action. Examples include training in techniques to recruit members of underrepresented communities, which would include raising senior staff awareness of issues relating to cultural diversity, and perhaps taking some steps towards making the 'feel' of offices and workplaces more diverse by attention to decoration, artwork and illustrations in posters, piped music and even food options in canteens. For existing staff, the encouragement of staff support networks (which might also affect gay and lesbian staff or other marginalized and underrepresented groups) has some merit: other establishments have considered holding events to celebrate diversity or taking explicit note of key religious and cultural festivals (see the Interfaith Calendar: a listing of primary sacred times for world religions: http://www.interfaithcalendar. org/). Such activities may be supported by equality and diversity advisory and steering groups and officers appointed to support the equality agenda (now increasingly being adopted as part of the Race Equality Strategy required by the Race Relations Amendment Act 2000), and the production of cultural awareness tools, such as booklets explaining the specific cultural needs of different groups, and distributed to all front-line staff.

In recent years there have been a number of initiatives to bring about change in the NHS, aimed at correcting established patterns of underrepresentation, under-promotion, discrimination and the experience of racialized bullying.In particular, the model of the 'Positively Diverse' programme, which began in Bradford, has become accepted as 'best practice' and been rolled out across the NHS. The programme, now managed by NHS Employers, has developed an integrated change management process, based on the experience of the original 12 pilot sites and over 290 subsequent NHS organizations who have joined the scheme. Following the outline procedures of the field book, there are six key stages to be undertaken which should lead to a better outcome for all staff. Indeed, it is stated that Positively Diverse organizations are already reaping benefits in terms of reduced staff turnover, sickness absence and better overall staff morale and performance (see http://www. nhsemployers.org/excellence/excellence-449.cfm). Operating in tandem with this initiative is the implementation of the Improving Working Lives programme. Under this policy, it is expected that by March 2006 all NHS employers will have achieved the 'Practice Plus' level of compliance with the standards set out (http://www.nhsemployers.org/excellence/excellence-400. cfm) including a constantly revised set of targets for 'valuing diversity' and adherence to the agreements on international recruitment. Clearly, while this depends on self-report and periodic audit, such a mechanism is an effective way of encouraging (and, if necessary, forcing) trusts to incorporate and adhere to best practice models in human resource management, including measures to protect staff from racial harassment and discrimination.

Finally, we must not assume to imply that minority ethnic or migrant workers are themselves always passive victims or recipients of discrimination and compensatory interventions. There is a significant presence of senior staff who have overcome obstacles and become role models for later entrants and examples of significant contribution to the NHS and national life. Mary Seacole was not the only national icon of black nursing, and while Lord David Pitt may have been the first Caribbean-born doctor to be elevated to the House of Lords, he is not the only one to be given such an honour. Other health care workers of BME origin have also found their way into politics and high places, including the late-lamented Lord Michael Chan, a former paediatrician. It would be invidious to single out persons now living, but a research study of some of these found a number of common themes in their stories of success. Vina Mayor (unpublished thesis: also *Nursing Standard* (2004) **18** (3): 104 May) interviewed nearly ninety 'successful' nurses from BME backgrounds, and identified a number of common themes in their personal histories. None said that it had been easy, or denied meeting opposition, although some were more likely to attribute their problems to racism than others. All had experienced greater difficulty as they had reached higher grades, and most had invested considerable amounts of energy and personal commitment (and other resources) into study and searching out training opportunities, while accepting great stress and deprivation in their private lives. If it had not been for their own determination and search energy, few would have been given advice or access to training, and the growth of personal support networks had been a crucial resource. Others had focused on specialized areas of work, such as the haemoglobinopathies, where they might have found some element of specialized expertise in their own 'ethnic identity' – what Mayor describes as a 'niche market'. This, of course, risks marginalization as would the move into 'equal opportunities' posts, from which stereotyped (even if high profile) positions it is sometimes hard to escape. The worst response, however, is to rely on conflict avoidance and a low profile, and a hope that 'someone, somewhere' will recognize the merits of the individual. It should not be necessary for mentorship under the aegis of positive action to be provided to ensure that the skills and potential of such high quality staff are released and put to work for the NHS (Szczepura et al. 2000).

A healthy health service depends upon a multicultural and diverse work-force, and could not survive in the UK or Europe without the contribution of internationally recruited staff. However, it is clear that these latter have been exploited, not least in achieving the former. As the populations of all states become part of the globalizing economy and travel becomes easier, monocultural practice becomes unacceptable, but no employer can continue to exploit migrants indefinitely. There have been a number of initiatives to improve the situation, both in respect of the recruitment and retention of minority ethnic and migrant staff, and to address issues such as their experience of racial harassment and discrimination. Similarly, there are a growing number of agreements and conventions to improve the lot of migrant staff and to reduce the dependence of advanced economies (so-called 'First World' nations such as the UK, USA and Europe) and level of exploitation of 'Third World'-sending countries. However, it would be unrealistic to expect health care staff not to migrate in pursuit of personal and career betterment, and therefore it is important that such workers are protected from discrimination and enabled to achieve their potential – and that their skills and insights are used to improve health care providers' ability to meet the needs of migrant and minority-culture service users. This may, indeed, require recourse to 'positive action' and changes in established ways of working and managing staff, but these changes may not be bad for all staff, and might draw attention to other individuals or groups whose merits have been overlooked, as well as reducing strains and stresses in the workforce, as may for example arise from other non-racialized forms of bullying or neglect. In other words, anti-racist practice may simply be fundamentally best practice in what should be basic professional practice.

Note

1. 6.8 per cent ethnic minority people are unemployed, compared with only 3.4 per cent white people. Black Caribbean men are the group most likely to be unemployed, with 9.8 per cent of the population seeking work (Ethnic Minority Employment Task Force: www.emetaskforce.gov.uk/keys.asp).

References

Alexis, O. and Vydelingum, V. (2004) The lived experience of overseas black and minority ethnic nurses in the NHS in the south of England. *Diversity in Health and Social Care*, 1 (1): 13–20.

Allan, H. T., Larsen, J. A., Bryan, K. and Smith, P. A. (2004) The social reproduction of institutional racism: internationally recruited nurses' experiences of the British health service. *Diversity in Health and Social Care*, 1 (2): 117–26.

Archibong, U. and Giga, S. (2005) *Positive Action in the NHS* (London: NHS Employers).

Beishon, S., Virdee, S. and Hagell, A. (1995) *Nursing in a Multi-Ethnic NHS* (London: Policy Studies Institute).

Bowler, I. (1993) Stereotypes of women of Asian descent in midwifery. *Midwifery* 9 (1): 7–16.

Coker, N, (ed.) (2001) *Racism in Medicine: An Agenda for Change* (London: King's Fund).

CRE (1983) *Ethnic Minority Hospital Staff* (London: Commission for Racial Equality).

Culley, L. (2001) Equal opportunities, policies and nursing employment within the British National Health Service. *Journal of Advanced Nursing* 33 (1): 130–7.

Dimond, B. (2004) Race relations in the UK: the implications for health and social care of recent changes in the law. *Diversity in Health and Social Care* 1 (1): 7–10.

Dreachslin, Janice L. et al. (2000) Workforce diversity: implications for the effectiveness of health care delivery teams. *Social Science and Medicine* 50 (10): 1403–14.

Gavin, M. and Esmail, A. (2002) Solving the recruitment crisis in UK general practice: time to consider physician assistants?' *Social Policy and Administration* 36 (1): 76–89.

Gerrish, K., Husband, C. and Mackenzie, J. (1996) *Nursing for a Multi-ethnic Society* (Buckingham: Open University Press).

Godfrey, K. (2004) Inequality in our sights. *NHS Magazine*, 14–15 (May) *http:// www.nhs.uk/nhsmagazine/archive/may04/feat10.asp*

Home Office (2005) *Improving Opportunity, Strengthening Society: The Government's Strategy to Increase Race Equality and Community Cohesion* (London: Home Office).

International Dialogue on Migration (2005) *Health and Migration: Bridging the Gap* 6 (Geneva: International Organisation for Migration).

Johnson, M. R. D. (1988) Mobility denied: Caribbean minorities in the UK labour market. In *Lost Illusions* (eds M. Cross and H. Entzinger) (London: Tavistock), pp. 73–105.

Lee-Cunin, M. (1989) *Daughters of Seacole* (Batley: West Yorkshire Low Pay Unit).

Matiti, M. R. and Taylor, D. (2005) The cultural lived experience of internationally recruited nurses. *Diversity in Health and Social Care* 2 (1): 7–16.

Owen, D. (1994) *Black People in Great Britain: Social and Economic Circumstances* (Coventry: National Ethnic Minority Data Archive Census Statistical Paper 6).

Szczepura, A., Miles, P., Johnson, M. R. D., Watson, N. and Pawar, A. (2000) *An Evaluation of the 1998 Development Programme for Black and Minority Ethnic Managers in the West Midlands NHS* (Coventry: Centre for Health Services Studies, University of Warwick).

Taylor, B. (2005) The experiences of overseas nurses working in the NHS. *Diversity in Health & Social Care* 2 (1): 17–28.

Thomas, David A. (2001) The truth about mentoring minorities: race matters. *Harvard Business Review* (2001) 79 (4): 98–107.

Thomas, M. and Morton-Williams, J. (1972) *Overseas Nurses in Britain* (London: Political and Economic Planning).

Resources: websites

Equality and diversity: Department of Health web pages *http://www.dh.gov.uk/ PolicyAndGuidance/HumanResourcesAndTraining/ModelEmployer/EqualityAnd Diversity/fs/en*

New Zealand Ministry of Health: Toolkits and the Treaty of Waitangi *http:// www.newhealth.govt.nz/toolkits/tow.htm* (accessed 24 Jan. 2006)

NHS Employers: Positively Diverse *http://www.nhsemployers.org/excellence/excellence-449.cfm*

Practical Guide to Ethnic Monitoring in the NHS and Social Care *http://www.dh.gov.uk/assetRoot/04/11/68/43/04116843.pdf*

Positive Action in the NHS (DoH 2005) *https://www.nhsemployers.org/restricted/downloads/download.asp?ref=561&hash=58ae749f25eded36f486bc85feb3f0ab*

Leadership and Race Equality: Mentoring Guidelines (London: DoH 2004) *http://www.modern.nhs.uk/1115/21174/BMEguidelines.pdf*

Sharing the Challenge, Sharing the Benefits: Equality and Diversity in the Medical Workforce (DoH, 2004) *http://www.dh.gov.uk/assetRoot/04/08/38/83/04083883.pdf*

Equalities and Diversity Strategy and Delivery Plan to Support the NHS (DoH, 2003) *http://www.dh.gov.uk/assetRoot/04/06/95/47/04069547.pdf*

Equality and Diversity in Local Government in England (London: Office for Public Management; Office of the Deputy Prime Minister 2003) *http://www.local.odpm.gov.uk/research/crosscut/equality/rprt.pdf*

Improving Working Lives: Tackling Racial Harassment in the NHS: Good Practice Guidance (DoH 2001) h*ttp://www.dh.gov.uk/assetRoot/04/07/45/11/04074511.pdf*

Working Lives: Programmes for Change: Positively Diverse (DoH, 2001) *http://www.dh.gov.uk/assetRoot/04/03/50/06/04035006.pdf*

Tackling Racial Harassment in the NHS: Evaluating Black and Minority Ethnic Staff's Attitudes and Experiences (DoH, 2001) *http://www.dh.gov.uk/assetRoot/04/07/45/24/04074524.pdf*

The Vital Connection: An Equalities Framework for the NHS: Working Together for Quality and Equality (DoH 2000) *http://www.dh.gov.uk/assetRoot/04/03/50/54/04035054.pdf*

CHAPTER 6

Building Research Capacity in Health Services

JO COOKE, JO MIDDLEMASS AND GILL SARRE

Why should we build capacity?

Research capacity building (RCB) has a major part to play in producing high quality health care, and has gained international recognition in this regard (NAPCRGC 2002; Mickan 2002). It does this by increasing the ability and opportunities to do research alongside practice, by identifying problems and finding solutions and by discovering better ways of providing health care. The ultimate aim of RCB is to support health improvement in the populations in receipt of services (Lansing and Dennis 2004; Sitthi-Amorn et al. 2000).

The Department of Health within the UK has adopted the definition of research capacity building as 'a process of individual and institutional development which leads to higher levels of skills and greater ability to perform useful research'. (Trostle 1992: 1321). Initiatives to build research capacity include developing research for practice, where research is conducted by academics to inform practice decision-making; research with practice, which encompasses research being conducted in collaboration with academics and practice; and research by practice, where ideas are initiated and research is conducted by practitioners (Mant 1997; Marks and Godfrey 2000). This chapter will focus particularly on initiatives, working examples and the theoretical underpinning of building research capacity with and by practice. Our position is that by emphasizing this more participatory approach of involving practitioners and services in capacity development, the interventions developed add value to both research and practice, and therefore impact on the 'usefulness' of research being developed.

Where should capacity building be focused?

Capacity development has traditionally focused on professional groups with a low research-skills base and contexts where research is not traditionally part of the practice culture. The professional groups who have a poor skills base include nurses, allied health professionals (AHP) and social care practitioners

(Campbell et al. 1999; DoH 2000a; Ross et al. 2002; Cooke et al. 2002). The need for capacity building in nursing and AHP was recognized in a report written for the Higher Education Funding Council for England and the Department of Health, which highlight a lack of funding for these professionals to undertake research (HEFCE 2001). In a strategy to support Research and Development (R&D) for nursing, the Department of Health pointed to difficulties in supporting training and research skills development in nurses (DoH 2000b). Experienced nurses lack opportunities for research training, have difficulties finding protected time and resources to fund research, and find workload pressures a barrier to undertaking research. The Report also acknowledged that undergraduate programmes mainly focus on professional competences rather than research skills. These issues are mirrored in other professional groups, such as social workers, where research is not a realistic career option, is not central in training, and is not important in influencing career progression (Cooke et al. 2002). In terms of health care contexts, primary care has been identified as having a poor capacity for undertaking research. This is paradoxical in relation to need and service provision, as over 90 per cent of NHS contacts are in primary care (Mant 1997; Campbell et al. 1999; Harrison 2005) but only 7 per cent of the annual NHS DoH R&D spend supports primary care research (Mant 1997; Campbell et al. 1999; DoH 1999).

The National Working Group on R&D in primary care (Mant 1997) made a strong case for the involvement of primary care practitioners in R&D and suggested that this would lead to better quality care through the development of a self-critical professional culture and more rapid dissemination and uptake of research evidence. This premise has been supported by evidence in the international literature (Mant et al. 2004). The NHS R&D Strategic Review Primary Care (DoH 1999) strongly supported the conclusions drawn in the Mant Report and further recommended that primary care organizations should develop R&D strategies which would bring service development closer to research and teaching, and suggested that primary care should have better access to R&D funding to improve this.

Work around building capacity in developing countries has focused on issues to do with priority setting and problem solving in order to generate knowledge where it is most required (CHRD 2002; GFHR 2000). It also includes issues around empowerment and learning in the spirit of engendering self-reliance and sustainability (GFHR 2000). Whilst these issues are particularly important for developing countries, they are also pertinent themes to inform capacity building in all health care settings.

Policy and research capacity building

Most developed and many developing countries have produced policies to support RCB which are usually directed under some form of R&D strategy or strategic body. In the UK there is a National Coordinating Centre for Research Capacity Building. In the USA this task is directed by the Agency for Healthcare Research and Quality (AHRQ) and in Australia research capacity is included in the Primary Health Care Research Evaluation and Development strategy (PHCRED). National plans for building capacity have generally focused on the following areas:

Building the research workforce. This support generally takes the form of fellowships and bursaries to facilitate research career progression. In the UK this includes researcher development, post-doctoral and career scientist awards. Similar fellowships are offered in other developed and developing countries.

Building infrastructure and networks. This is particularly represented in primary care. In the USA, AHRQ provides grants to assist new or established primary care practice-based research networks. A strong interest in building primary care networks has evolved in the UK, leading to the UK Federation of Primary Care Research Organisations. However, other network structures have also developed based on need, characterized by low research activity and/or gaps in knowledge. Currently in the UK, efforts are being made to develop a national coordinated set of networks based around disease-specific areas including cancer, mental health, medicines for children, diabetes, stroke and Alzheimer's disease. In the USA funding is available from the Building Research Infrastructure and Capacity Program (BRIC) to build research capacity in states that have not traditionally been involved in health service research.

Investing in research support. In the UK this includes a network of Research and Development Support Units (RDSU) to support practitioners undertaking research. Support structures often link with other capacity-building initiatives including grants and fellowship schemes. In the USA, for example, grants are focused on academic institutions that offer advanced training to people with a strong interest in health services research who want to prepare for research careers and apply for funding.

Responsive funds to support projects. Grants to fund projects can stimulate research activity and interests. For example, in Australia the PHCRED offer grants to primary care practitioners to submit project protocols and link these to support structures to enable capacity building. Currently the UK does not have responsive funding from central government (DoH 2005a).

Developing and strengthening academic infrastructure. The strategy for developing primary care in Australia focuses strongly on building capacity in primary care academic institutions. The North America Primary Care

Research Group also supports this type of RCB investment in order to provide enough effective mentorship and leadership in primary care (NAPCRG
2002). In the UK, the research capacity strategy specifically invests in academic units to support research activity.

Principles of capacity building

Before describing in detail how some of these policy initiatives have been
translated into effective RCB interventions, it is important to describe some
principles of capacity building that might better inform this translation for
practice. These principles have been developed through an exploration of the
literature and dialogue between Trent RDSU, the NHS and the social care
organizations it supports, through a series of workshops and consultative
events to check their validity and workability. The principles are: developing
skills and confidence; supporting linkages and partnerships; ensuring the
research is 'close to practice'; developing appropriate dissemination; investing
in infrastructure; and building elements of sustainability and continuity
(Cooke 2005).

1. Developing appropriate skills, and confidence, through training and creating opportunities to apply skills

A core element of any RCB strategy should be the development of research
skills in both practitioners and researchers. Skills can be developed through
training (DoH 2004a; NAPCRG 2002; Del Mar and Askew 2004) and the
application of skills in practice (Cooke et al. in press). Linking training and
practice is important because it enhances confidence, and it also helps to
consolidate learning. It can be supported by mentorship and supervision
(NAPCRG 2002; Del Mar and Askew 2004), where novice researchers have
access to and advice from more experienced researchers throughout the
research process, enabling better decision-making and higher quality research.

Research practitioner skills should be placed in the context of career
development and opportunities to apply and extend skills. Policy and position
statements (DoH 2004b; NAPCRG 2002; Pitkethly and Sullivan 2003)
support the concept of career progression or 'careers escalator'. Difficulties
have been identified in the UK, however, around workforce flexibility and
how to support careers that include a balance between research, teaching
and practice in health and social care. The Strategic Learning and Research
Committee (StLaRC) (Butterworth 2004), for example, emphasizes different
employment rights for research practitioners when they tread the path
between academia and practice. The Report highlights the need for clear
employment and career pathway models that include better working between
higher education institutions and health and social care providers. Additionally they suggest joint appointments as a way forward.

There is some empirical evidence that research skill development increases research activities (Hakansson et al. 2000) and enhances positive attitudes towards conducting and collaborating in research. Bacigalupo et al., highlight statistical differences in relation to research skills training and attitudes to getting involved with research amongst primary care practitioners (Bacigalupo in press). Compared to the rest of the primary care workforce, those practitioners who had a masters degree preferred to conduct their own projects and to collaborate more with experienced researchers.

2. Supporting useful research 'close to practice'

RCB should generate research that is 'useful' (Trostle 1992), leading to health gain and health improvement (NAPCRG 2002). This principle proposes that 'useful' research is that which is conducted 'close' to practice because it helps to produce more relevant research, and because of the knock-on effects that conducting research has on practitioners and services.

Many argue that the most relevant and useful research questions are those generated by, or in consultation with, practitioners and services (NAPCRG 2002; Mant 1997; Smith 1997) and service users (NHS SDO 2000; Hanley et al. 2000). The underlying premise is that these research questions are based on what is important to patients and results are therefore more likely to be used. Others suggest that research questions should be based on problem solving and setting priorities that have been developed by identifying service needs (Lansing and Dennis 2004). The current R&D strategy in the UK, for example, has been based on local need and national priorities (DoH 2000a), where programmes of research evolve from listening exercises related to service need, and much of the international literature for developing countries strongly advocates priority setting as an essential element to capacity building. Others have also highlighted that the 'immediate' usefulness of research is related to its take up in practice (Frenk 1992). If RCB activities are to influence the quality of services, selecting projects whose findings inform practice seems important.

The 'close to practice' principle may not only have implications for how research questions are developed, but also for the choice of methodologies adopted. Some methodologies are based themselves on problem-solving approaches and have a strong educational component. These include, for example, action research approaches and participatory inquiry methodologies (Sitthi-Amorn et al. 2000; Cooke et al. 2002; Hurst 2003). The current service delivery organization programme acknowledges the usefulness of these approaches to health services research and the impact on practitioners and services; others have highlighted these research approaches as having a real potential for building capacity and interest (Hurst 2003).

Getting practitioners involved with research questions from the start may also be capacity building in itself. There is some evidence that practitioners are more likely to engage and undertake research if they see its relevance to their own practice or policy, and so become co- workers and collaborators on projects (Cooke 2002; Bacigalupo et al. in press). Once they have had this experience, they are also more likely to want to lead and collaborate on other projects (Bacigalupo et al. in press).

Building research capacity 'close to practice' is also 'useful' because of the skills of critical thinking it engenders in practitioners that can also affect practice decision-making (Del Mar and Ashew 2004). Practitioners in a local bursary scheme, for example, said they were more able to take an evidence-based approach in their everyday practice, had more insight into their personal practice and felt stimulated in doing this work (Lee and Saunders 2004).

The link between the use of evidence in practice and the generation of evidence for practice is an important one, but in the context of UK policy there are some tensions. Clinical effectiveness and support to promote evidence-based practice (EBP) is funded from a different pot to that for research. As a consequence, research and EBP are governed and supported from different places within NHS organizations, resulting in a lack of joined-up thinking and activity. Whilst protecting funding for research is important to promoting research activity separate from clinical work, the unintended consequence may be that the research–practice divide is perpetuated.

3. Linkages, partnerships and collaborations

The notion of building partnerships and collaborations is integral to capacity building as it is the mechanism by which research skills and practice knowledge are exchanged, developed and enhanced (Griffiths et al. 2000). The linkages that enhance RCB can exist between:

- universities and practice (DoH 1999; DoH 2004; Gillibrand et al. 2002; Rowlands et al. 2004). Many research capacity initiatives link universities and health services. These include, for example, RDSUs and academic units that work with practitioners to conduct research and build capacity, as well as examples of more formal and established links such as joint posts held by universities and services;
- novice and experienced researchers (NAPCRG 2002; Pitkethly and Sullivan 2003; Thomas and While 2001). This can enhance capacity through methods such as mentorship and supervision;
- different professional groups and different health and care provider sectors (Rowlands et al. 2004; NHSSDO 2000). Health care research should mirror care pathways, and the ability to conduct research to support this involves developing partnerships between practitioners and different provider sectors, for example between health and social care and different professional groups;

- service users, practitioners and researchers (NHSDO 2000; Hanley et al. 2000). Tied to the 'close to practice' principle, capacity can be developed by investing in links between researchers and service users. However, this involves training and support for service users as well as for practitioners in different countries (Del Mar and Askew 2004; Rowlands et al. 2004). Increased learning and more generalizable research can be conducted between countries. Forging these links builds a potential for this work to be undertaken;
- health and industry (NAPCRG 2002; Davies 2005; DoH 2004b). Current UK policy supports the development of a mutually beneficial partnership between industry and research to produce research for patient benefit.

The underlying rationale for forging linkages and partnerships is that intellectual capital (sharing knowledge) and social capital (building relationships) can be encouraged, which enhances the ability to do research (Fenton et al. 2001).

4. Research capacity building should ensure appropriate dissemination

Research is only useful if it is communicated effectively to where it can have an impact. For this reason a key principle in capacity building should be that research is appropriately disseminated. This includes writing for publication in peer-reviewed journals, and giving conference presentations to academic and practice communities. Often these are used as measures in themselves to demonstrate that capacity building has taken place, and the research it has produced is of a high quality (Del Mar and Askew 2004). However, this principle extends beyond the more traditional view of dissemination. The litmus test that ultimately determines the success of capacity building is that it should impact on practice, and on the health of patients and communities (Smith 2001; CHRD 2002). Smith argues that the strategies of dissemination should include a range of methods that are fit for purpose, and include traditional dissemination, but also instruments and programmes of care implementation, protocols, lay publications, and publicity through factsheets, the media and the internet. When planning RCB interventions, this more diverse approach should be considered. It may be worth linking different dissemination strategies to impact assessment to help inform future dissemination strategies around RCB.

5. Research capacity building should include elements of continuity and sustainability

Sustainability is an important factor to consider in terms of impact and safeguarding enthusiasm in budding researchers, and is linked to the culture of an organization and strong and supportive leadership. Sustainability refers to the maintenance and continuity of newly acquired skills and organizational structures to undertake research. The Council on Health Research for Development (2002) highlights the importance of sustainability and notes that it is easier to build than to utilize and maintain capacity. Crisp et al. suggest that capacity can be sustained by applying skills to practice (Crisp et al. 2000) and can be provided through accessing funding opportunities, through maintaining and nourishing effective partnerships and through ensuring that skills and expertise are acknowledged and used in an organization.

RCB interventions focusing at a policy and institutional level are most effective in producing sustainable change (Lansang and Dennis 2004; White 2002). White argues that sustainable research capacity is dependent on both operational and strategic dimensions at an organizational level. Poor management can undo years of careful capacity building growth (White 2002). Research capacity goals need to be relevant to, and embedded within, organizational goals and decision-making, and be important enough for organizations to invest in effective research management and strong leadership. If an enabling and sustaining environment is not developed, researchers will simply leave and investment in capacity will be lost to organizations.

6. *Appropriate infrastructures enhance research capacity building*

Infrastructure is composed of structures and processes that are set up to enable the smooth and effective running of research projects. At a team level, for example, project management skills are essential to enable projects to move forward, and should be suitably supervised with academic and management support.

Many have recognized the importance of finding time and space to do research. Structural and organizational methods that support this include the identification of protected time and backfill arrangements as well as requisite funding (Sarre 2003). Making research work 'legitimate' by including it as part of job descriptions for certain positions may also be beneficial, not only by reinforcing research as a core skill and activity, but also for reviewing it in annual appraisals which can then be tools for research capacity evaluation.

Organizational infrastructure to help direct new practitioners to research support has also been highlighted (DoH 2004a). This is particularly the case in light of the research governance framework (DoH 2005b; DoH 2001). Developing administrative and support staff to help researchers through this process is important to enable research to be undertaken. (Shaw 2004).

The report on the evaluation of the pilot PCT (RM&G) sites published by the Department of Health (DoH 2002) notes that the introduction of governance systems and management could have a positive impact on research culture within the NHS. For example, the necessity for NHS organizations to know about and record research activity and researcher involvement was seen as an opportunity for networking and utilizing research skills. Although there was concern expressed from the outset that the implementation of the Research Governance Framework had the potential to create barriers to conducting research (George et al. 2002), there has also been a significant expectation that the increased awareness of research and the development of infrastructure would have a positive impact on the development of research culture, capacity and activity (Bryar 2002; Newell and Plews 2002). The reality of implementing systems to deal with the complexities of the research governance regulations has proved problematic, particularly in primary care where the relative lack of research management expertise and infrastructure has resulted in what are perceived as disproportionately bureaucratic systems. Recent discussion in the literature has focused on the detrimental impact of both ethical review and NHS approval systems, and there is evidence of serious delays in getting research projects started (Hill et al. 2005). There is also a suggestion that it is deterring researchers, particularly those who are inexperienced, from undertaking research (RCN 2005). The impact on student research has been perceived as a particular issue. Ellis and Peckover argue that there are tensions between the overall aims of the Research Governance Framework and the development of research skills at a Masters degree level (Ellis and Peckover 2003). Bentley and Enderby (2005) compared numbers of applications to local research ethics committees in South Yorkshire over two successive years and found a decrease of 40 per cent in overall applications in 2004–5 compared to 2003–4. During the same period, applications to MRECs remained constant, suggesting that it is smaller, local research studies that are being deterred and therefore there is a detrimental effect on research capacity at the grassroots level.

There has been strong support for governance procedures to be more proportionate to risk (DoH 2004; Meerabeau et al. 2004) and to encourage streamlining of research approval processes (Recommendations from the NTRAC Workshop 2005). Recent initiatives to improve operational guidance, such as that provided by the NHS R&D Forum, aim to reduce inconsistency and bureaucracy.

Despite the somewhat hostile reaction to some aspects of the research governance implementation process, there is evidence that benefits to research capacity-building have arisen through the development of infrastructure and supportive partnerships. Although they identified considerable barriers to students and their supervisors, Ellis and Peckover (2003) argue that the implementation of the Research Governance Framework has encouraged a more collaborative approach between academic and NHS organizations, and that greater consideration is given to ensuring that student research 'fits' with the national and local R&D agenda, and is therefore close to practice. The shared arrangements for primary care organizations, supported by revenue funding from the Department of Health, has resulted in the development of some fruitful partnerships, drawing together expertise across primary care,

Box 6.1   Examples of training needs assessments

Bolton PCO instigated a needs assessment by inviting interested staff to a lunchtime seminar to explore their training and support needs relating to the development of R&D capacity. Small group-led discussions explored the following topics: What skills do I have already? What do I need to know to fulfil my role around R&D? How can the gaps be filled? What are the barriers? How can the PCT best overcome any of these? How will I know if it worked?

The results of this consultation helped to identify the support and training required to meet the quality improvement for the trust through research and development. This included increasing managerial support for researchers; incorporating research on people's job descriptions; and personal development plans and within service specifications, thus providing a legitimate remit, with a resource allocation, for research activity.

Barnsley PCO undertook a needs assessment of all its staff (both health and social care) to identify training needs and expertise across the trust. Information was collected via a questionnaire. This informed a training strategy that included providing research fellow support, and planning training and resources. An Introduction to Research course was designed and conducted in a community setting. A Small Projects Fund was set up to pump-prime pilot research projects in order to improve the opportunities for researchers to apply for external funding for future research work, and funding was provided to support practitioners on Masters degrees, including backfill support (see Bacigalupo et al. 2006, for further details).

secondary care and social care organizations (Sarre 2002; DoH 2002). The sharing of research skills and expertise across organizational boundaries can contribute to the development of research capacity through increased opportunities for training and wider involvement in research (Shaw et al. 2004). Barnsley Health and Social Care R&D Alliance is an example of a successful strategic research partnership that has been built on the foundations of research management and governance (RM&G) arrangements with the support of the Trent RDSU (see Box 6.1).

Developing multiple strategies for capacity building

Many authors agree that RCB should take place at an individual and organizational level (Marks and Godfrey 2000; Del Mar and Askew 2004; Sarre

2002), in teams (Smith 1997; Carter et al. 2002), and networks (Griffiths et al. 2000). Many support a multidimensional approach to capacity building including work with individuals, teams and through infrastructure development as well as promoting a research culture in organizations where research is a valued, expected and enjoyable activity. Examples are given below of interventions that have worked at different structural levels.

Organizations

The Department of Health has recognized the importance of environment within organizations when supporting research capacity and promoting a culture that produces high-quality research. Research culture is a difficult concept to describe although most people would recognize it – or the lack of it – in an individual organization. One NHS trust worked with a local university in the North of England to measure research culture in order to plan RCB (Whitford et al. 2005). 'Culture' was measured using a questionnaire in three sections, including biographical questions, level of research engagement/training needs and the R&D Culture Index. The Culture Index comprised 18 statements with a four-point Likert scale ranging from 'strongly agree' to 'strongly disagree'. Staff were asked to respond to the statements and identify the five statements that they perceived to most strongly contribute to an R&D culture. Having access to R&D support and training opportunities were identified as the two key contributors to the development of an R&D culture. Key statements selected that were seen to contribute to a culture of R&D related to the working environment and organizational infrastructure rather than personal skills and attributes.

A key element, then, to building a culture in an organization is to systematically plan and implement a research training strategy. Ideally this should be based on a needs assessments. (See Box 6.1 for an example of needs assessment undertaken in practice.) Accessible training and support is necessary to bring general research and development skills up to a minimal level, while extending those among specific members of staff. Training can be provided by in-house training, support from RDSUs and by creating links with local universities. Funding for protected time and course fees enhances the ability to implement research training strategies

The north of England culture study also highlighted the importance of R&D support (Whitford et al. 2005). This can be obtained through developing effective supportive infrastructure within organizations. An example of this is given in Box 6.2.

The literature also points us to factors that influence RCB within organizations, for instance, support for the research agenda at the highest level within the organization (Crisp et al. 2000; White 2002) and good management (Robertson et al. 2005). A project undertaken across 39 PCTs in the former Trent region during 2002–3 (Sarre 2003) identified a range

---

Box 6.2   Developing supportive infrastructure: developing research facilitator posts

Research facilitator posts were created as part of an initiative to build up the capacity and quality of research within the county of Lincolnshire (UK). In this example the research facilitators were all clinicians, working half-time in the clinical role and half-time helping to build up research capacity within their organization. They all worked to a joint countywide research strategy agreed by the overarching Research and Development Group (with membership from all health organizations within the county). The core organizations of the research group also shared the same research management and governance arrangements with one of the Primary Care Organizations (PCO) taking the lead role.

The research facilitators worked closely with: Partnership Research Management and Governance structures; Clinical trial networks; the Medical Research Council; the local RDSU; academic institutions; general practitioners and their staff; community nurses including district nurses, health visitors and school nurses; therapists including physiotherapists and occupational/speech therapists; PCO employed non-clinical staff; dentists, optometrists and community pharmacists; social services; and members of the public.

There were a number of proven benefits to these posts including: research that meets the organizations' needs and research questions; more quality research being undertaken, both collaboratively and as lead researchers; more joint working both interdisciplinary and across organizations; more working with academic units including joint appointments; more collaboration in multicentred trials in primary care; increased research funding both by identifying funding streams and by applying or assisting others to apply; increased numbers of intellectual property identified and exploited on behalf of the researcher and trust.

---

of factors that appear to be positively associated with the development of organizational research culture:

- strong organizational support at senior management level;
- incorporation of R&D into the business of the organization at a strategic level;
- commitment to partnership approaches and working;
- strong R&D leadership from the top;
- supporting local champions;
- access to support, information, training, networks and advice.

Some allocated resources

In this same study, the benefits to developing a research culture included: encouraging innovation in the organization, supporting effective staff performance and professional development, and helping to meet organizational objectives (including improving the quality of care and supporting the use of evidence in practice). It was also thought to have an impact on the recruitment and retention of high quality staff. Additionally, developing a research culture was seen to have a positive effect in enhancing organizational reputation and pride. These factors may be important to 'sell' the idea of building a research culture in organizations to senior managers.

Teams

Jowett et al. (2000) found that GPs were more likely to be research-active if they were part of a practice where others were involved in research. Guidance

---

Box 6.3   Trent RDSU Designated Research Team (DRT) in primary care

The Designated Research Team (DRT) scheme builds on a programme providing a team with funding (£30,000 over two years) to enable protected time for up to three team members to do research, and which also funds training, research consultancy, and user involvement where appropriate. Teams are structured in a variety of ways, but each team should include at least one member who is a novice researcher and someone who is based in an academic department. Multiprofessional teams are encouraged. Support is provided through mentorship from RDSU staff and apprenticeship from the academic collaborator. Teams are held accountable for their progress through six-monthly reporting to the RDSU on goals negotiated with them at the beginning of the contract.

The approach is particularly strong in building and sustaining skills in practitioners. Establishing and maintaining links between academia and research networks seem a major contributory factor to success, as well as the notion of 'learning by doing' supported by mentors. The environment in which the team is situated is also crucial to the team's success. Having support from managers in highly significant in terms of legitimizing research activity. The approach has noted that providing funding for protected time does not always mean research is undertaken. The availability of backfill arrangements is crucial to protecting research time.

---

from a number of national bodies highlights the need for multiprofessional and interprofessional involvement in conducting useful research for practice, which implies there is a need for an appropriate mix of skills and practice experience within research teams to enable this (Raghunath and Innes 2004). High-profile researchers or well-funded research teams are relatively easy to identify and are more likely to have published in peer-reviewed journals or appear on a database such as the National Research Register. In comparison, unfunded, low-profile individual researchers who should be the target of trusts' support and investment may remain 'hidden'. An example of the promotion of research teams is given in Box 6.3.

Networks

As previously mentioned, one international policy response to building research capacity is the development of research networks. In the UK this is particularly true in primary care, but more recent developments have focused on different disease group networks.

Primary care networks have developed in two main categories (Fenton et al. 2001):

- those that support practitioners doing their own research, where research practitioners develop their research and evidence-based practice skills, and where members meet to discuss ideas and gain academic support; and

---

Box 6.4   WeLReN: supporting top-down and bottom-up approaches to plan activity in a research network

A whole systems approach was adopted by WeLReN. WeLReN developed their plan around different programmes of work, including projects led by academics and practitioners. For all these projects, patients and practices were recruited via the network. Top-down projects are led by academics and experienced researchers, and are usually externally funded. Bottom-up projects are supported through local bursary money. Coalition projects that are developed at a yearly event selected by the network participants are based on a policy theme that matches local need and interest. These coalitions include experts and multiprofessionals with a range of research experience. A team emerges to undertake a coalition project, funded through the network, and supported by training and workshops to help those involved progress through the research cycle. Twenty-four per cent of the practices in the area are actively involved in a research project yearly, and 2.4 per cent of general practices are involved in directly running a project.

- research participation networks, where practitioners participate in joining forces to recruit patients. More recent UK NHS-wide initiatives have focused on recruitment networks, particularly in relation to Randomized Control Trials.

Networks are likely to be most effective when relationships within them are beneficial to the individual practitioner and the network organization (Fenton et al. 2001). This can be achieved by using bottom-up and top-down approaches, where activity is shaped both by members of the network and by network managers/leaders and academics. A good example of working in this participatory manner was developed by WeLReN (see Box 6.4) (Thomas and While 2001). Many networks operate bursary schemes or seed-corn funding to nurture new research ideas (Pitkethly and Sullivan 2003) and support or provide training to develop research skills in their members. Many include both academic and practice memberships and leadership.

Individuals

Networks, organizations and teams can support and develop individuals within them through training, mentorship, funding opportunities, supporting protected time, and recognizing and utilizing research skills. However, certain RCB interventions particularly focus on developing individuals through nurturing research careers. In the UK, but also in many other countries, this involves developing fellowship schemes to help career progression from doctoral, to post-doctoral, to scientific career awards. These fellowships can focus on particular professional groups where research skills are at a low level, for example nursing and AHP. Fellowships are an important element in shaping the research workforce, but it is important not to see them in isolation from other RCB initiatives that support research culture and activity. Many practitioners need mentoring and support to be able to reach the standard at which they may successfully take advantage of such opportunities.

Conclusion

In conclusion, this chapter has discussed what is meant by RCB, and has explained its relevance and contribution to the development of high quality services. It has described a theoretical framework based around six principles of RCB, and some examples grounded in practice have been included. A point to bear in mind when supporting research capacity building is that its purpose is to produce usable research. This is likely to occur when research is carried out with or by practitioners, when a research culture is nurtured and when research and practitioners who have a positive impact on services are developed.

References

Albert, E. and Mickan, S. (2002) 'Closing the gap and widening the scope: New directions for research capacity building in primary health care'. *Australian Family Physician* **31** (12): 1038–41.

Bacigalupo, R., Cooke, J. and Hawley, M. (2006) 'Research activity, interest and skills in a health and social care setting: a snapshot of a primary care trust in Northern England', *Primary Care Research and Development*. **1**: 68–77.

Bryar, R. (2002) 'The promise of research governance: building research and development capacity and clinical research in primary health care', *Primary Health Care Research and Development* **3**: 137–8.

Butterworth, A. (2004) *Developing and Sustaining a World Class Workforce of Educators and Researchers in Health and Social Care: A Report to the Strategic Learning and Research Committee* (London: NHSU).

Campbell, S. M., Roland, M., Bentley, E., Dowell, J., Hassall, K., Pooley, J. et al. (1999) 'Research capacity in UK primary care', *British Journal of General Practice* **49**: 967–70.

Carter, Y. H., Shaw, S. and Macfarlane, F. (2002) 'Primary Care research team assessment (PCRTA): development and evaluation: Occasional paper'. *Royal College of General Practitioners* **81**: 1–72.

Cooke, J., Owen, J. and Wilson, A. (2002) 'Research and development at the health and social care interface in primary care: a scoping exercise in one National Health Service region', *Health and Social Care in the Community* **10** (6): 435–44.

Cooke, J. (2005) *Developing a Framework of Indicators to Measure the Art and Science of Research Capacity Building* (Belfast: RCN).

Cooke, J., Nancarrow, S., Hammersley, V., Farndon, L. and Vernon, W. (2006) 'The "Designated Research Team" Approach to Building Research Capacity in Primary Care', *Primary Health Care Research and Development* (in press).

Community Practitioners' and Health Visitors' Association, the Royal College of Midwives, the Royal College of Nursing (2005) *Position Paper on the Implementation of Research Governance Procedures. http://www.man.ac.uk/rcn/rs/RCMRCNCPHVFeb05.htm*

Council on Health Research for Development (2002) *Revisiting Capacity Development: Learning Brief* (Geneva: Council on Health Research for Development).

Crisp, B. R., Swerissen, H. and Duckett, S. J. (2000) 'Four approaches to capacity building in health: consequences for measurement and accountability', *Health Promotion International* **15** (2): 99–107.

Davies, S. (2005) R&D for the NHS: Delivering the research agenda', in: *How to Build Research Capacity in the NHS: Understanding the Strategies that Work* (London: National Coordinating Centre for Research Capacity Development).

Del Mar, C. and Askew, D. (2004) 'Building family/general practice research capacity', *Annals of Family Medicine* **2** (Supplement 2): 535–40.

Department of Health (1999) *Strategic Review of the NHS R&D Levy: The Clarke Report* (Central Research Department, Department of Health).

Department of Health (2000a) *Towards a Strategy for Nursing Research and Development* (London: Department of Health).

Department of Health (2000b) *Research and Development for a First-Class Service* (Leeds: DoH).

Department of Health (2001) *Research Governance Framework for Health and Social Care* (London: Department of Health).

Department of Health (2002) *Development of Research Management and Governance in Primary and Community Care*: Information for Primary Care Trusts: *http://www.dh.gov.uk/assetRoot/04/06/69/25/04066925.*

Department of Health (2004a) *Research Capacity Development Strategy* (London: Department of Health).

Department of Health (2004b) *Research for Patient Benefit* (London: Department of Health).

Department of Health (2005a) *Research Governance Framework for Health and Social Care* (London: Department of Health).

Department of Health (2005b) *Best Research for Best Health: A New National Health Research Strategy. The NHS Contribution to Health Research in England: A Consultation* (London: Department of Health).

Ellis, L. and Peckover, S. (2003) 'Research governance and postgraduate nurse education: the tensions and solutions', *Nurse Researcher* **11** (1): 32–45.

Fenton, F., Harvey, J., Griffiths, F., Wild, A. and Sturt, J. (2001) 'Reflections from organization science of primary health care networks', *Family Practice* **18**: 540–4.

Frenk, J. (1992) 'Balancing relevance and excellence: organisational responses to link research with decision making', *Social Science and Medicine* **35** (11): 1397–404.

George, A. J. T., Gale, R., Winston, R. and Korn, D. (2002) 'Research governance at the crossroads', *Nature Medicine* **8** (2): 99–101.

Gillibrand, W. P., Burton, C. and Watkins, G. G. (2002) 'Clinical networks for nursing research', *International Nursing Review* **49**: 188–93.

Global Forum for Health Research (2000) *The 10/90 Report on Health Research 2000* (Geneva: Global Forum for Health Research).

Griffiths, F., Wild, A., Harvey, J. and Fenton, E. (2000) 'The productivity of primary care research networks', *British Journal of General Practice* **50**: 913–15.

Hakansson, A., Henriksson, K. and Isacsson, A. (2000) 'Research methods courses for GPs: ten years' experience in southern Sweden', *British Journal of General Practice* **50** (459): 811–12.

Hanley, J., Bradburn, S., Gorin, M., Barnes, M., Evans, C. and Goodare, H. B. (2000) *Involving Consumers in Research and Development in the NHS: Briefing Notes for Researchers* (Winchester: Consumers in NHS Research Support Unit).

Harrison, R. A. (2005) 'Barriers and opportunities to developing research capacity in primary care trusts: the views of staff attached to a primary care trust', *Primary Health Care Research and Development* **6**: 185–9.

Hill, J., Foster, N., Hughes, R. and Hay, E. (2005) 'Meeting the challenges of research governance', *Rheumatology* **44**: 571–2.

Hurst, J. (2003) 'Building a research conscious workforce', *Journal of Health Organization and management* **17** (5): 373–84.

Jowett, S., Macleod, J., Wilson, S. and Hobbs, F. (2000) Research in Primary Care: extent of involvement and perceived determinants among practitioners for one English region', *British Journal of General Practice* **50**: 387–9.

Lansing, M. A. and Dennis, R. (2004) 'Building capacity in health research in the developing world', *Bulletin of the World Health Organisation* **82** (10): 764–70.

Lee, M. and Saunders, K. (2004) 'Oak trees from acorns? An evaluation of local bursaries in primary care', *Primary Health Care Research and Development* **5**: 93–5.

Lester, H., Carter, Y. H., Dassu, D. and Hobbs, F. (1998) 'Survey of research activity, training needs. departmental support, and career intentions of junior academic general practitioners', *British Journal of General Practice* **48**: 1322–6.

Mant, D. (1997) *National Working Party on R&D in Primary Care: Final Report* (London: NHSE South and West).

Mant, D., Del Mar, C., Glasziou, P., Knottnerus, A. and Wallace, P. C. (2004) 'The state of primary-care research', *The Lancet* 364: 1004–6.

Marks, L. and Godfrey, M. (2000) *Developing Research Capacity within the NHS: A Summary of the Evidence* (Leeds: Nuffield Portfolio Programme Report, no. 12).

Meerabeau, L., Ruston, A. and Clayton, J. (2004) 'The research governance framework for health and social care: implications for developing research in primary care', *NTResearch* 9 (6): 421–9.

Newell, R. and Plews, C. (2006) 'Research governance, research awareness, and research activity', *Clinical Effectiveness in Nursing* 6: 53–4.

NHS Service Delivery Organisation (2000) *NHS Service Delivery and Against National R&D programme: National Listening Exercise* (London: NHS SDO).

North American Primary Care Research Group Committee on Building Research Capacity and the Academic Family Medicine Organisations Research Sub-Committee (2002) 'What does it mean to build research capacity?' *Family Medicine* 34 (9): 678–84.

Pitkethly, M. and Sullivan, F. (2003) 'Four years of TayRen: a primary care research and development network', *Primary Care Research and Development* 4: 279–83.

Raghunath, A. S. and Innes A. (2004) 'The case of multidisciplinary research in primary care', *Primary Care Research and Development* 5: 265–73.

Robertson, S., Hornby, C. F. and Jones, R. (2005) 'Joint working to develop R&D capacity in three rural primary care trust', *Primary Health Care Research and Development* 6 (1): 1–4.

Ross, F., Vernon, S. and Smith, E. (2002) 'Mapping research in primary care nursing: current activity and future priorities', *Nursing Times Research* 7 (1): 46–59.

Rowlands, G., Crilly, T., Ashworth, M., Mager, J., Johns, C. and Hilton, S. (2004) 'Linking research and development in primary care: primary care trusts, primary care research networks and primary care academics', *Primary Care Research and Development* 5: 255–63.

Sarre, G. (2002) 'Capacity and activity in research project (CARP): supporting R&D in primary care trusts'.

Sarre, G. (2003) *Trent Focus Supporting Research and Development in Primary Care Organisations: Report of the Capacity and Activity in Research Project (CARP)* (Nottingham: Trent Focus).

Shaw, S. (2004) 'Developing research management and governance capacity in primary care organizations: transferrable learning from a qualitative evaluation of UK pilot sites', *Family Practice* 21 (1): 92–8.

Shaw S., Macfarlane F., Greaves, C. and Carter, Y. (2004) 'Developing research management and governance capacity in primary care organizations: transferable learning from a qualitative evaluation of UK pilot sites', *Family Practice* 21 (1): 92–8.

Sitthi-Amorn, C., Somrongthong, R., Reeder, J. C. and Simon, J. (2000) 'Strengthening health research capacity in developing countries: a critical element for achieving health equity', *British Medical Journal* 321 (7264): 813–17.

Smith, L. F. P. (1997) 'Research general practices: what, who and why?' *British Journal of General Practice* 47: 83–6.

Smith, R. (2001) 'Measuring the social impact of research', *British Medical Journal* 323 (7312): 528.

Task Group 3 (2001) *Research in Nursing and Allied Health Professionals* (London: HEFCE).

Thomas, P. and While, A. (2001) 'Increasing research capacity and changing the culture of primary care towards reflective inquiring practice: the experience of West London Research Network (WeLReN)', *Journal of Interprofessional Care* **15** (2): 133–9.

Trostle, J. (1992) 'Research capacity building and international health: definitions, evaluations and strategies for success', *Social Science and Medicine* **35** (11): 1321–4.

White, F. (2002) 'Capacity-building for health research in developing countries: a manager's approach', *Pan American Journal of Public Health* **12** (3): 165–72.

Whitford, D. L., Walker, C. and Jelley, D. (2005) 'Developing R&D capacity in a primary care trust: use of the R&D culture index', *Primary Health Care Research and Development* **6** (1): 17–23.

CHAPTER 7

Regulation of Herbal Medicine and Complementary Medicine

ANDREW STABLEFORD

It is a rather surprising fact that 80 per cent of the world's population is dependent for its primary health care on traditional medicine systems (WHO 1998) and the World Health Organization (WHO) is committed to maintaining or improving this position. There is a distinction, however, between the Third World where there is often complete dependency upon traditional medicine and the West where the recent use of western allopathic medicine is regarded as mainstream and traditional medicine had until recently largely disappeared or at best was regarded as a fringe activity. There has been a dramatic revolution that has been accelerating over the past two decades, and that no one confidently predicted, in the resurgence of interest from the public in traditional or complementary and alternative medicine (CAM). As a fringe activity, complementary medicine was able to maintain an uneasy but insignificant relationship with allopathic medicine. Complementary medicine had been the preserve of an eccentric minority and its presence could be ignored or tolerated by the general public. Recent figures attest to a change in the situation in recent years. The Prince of Wales Trust (2003) reports the following statistics. Twenty per cent of the UK population uses complementary medicine (i.e. more than five million people within the last year). There are over 49,000 complementary medicine practitioners of different kinds in the UK, as opposed to 36,000 general medical practitioners (GPs). Fifty-eight per cent of GPs have provided access to some kinds of complementary medicine for their patients and 75 per cent of the public wish access to complementary medicine on the NHS. The rise in use of CAM reflects the public's growing dissatisfaction with conventional orthodox medicine. The most commonly reported reasons for the use of complementary medicine are its affordability and its affinity with the philosophical ideals of the public. It is seen as less paternalistic than western allopathic medicine and allows more individual control over health care and, although western allopathic medicine has demonstrated its effectiveness at dealing with acute and life-threatening conditions, it has by definition proved ineffective for dealing with a wide

114

range of chronic conditions endemic within modern society. With such a booming industry it is inevitable that questions are being raised regarding safety, efficacy, quality and practitioner status.

With the numbers of practitioners, therapists and consumers rising, concerns about the professional training, standards and safety of alternative and complementary therapists have been forced into the public domain and there have been increasing pressures to bring Complementary and Alternative Medicine (CAM) under statutory control and regulation. There is, however, considerable confusion about what constitutes CAM and about the professional standing of its practitioners and how they should be regulated. In reality CAM embraces a large and diverse range of therapies, some of which have well developed structures for self-regulation and are supported by a substantial and systematic body of knowledge and evidence and others of which are fragmented, having little structure or regulation. There is an implicit association in the popular conception between the terms complementary medicine, holistic medicine, natural medicine and traditional medicine and an assumption that these are different from mainstream medicine and that by definition they are intrinsically safe.

The World Health Organisation defines traditional medicine as 'referring to health practices, approaches, knowledge and beliefs incorporating plant, animal and mineral-based medicines, spiritual therapies, manual techniques and exercises, applied singularly or in combination to treat, diagnose and prevent illnesses or maintain well-being'. Traditional medicine systems are used extensively in Africa, Asia and Latin America in particular and are based upon indigenous and relatively unchanged ancient practices. In the developed countries, adaptations of traditional medicine systems are generally used which are termed complementary or alternative. Although both terms are widely used, neither is popular within the CAM professions who generally do not regard themselves as being either complementary or alternative but as stand-alone medical disciplines. Many CAM professions developed towards the end of the 19th century, particularly in North America. Medical doctors who were concerned by the ineffectual and in many cases dangerous practices of medicine at that time developed alternative approaches to healing based upon 'natural' procedures and encompassing the new and emerging medical sciences. From these roots grew the now widely known and practised disciplines of naturopathy, osteopathy, chiropractic and herbal medicine.

The herbal medicine practised in the UK today originated in America as a system called 'physiomedicalism' that was an integration of modern medical understanding, natural therapeutics and the use of the botanic healing system of the indigenous native Americans. Physiomedicalism was introduced into the UK in the 19th century with the arrival of those Americans trained in botanic medicine who had been harried in the USA by the orthodox medical profession. The system was adopted in the UK as the primary form of herbal medicine practice and still forms the basis of practice in this country today and in the developed world, for example, in Europe, North America,

Australia and New Zealand. Traditional herbal medicine as such does not exist in the UK as it was a largely verbal tradition and also was based largely upon pragmatic treatment with little in the way of a substantive body of therapeutic understanding. Herbal medicine in the West is not a traditional and definitive system but one that has developed and evolved with the changes in society and advances in medical understanding. In preceding generations, it was used effectively to treat the pandemic infective conditions that blighted industrial society. Today herbal medicine is used to treat the complex conditions that have taken their place, in particular the diseases induced by stress and immunological disturbance. It has a dynamic pharmacopoeia which adapts to trends within the profession. Traditionally it was composed largely of North American and English plants but now contains plants from throughout the world and increasingly it is encompassing those from the Chinese and Ayurvedic traditions. In some countries such as Australia, New Zealand and South Africa, western style herbal medicine is practised but alongside it there may also be a herbal medicine tradition practised by the indigenous people using local plants. In the UK a distinction is now made between western herbal medicine, the traditional form of herbal medicine and a number of relatively new herbal disciplines which derive from the Chinese, Japanese, Tibetan and Ayurvedic traditions. All of these approaches, including western herbal medicine, incorporate practices other than herbal medicine, such as manipulation or massage using herbs or essential oils and dietary and other advice. Acupuncture is seen as a traditional Chinese practice, but again it is a discipline which is evolving and developing and becoming westernized in its mode of practice. The nature of modern western society with its sociocultural and economic pressures and complex inter-personal relationships has resulted in a society where people are ill in complex ways and the manifestation of illness is often quite different from that of undeveloped countries where ill health is much more related to factors of poor or inadequate diet and hygiene and to infectious diseases, problems that have been largely overcome in the West. CAM therapies have evolved and devel-oped in accordance with the demands of society and in the absence of therapeutic effectiveness of allopathic medicine.

A distinction must also be made between herbal medicine as a CAM profession and biomedicine. Biomedicine is the result of a worldwide explo-sion of research into medicinal plants and the development of the production and commercialization of natural plant products. Australia has become the global hub of international biomedicine and is developing an area known as 'Cellulose Valley' in Lismore on the north coast of New South Wales. Cellulose Valley is focused on developing quality-assured value-added natural plant products. Biomedicine conceptualizes medicinal herbs by their phar-macological constituents and has no regard for the quality of herbal medicine actions and their use within a context of 'holism'. It does not espouse the traditional philosophies and practices of herbal medicine and is not part of the CAM movement. The pharmacological approach and economic scale of the research and development of biomedicine are appropriate to the orthodox licensing regulations of the drugs industry and this is a completely different situation to that of the use of traditional herbal remedies.

Traditional herbal medicine differs from biomedicine, both in the nature of the remedies used and in the rationale on which they are prescribed. Herbal medicine uses the whole medicinal plant or its extract which may contain a great many natural constituents and, even more when given in combinations of herbs. The use of the whole herb means that the constituents work in conjunction with each other and are buffered so that the adverse or extreme action of one constituent is moderated by others in the plant. Within the professional practice of herbal medicine as opposed to over-the-counter (OTC) or self-administered practice, there has been a tradition of using a system of herbal medicine based upon the formulation of complex and sophisticated combinations of medicines made from tinctures or alcohol-based extracts of plants. Tincture formulations allow the administration of combinations of herbal medicines easily and conveniently prepared for individual patients and contain relatively small amounts of each herb. There is a growing trend within the profession in the use of very low dosage and non-material or 'energetic' application of herbal medicines in this form. This application has some similarities to homeopathy, although not embracing the Hahnemann doctrine of 'like cures like'. Putting aside questions of the validity of this approach or indeed the effectiveness of herbal medicine as a whole, the fact is that within professional herbal medicine the quantities prescribed are small and a quite different situation applies to that of the OTC trade where the ingestion of relatively larger quantities of herbal medicines in the form of tablets or capsules presents a greater potential hazard.

This distinction between the profession and the OTC herbal medicine trade is not well understood or recognized outside the herbal medicine profession and is part of the reason why OTC herbal medicines and practitioner-prescribed medicines are evaluated by the same criteria. There is also a distinction between biomedicine and traditional herbal medicine in terms of the therapeutic principles that drive them. Biomedicine is aligned with orthodox, allopathic medicine that generally seeks to control symptomatic manifestations of illness. Herbal medicines can be highly effective when applied in this way; in fact, 25 per cent of modern medicines are made from plants first used traditionally. This approach has more in common with the OTC trade or self-administration of herbal medicines and has been part of the traditional pragmatic use of herbal medicines for many centuries. Professional herbal medicine, however, sees the symptoms of illness as being the starting point to understanding the processes that underlie illness and it is for this underlying disharmony that the medicine is prescribed. Very little research has been undertaken on whole medicinal plants because the drug approval process does not accommodate undifferentiated compounds of constituents. It is clearly highly problematical to analyse the effectiveness and safety of complex combinations of herbal medicines based upon the same guidelines that control the drugs industry, particularly when the therapeutic intentions are indirect.

Concerns about the safety of herbal medicines have been further fuelled by the perceived potential for problematical interactions between herbal medicines and prescribed drugs. The herb hypericum has been particularly mentioned as an illustration of the potential problems. Hypericum inducts the cytochrome P450 enzyme system (Juckett 2004) and interferes with the metabolic processing of a number of drugs, for example antidepressants (SSRIs), oral contraceptives, cyclosporin, anticonvulsants, digoxin, theophyllin and warfarin (Broughton and Denham 2000). As a result of the uncertainties of its use, hypericum has been banned from OTC sale in the Republic of Ireland. The reality is that the true net physiological and clinical effects of combining substances can be extremely difficult to evaluate and applies as much to the concurrent consumption of a wide variety of plants as vegetables as it does to herbal medicines, if not more so as the quantities concerned are generally much greater. Problematical effects of interactions may apply to the prolonged ingestion of high-dose standard extracts of herbs but not to the relatively low doses used in normal herbal medicine practice. True interactive effects are less common than are reported in the media and by the medical community (Wicke 2004).

There are considerable disparities between countries in terms of legislation for and tolerance of CAM practitioners. This is of particular concern within the EU where parity of legislation is part of the ethos of the union. In many countries the practice of medicine is the preserve of the qualified medical practitioner and any form of medical treatment is regulated under statutory control. In reality, following the surge in popular demand, CAM is practised by unregulated practitioners in these countries despite statutory regulation and demonstrates that the law is no longer representative of public attitude or necessarily in their interests. The legal situation in the UK is that practitioners of CAM practise under 'common law' and are subject to the rules of law that apply to all citizens, for example laws that cover false and misleading statements, professional negligence and criminal assault and injury. The only statutory controls are those detailed under the Pharmacy and Medicine Act (1941) that states that 'advertisement' written or oral shall not be made claiming remedies for the following list of disorders; Brights disease; cancer; cataract; diabetes; epilepsy; fits; glaucoma; locomotor ataxy; paralysis; and tuberculosis. In addition, there are prohibitions from the practice of midwifery, dentistry, veterinary medicine and the treatment of sexually transmitted diseases. Under common law, practices are tolerated unless specifically prohibited and CAM practitioners have been largely free to practise providing that they do not claim to be members of a regulated profession with a protected title (for example, a medical doctor), practise a protected discipline such as dentistry, midwifery or veterinary medicine or supply prescription-only drugs. In the UK, the only CAM practitioners regulated by specific legislation are osteopaths and chiropractors. The Osteopaths

Act came into force in 1993 and the Chiropractors Act in 1994. In statutory regulation, it is the practitioners who are regulated rather than the practice and it does not prevent osteopathic or chiropractic techniques being used by other practitioners or therapists provided that they do not claim or imply that they are osteopaths or chiropractors. The protected titles of osteopath and chiropractor make it clear who is statutory-qualified and who can be on the professional register.

The history of the relationship between the medical establishment and Parliament and CAM in the UK is exemplified by the experience of herbal practitioners, the longest-standing CAM practitioners in the UK. Following fierce opposition from doctors and pharmacists, the right of herbalists to practise was upheld in English law by Henry VIII's Herbalists Charter in 1543 and this has formed the basis of the practice of CAM in the UK ever since. In 1941 Parliament passed a bill that rendered the practice of herbal medicine illegal. A heroic campaign fought by an alliance between herbal medicine manufacturers and herbal practitioners led to the overturn of the bill and the provision for the rights of the herbal practitioner within the Medicines Act 1968 Section 12, paragraphs 1 and 2 and Section 56, paragraphs 1 and 2. Section 12(1) specifies that herbal medicines are exempt from licensing if they are supplied subsequent to a personal consultation and Section 12(2) exempts herbal medicine from licensing provided that they are produced according to standard traditional and non-industrial methods and that no claims for the use of the remedy are made on the labelling. Section 56 expands on the provisions of Section 12. Statutory Instrument 2130 1977 lists a number of herbs 'in respect of which the exemptions conferred by Section 56 of the Medicines Act 1968 do not have effect'. This serves to remove certain potentially hazardous herbs from public access and specifies that they may only be prescribed following consultation or supplied under the supervision of a pharmacist. There is also a specification regarding the maximum permitted dosages and the daily dosages for each herb. These provisions serve to recognize the status of the herbal practitioner but unfortunately fail to give a clear definition of who or what that practitioner is.

In 1994 a sudden announcement was made by the Medicines Control Agency (MCA), now renamed the Medicines and Healthcare products Regulatory Agency (MHRA), that existing European legislation was to be implemented that removed the rights imposed by the Medicines Act 1968 for herbal practitioners to dispense unlicensed herbal medicines and that effectively would have removed the basis of the practice of herbal medicine in the UK. The subsequent public outcry was huge and the Department of Health was forced to back down. The MCA effectively found a loophole by saying that herbal medicines were traditionally not industrially produced and that the EU Medicines Law only applied to medicinal products that were industrially produced. The interest in and support of the UK public for CAM had been seriously underestimated. As a consequence of this campaign the organizations representing both herbal practitioners and herbal manufacturers were strengthened in their links and cooperation, particularly through the formation of the European Herbal Practitioners Association (EHPA). The vulnerability of the profession and the prospect of the loss of the continuing availability of herbal medicines were clearly exposed and it became apparant that the rights of herbal practitioners would need to be protected under legislation if they were to be safe from EU legislation.

The UK is at the forefront of recognition of and legislation for CAM. The latest and current move towards statutory regulation of CAM practitioners originates from the House of Lords Select Committee on Science and Technology's Report on Complementary and Alternative Medicine (House of Lords 2000) and the Government's Response (Department of Health 2001). The report acknowledged the widespread and increasing use of CAM and the fact that CAM consists of a considerable and diverse range of therapies that vary greatly in terms of evidence base and quality of practitioner training and lack of an effective regulatory system. With some therapies, the public may be at risk from practitioners with inadequate or inappropriate training. Higher-risk practices are those that use spinal manipulation such as osteopathy and chiropractic, which are already regulated, invasive techniques such as acupuncture or the ingestion of substances as in herbal medicine. The committee proposed that the CAM therapies should be classified into three groups. Those within Group 1 included the most organized CAM professions which have a significant evidence base, a voluntary system of regulation and competent levels of practitioner training and where NHS provision is increasing. The professions allocated to Group 1 were herbal medicine, acupuncture, homeopathy, chiropractic and osteopathy. Therapies assigned to Group 2 were regarded as being more supportive in a complementary way to conventional medicine and requiring further research and development of their regulatory structures. The therapies assigned to Group 3 were regarded as having an inadequate evidence base to be clinically useful. Herbal medicine was defined as 'a system of medicine which uses various remedies derived from plants and plant extracts to treat disorders and maintain good health'. Whereas western herbal medicine was assigned to Group 1, Maharishi Ayurvedic medicine was assigned to Group 2 and Ayurvedic medicine, Chinese herbal medicine and traditional Chinese medicine were assigned to Group 3.

The House of Lords Select Committee recommended in its report that herbal medicine and acupuncture should be brought under a statutory regulatory framework:

> 'It is our opinion that acupuncture and herbal medicine are the two therapies which are at a stage where it would be of benefit to them and their patients if the practitioners strive for statutory regulation under the Health Act 1999, and we recommend that they should do so' (paragraph 5.53).

The House of Lords Select Committee (1999–2000) identified three clear advantages of statutory regulation. Firstly, there would be a legal, single register of practitioners which would ensure that the public had clear access to appropriately qualified, trained and competent practitioners. Secondly, there would be a legal protection of title for professional practitioners, making it clear who was qualified and registered and who wasn't. Thirdly, there would be legal underpinning of the regulatory body's disciplinary procedures ensuring that appropriate action, for example removal from the register, could be taken against practitioners who were demonstrated as incompetent or unfit to practise. The report stated that the advantages of statutory self-regulation over voluntary self-regulation were that there would be legal underpinnings to ensure that the necessary outcomes were met.

The Government Response (Department of Health 2001) agreed with the recommendations of The House of Lords Select Committee on the statutory regulation of acupuncture and herbal medicine. As a first step in the process, two independent working parties were set up to develop recommendations for the statutory regulation of herbal medicine and acupuncture, the Herbal Medicine Regulatory Working Group (HMRWG) and the Acupuncture Regulatory Working Group (ARWG). Both regulating bodies were a joint establishment of the Department of Health and the Prince of Wales' Foundation for Integrated Health and, in the case of the HMRWG, also the European Herbal Practitioners Association (EHPA).

The EHPA was founded in 1993 when it became clear that the legislative framework under which herbal medicine was practised was likely to change, in particular with the development of the European Union (EU) and the need to present a united front. The British Herbal Practitioners Association (BHPA) was formed to represent the different professional herbal practitioner associations in the UK, and the EHPA joined the BHPA, along with Irish and Danish herbal associations, to represent herbal medicine in Europe. The EHPA is primarily concerned with acting as an umbrella organization to represent the interests of both practitioners and the industry and to develop and maintain standards of training and education in herbal training institutions and to provide facilities for accreditation of courses. The EHPA is also concerned with negotiations with the Medicines and Healthcare products Regulatory Agency (MHRA) on reviewing the standards of safety and quality of unlicensed herbal medicines in the UK and with the Directive on Traditional Herbal Medicinal Products (DTHMP) in the EU.

The Prince of Wales' Foundation for Integrated Health was established as a charity in 1997 at the personal initiative of His Royal Highness, The Prince of Wales. The Foundation published a list of recommendations in a discussion document, 'Integrated Health care: A Way Forward for the Next Five Years?' (1997) which forms the basis of their programme of work. The Foundation is committed to the development and integrated delivery of safe, effective and efficient forms of health care by facilitating collaboration between all forms of health care. They are committed to increasing access to complementary health care and believe that it should be accessible for all those who need it through integration with conventional medicine. They are also committed to developing a common basis for all health care education, training and programmes of continuing professional development for all health care practitioners. They promote the encouragement of the complementary medicine professions to develop and maintain statutory or voluntary systems of regulations and have a five-year plan of work supported by a £1,000,000 grant from the King's Fund. Initiatives include support for the establishment of national herbal medicine and acupuncture statutory regulation working groups, individual programmes of work with the UK's 20 main complementary therapy professions and the provision of information resources, seminars and networking events.

The HMRWG and the ARWG were commissioned to examine the options for achieving statutory regulation of the herbal medicine and acupuncture professions as a whole and provide recommendations which would form a basis for wider consultation by the government and subsequently for the statutory regulation of the herbal medicine and acupuncture professions. The reports of the two bodies were published in September 2003 and have been used to produce the proposals for the most appropriate way forward as given in the government document 'Regulation of Herbal Medicine and Acupuncture: Proposals for Statutory Regulation' (Department of Health 2004). Following the publication of this document, there has been a three-month consultation period that closed on 7 June 2004, during which responses were encouraged from those within the CAM and medicine communities. The DoH have produced the document 'Statutory Regulation of Herbal Medicine and Acupuncture – Report on the Consultation' (2005) in which they summarize the reactions received. A total of 698 responses to the consultation were received and these included nine organizations representing acupuncture practitioners, 12 organizations representing practitioners of herbal medicine, nine organizations representing practitioners of Traditional Chinese Medicine (TCM), along with responses from other CAM organizations, NHS bodies, Health and Social Services Boards, professional associations for regulated health care professionals and statutory regulatory bodies. In addition, many replies were received from individual practitioners of herbal medicine, acupuncture, TCM and other CAM professions and members of the public. Other CAM organizations are particularly concerned with the outcome of the statutory regulation of herbal medicine and acupuncture as this will set the standard for the future regulation of other CAM professions.

There is widespread opposition to statutory self-regulation in many quarters of CAM and many would prefer the alternative of voluntary self-regulation. Voluntary self-regulation can be seen as having the advantage of maintaining autonomy and control over the traditions of a profession as well as protecting the diversity and standards of practice whilst still being subject to standard legislation. Within statutory self-regulation, the governing committees will be comprised of lay members (many of whom will be from other medical and health-related professions) and government departments as well as representatives of the professions and may result in a significant change in the power for self-determination over the interests of the CAM professions. There has been a strong opinion, particularly within some parts of the acupuncture profession, that the determination on the part of the DoH towards statutory self-regulation is because of the potential problems and hazards associated with the use of medicinal herbs in herbal medicine.

The key elements of the DoH proposals and the responses are as follows. The proposals put forward by the Herbal Medicine Regulatory Working Party (HMRWG) recommend the formation of a shared Complementary and Alternative Medicine Council (CAM Council) rather than individual councils to represent the interests of the different CAM professions. The new CAM council would represent both herbal medicine and acupuncture and would be available also for the inclusion of other complementary and alternative medicine professions in the future. The advantages were stated as being the possibility of forming a larger critical mass of practitioners that would have more influence and be better able to protect the interests of the public and practitioners, the prospect of promoting interdisciplinary work between herbal medicine and acupuncture practitioners and the minimizing of registration fees for practitioners by sharing administrative costs. The professions of herbal medicine and acupuncture have relatively small numbers and the experience of other professions is that practitioner fees are inversely proportional to the size of the body concerned. The report illustrates the cost differences to practitioners of different professions, for example at one extreme members of the Nursing and Midwifery Council with a registrant of some 650,000 pay an annual registration fee of £20 whereas members of the General Chiropractic Council with 1,950 registrants pay an annual registration fee of £1,250. Such large fees could mean that the many practitioners of CAM who work with relatively small turnovers would be unable to afford registration. The Acupuncture Regulatory Working Group (ARWG) preferred option was for separate councils. They were concerned that the complexity of a larger, inclusive body might become more costly and that the additional concerns that the herbal medicine profession has with the regulation of medicines might add additional finance burden which would be shared with the acupuncture profession. The DoH came to the decision that a joint CAM committee would be the best route forward, particularly as there are many instances where practitioners work in both the fields of herbal medicine and acupuncture. An alternative option given was the establishment of separate councils for herbal medicine and acupuncture but with a shared secretariat function to support both. This arrangement would enable the separate interests of the bodies to be upheld but would help reduce administrative costs. Both parties felt that it was inappropriate, given the lack of background of the CAM professions in mainstream health care, for herbal medicine and acupuncture to seek membership of the Health Professions Council (HPC) as, for example, in the case of chiropody. The DoH agreed with this proposal. The Council for the Regulation of Healthcare

Professionals (CRHP), which is accountable to Parliament, currently coordinates the existing professional self-regulatory bodies and the proposed new CAM Council would join this alongside the other members. The CRHP includes the General Osteopathic Council and the General Chiropractic Council which represent the osteopaths and chiropractors who have already gone through the statutory self-regulation process as well as the Nursing and Midwifery Council, General Optical Council, General Medical Council and General Dental Council. There is widespread agreement that other CAM professions might in the future join the CAM Council, in particular homeopathy in the relatively near future. It was suggested that there might be advantages in the future for examining whether the osteopathy and chiropractic professions might be brought within a wider regulatory body.

The DoH sought views on the proposal for three titles to be protected under statutory regulation; acupuncturist, herbal practitioner and Traditional Chinese Medicine practitioner. There was broad agreement on this issue with some concern from the Chinese medicine corner about the ambiguity of the title Traditional Chinese Medicine practitioner and a suggestion that it be changed to Chinese Medical Practitioner. Many respondents felt the inclusion of the term 'registered' in the titles would aid public understanding. The consultation document also set out a list of subsidiary titles that could be used by practitioners along with the protected title to denote their specialist tradition or main area of practice. There was a consensus that this would probably confuse the public and that perhaps specialist traditions could be referred to in the appropriate practitioner registers.

The DoH proposed that the new council would have the key functions of keeping a register of practitioners, determining standards of education and training, giving advice regarding standards of conduct and performance and administering professional procedures, for example, discipline. The professional bodies would work alongside the council and continue in their roles, taking responsibility for promotion to the public, development work and undertaking any other non-regulatory functions. The number and nature of the professional bodies may change in response to the new regulatory system and in conjunction with the requirements of the membership. There was general consensus in accepting these proposals. The only main concern was doubt about the appropriateness of the proposed council advising herbal medicine practitioners on the use of herbal medicines within their practice. The Prince of Wales' Foundation for Integrated Health suggested that this function could be carried out by a herbal medicines advisory group to the Medicines and Healthcare products Regulatory Agency.

The DoH proposed that the composition of members of the new council should be representative of the interests of patients and the public as well as those of the professions concerned. The suggestion was for the inclusion of 12 practitioner members who should be wholly or principally engaged in the practice of herbal medicine or acupuncture with at least one practitioner to represent western herbal medicine, Ayurvedic, traditional acupuncture, western medical acupuncture and traditional Chinese medicine. Ten other members would be lay members, including at least one person from each of the countries of England, Scotland, Wales and Northern Ireland and at least two people with educational expertise. Lay members may include members of other health and social care professions. It was further proposed that the Chair of the council should be a lay person to ensure equality and impartiality across the different professions and traditions. There was considerable disagreement with the proposals. Concern was expressed that the inclusion of lay persons who might be members of other health and health-related professions should be limited as there might be a conflict of interests. It was also suggested that specific representation among lay members was needed for patient support and consumer groups. There was also considerable concern that the practitioner membership should be proportional to the size of the group represented. Many traditions have a relatively small membership and their representation on the council may exert a disproportionate influence. The EHPA suggested that the smaller traditions should have observer-only status until receiving automatic representation when an agreed number of member practitioners was reached. Another suggestion was for a single council member to represent a group of minority traditions.

The proposal for collaborative regulation was one of the most contentious issues. The House of Lords Select Committee considered the position of orthodox healthcare practitioners who were concurrently practising CAM. Their position was as follows:

We recommend that if CAM is to be practised by any conventional health care practitioners, they should be trained to standards comparable to those set out for that particular therapy by the appropriate (single) CAM regulatory body (paragraph 5.83)

and:

All those who deliver CAM treatments, whether conventional health professionals or CAM professionals, should have received training in that discipline independently accredited by the appropriate regulatory body. (paragraph 6.33)

The DoH proposed that health care professionals who are currently regulated would continue to be regulated by their existing regulatory bodies and that those regulatory bodies would work closely with the proposed CAM council on educational issues to ensure the maintenance of standards. This is a thorny concern, particularly for many of those in the traditional acupuncture tradition. Many doctors, nurses and physiotherapists who are regulated by the General Medical Council, Nursing and Midwifery Council and the Health Professions Council respectively use western medical acupuncture within their practice. The standard of acupuncture practice used principally in symptomatic pain relief is regarded as lower and requiring significantly less training than that used by practitioners of traditional acupuncture. A large number of responses were received from the acupuncture professions in favour of dual registration and suggesting that all practitioners of herbal medicine and/or acupuncture should be required or be able to register with the proposed council. This is of particular importance for health care professionals registered with other councils in order to ensure that they are able to access the proposed protected title of 'acupuncturist' and are able to appear on registers of acupuncture practitioners. The success of close collaboration between the existing regulators and the proposed new council, particularly with regard to education and training, would depend upon the willingness of existing regulators to consult with and perhaps defer to the advice of the new council.

The DoH suggests that the committee structure of the new regulatory body should, in common with those of many other statutory bodies, consist of the following: an education and training committee dealing with qualifications for registration, registration procedures and CPD; an investigating committee dealing with initial complaints against individual practitioners; a professional conduct committee dealing with standards of conduct and disciplinary procedures; and a health committee dealing with the health issues associated with practitioners. In addition it was proposed that the new council should be free to establish further committees as appropriate. There was wide agreement from the profession and suggestions for new committees included a safety committee, a finance committee and a diversity committee.

There was also general agreement from respondents to the proposal that the Education and Training Committee should include both lay and practitioner members and that individual representatives from each of the herbal medicine and acupuncture disciplines would be included. There was some concern about the ratio of lay members to practitioner representatives and also that there should not be a disproportionate number of orthodox health care professionals. The majority were in favour of a lay chair. There was also general agreement with the idea of a separate registration committee, at least in the short term, that would be concerned with the specialist task of overseeing the registration of practitioners.

Under the DoH proposals for the registration of practitioners is the provision for a register consisting of two parts, one for herbal medicine practitioners and one for acupuncture practitioners with a provision for those who are practising both to opt for dual registration. The council would be involved in the accreditation of courses leading to the automatic acceptance of graduates onto the register. There would also be in place a core curriculum for herbal medicine and acupuncture and also the possibility of separate core curricula for individual traditions. There would be a system where practitioners applying for registration who did not train on accredited courses and also those qualifying overseas would be assessed individually against a set of national entry requirements. This is of particular importance for overseas practitioners; many Traditional Chinese Medicine practitioners may have trained and qualified in China and similarly many Ayurvedic practitioners will have trained and qualified in India or Sri Lanka. There was general agreement from the respondents to these proposals with some concern that overseas practitioners should satisfy adequate competency in the English language. There was also broad agreement to the arrangements proposed for registration for the transitional period until the council was fully functioning. The proposal was for a two year 'grandparenting' scheme whereby practitioners in practice prior to the opening of the register regardless of their affiliation to any professional association, practitioners in training in the UK during the transitional period and practitioners who trained overseas and wished to practise in the UK during the transitional period would all be accepted onto the register providing they met the following conditions: that they had engaged in lawful, safe and effective practice of the profession for which they sought registration for three out of the five years prior to the opening of the register or, where this requirement could not be met, that the applicant had undergone additional training or experience to satisfy the council's standards of proficiency for the relevant profession. Practitioners in practice prior to the opening of the register would be free to use their current professional titles until their cases had been determined by the council.

The question of the role of the new committee in the management of standards of conduct and performance was raised in the DoH proposals. There was wide agreement to the DoH recommendations that there should be reference to codes of practice to cover professional conduct, particularly with regard to patient confidentiality and informed consent and safe practice. The HMRWG also recommended that in the case of herbal medicine practitioners there should be a code of practice relating to the manufacture, preparation and dispensing of herbal medicines under Section 12(1) of the Medicines Act 1968 and the management of the dispensary by the herbal practitioner. There was also wide acceptance of the role of the council in determining CPD requirements for herbal medicine and acupuncture practitioners.

The final consideration proposed by the DoH concerned the model to be adopted by the new council in dealing with practitioners whose fitness to practise is impaired. The HMRWG and the ARWG have both suggested slightly different schemes. The HMRWG proposed a scheme where the Investigating Committee dealt with the initial complaint to determine if there was a case to answer and the nature of that case. The case would then be dealt with by the Professional Conduct and Competence Committee who would have responsibility for standards of conduct as well as holding disciplinary hearings. The Health Committee would deal with practitioners who might be unfit to practise due to health problems. The ARWG proposed a similar scheme, the difference being that the Investigating Committee has no role in referring to the Health Committee. The DoH proposed that an alternative, based upon the new model put forward by the General Medical Council (GMC), was also considered as an option. In the GMC scheme, the fitness-to-practise function is carried out in two stages, 'investigation' and 'adjudication'. The investigation stage is undertaken by the Investigation Committee which is composed of GMC members and its role is to determine whether a doctor's fitness to practise is impaired to the extent that further action is required. If this is the case, then the case is passed to the adjudication stage. The adjudication stage is carried out by a panel comprised wholly of non-GMC members who are empowered to assess all the elements of fitness to practise, competence, performance and health. A range of sanctions is then available to be imposed where fitness to practise is found to be impaired. Approximately two thirds of the respondents preferred one of the two working party suggestions.

Following the report on the responses to the consultation document, a draft order under section 60 of the Health Act 1999 will be prepared to establish the statutory system and lead to further consultation. The timing of these events is undetermined as the process has been indefinitely delayed by the publishing of the Shipman Report and the repercussions this will have for the regulation of all the health professions.

In the case of herbal medicine, there is a need for the parallel consideration of the regulation of herbal remedies made up to meet individual needs and supplied to the public after personal consultation as provided for under Section 12(1) of the Medicines Act 1968. Without the protection of legislation for the supply of unlicensed herbal remedies, the position of the herbal practitioner is untenable. The government has agreed that future regulatory arrangements relating to products used by herbal practitioners should safeguard standards but also recognize practitioner use. It is clear that the issue of statutory regulation is complementary to the wider European negotiations on the Directive on Traditional Herbal Medicine Products (DTHMP).

Following the collapse in 1994 of the implementation of the EU Medicines Law by the UK Medicines Control Agency (MCA), the situation in the UK for herbal practitioners has been perilous and the EHPA has campaigned to ensure that there is a long-term resolution of the problem. The Directive on Traditional Herbal Medicinal Products (DTHMP) was originally promoted by the UK government in conjunction with the EHPA to provide a means of licensing 'over-the-counter' (OTC) herbal medicinal products within the EU. Under these proposals herbal medicines which are for self-prescription will be exempt from the stringent requirements such as double-blind trials, animal testing, etc., provided that they satisfy certain requirements, i.e. that there is a history of safe and effective use of 30 years within the EU and that there is well-documented experimental and clinical evidence for their safety and usage. The proposals also include legislation to cover labelling which is to provide information concerning use and appropriate warnings, quality control procedures including supply audit, pharmacovigilance procedures and product recall and the use of procedures for the identification and authentication of raw herb materials.

The MHRA has also produced a consultation document on updated proposals for a new Herbal Medicines Advisory Committee, document

MLX318 (MHRA 2005). It was proposed that the committee would be composed of experts in herbal medicine practice, general practice, toxicology, pharmacy, pharmacology, hospital physicians and pharmacovigilance and would serve to submit advice to the proposed new Commission that would be formed by amalgamating the functions of the present Medicines Commission and the Committee on the Safety of Medicines for human use.

The DTHMP does not affect the provisions of Section 12(1) of the 1968 Medicines Act for one-to-one prescription of unlicensed herbal medicines by herbal practitioners. The MHRA produced the consultation document MLX299 on 'Proposals for the reform of the regulation of unlicensed herbal remedies in the United Kingdom made up to meet the needs of individual patients' (MHRA 2005). This document sought views on a number of proposals and ideas for regulatory reform. The main proposal was to strengthen the current arrangements by updating legislation to restrict potent herbs unsuitable for OTC dispensation, to usage by registered practitioners. It is also proposed to extend the scope of Section 12(1) to allow registered practitioners to supply traditional remedies of non-plant origin providing that they are safe and subject to appropriate quality assurances. This is of particular importance for practitioners of traditional Chinese and Ayurvedic medicine systems where remedies of animal and mineral origins are frequently used. There would also be a range of pharmaceutical standards of Good Manufacturing Practice (GMP) to cover issues of quality, safety and labelling. The results of the consultation process have been published in the 'Summary of responses to consultation document MLX299' (MHRA 2005b). There was general acceptance among the bodies representing herbal practitioners that change in legislation is inevitable, given the current circumstances. A number of orthodox bodies felt that the proposals did not go far enough in ensuring the safety of herbal medicines. Concern was expressed by those representing herbalists who work from retail premises and prepare medicines for patients over the counter and also from naturopathic practitioners, many of whom dispense herbal medicines, that they would be excluded from the regulations as being unregistered herbal practitioners. Herbalist interests generally took the view that only registered herbalists should be allowed to practise and that those from other professions wishing to practise should meet the same standards as herbalists if they were to be allowed to practise herbal medicine. The situation with regard to practitioners of homeopathy and aromatherapy was also uncertain and the proposals for pharmaceutical standards (GMP) were unnecessary for their particular activities. There was wide support for the proposal to enable a registered herbal practitioner to commission remedies made to the herbalist's specification by a holder of a Manufacturer's Licence.

In the UK, the Traditional Herbal Medicines Registration Scheme will provide a continual assessment of remedies, issue registrations, police yellow-card adverse reactions, inspect manufacturers and create the Herbal Medicines Advisory Committee. Products requiring registration are all unlicensed herbal remedies currently sold under section 12(2) of the Medicines Act and they are required to comply by April 2011. Any new products brought onto the market after April 2004 must comply by 30 October 2005.

The regulatory status of CAM varies considerable from country to country. With regard to herbal medicine, the developed countries have hardly any legislative criteria to establish traditionally used herbal medicines as part of their drug legislation. For many, herbal medicines are regulated under legislation for food substances. The majority of countries regard the regulation of CAM products and practitioners separately.

Within the EU, the DTHMP will ensure conformity of legislation to control the herbal products market. The situation with regard to CAM practitioners varies considerably, however, from member country to member country. Unlike the UK, it is common practice in many countries for some form of CAM to be practised by allopathic medical practitioners. The legal position of CAM practitioners who are not allopathic physicians is not always clear. Some countries require all medical intervention to be under the supervision of a qualified registered physician but in others there is no requirement to have a degree in medicine in order to practise medicine but only a registered doctor may give clinical examinations, diagnoses or apply specific therapy.

In France, herbal and homeopathic medicine are very popular with a very strong OTC tradition. A 1987 survey (WHO 2001) found that 36 per cent of allopathic doctors, mainly general practitioners, used at least one CAM therapy in their medical practices. The French social security system qualifies allopathic doctors who use CAM as 'doctors with a particular type of practice'. Under French law, all persons engaging in the diagnosis and treatment of illness must have a licence to practise medicine, a requirement for which is to be a member of the professional society of physicians. Despite the legislation, non-allopathic practitioners practise a wide range of CAM therapies and, although they risk prosecution, in reality the courts are becoming more tolerant. In Germany there is a similar high regard for CAM and the most frequently sought-after treatments are, in order of popularity, homeopathy, acupuncture, procaine injection therapy, chiropractic, ozone and oxygen therapy, herbal medicine, humoral pathology, massage and cell therapy (WHO 2001). Unlike France, there is no legal monopoly on the practice of medicine and licensed non-allopathic practitioners may practise medicine and all licensed medical practitioners are allowed to use complementary medicine. Three quarters of allopathic physicians do in fact use CAM (WHO 2001). There are many organizations for practitioners and patients of CAM. In Italy CAM is similarly popular with 24 per cent of the population having used CAM at least once (WHO 2001). Only registered allopathic physicians are allowed to practise CAM therapies and where these are used the physicians are responsible for any consequences to their patients. Chiropractic has been accepted as a profession even though it is not licensed and chiropractors are regarded as medical auxiliaries rather than medical specialists and must work under the supervision of an allopathic physician. Although non-allopathic CAM practitioners can be prosecuted, this seldom happens. The situation is similar in Spain where the practice of medicine in all forms is the preserve of the registered allopathic physician.

The popularity of CAM in Australia is as great as that in the UK with a very similar range of practitioners. Until the State Medical Acts were passed, there was no regulation of CAM practitioners and they practised under common law as in the UK. The regulation of CAM practitioners is now under the control of individual states. Osteopathy and chiropody are regulated in all states. The state of Victoria has set up a regulatory system for practitioners of traditional Chinese medicine and the states of Queensland and New South Wales are anticipated to follow suit. The federal government has set up a fund to assist in the development of a 'national uniform registration system' for practitioners of acupuncture, herbal medicine and naturopathy. The purpose of the register is to determine those in professional practice who will be exempt from charging the goods and services tax (GST). Herbal medicines in Australia are regulated under a national regulatory system administered by the Therapeutic Goods Administration (TGA). The TGA includes an Office of Complementary Medicine which deals specifically with CAM, and a specialist committee, the Complementary Medicine Evaluation Committee, provides the TGA with specialist information and advice on CAM products.

New Zealand also follows the UK situation regarding CAM regulation with little in the way of statutory control apart from the Chiropractors Act of 1982 that determined statutory regulation of chiropractors with the requirement of specific training courses and a professional register. Other CAM practitioners register with voluntary, self-regulated professional bodies, many of which are affiliated to umbrella organizations such as the New Zealand Charter of Health Practitioners. The situation is due to change with the implementation of the Health Practitioners Competence Assurance Bill (HPCA). The HPCA Bill provides for the statutory regulation of professions which may pose a 'risk of harm to the public' or where it is otherwise in the public interest that the profession be regulated. Initially the bill will bring the current unregulated CAM profession of osteopathy into regulation and provide a mechanism that will enable other CAM professions to be regulated without the need for separate acts of parliament. New legislation is in the pipeline for the regulation of all medicines, dietary supplements and complementary health care products in the proposed Trans-Tasman Therapeutic Goods Agency (TTTGA) for the Regulation of Therapeutic Products. This is a joint initiative of both the New Zealand and Australian governments. Under the proposals, new legislation will apply to the control of therapeutic products in both countries and these will vary in stringency according to whether the products have a high-risk profile, such as prescription medicines, or a low-risk profile, such as dietary supplements. The effect of legislation on traditional Maori medicine is unclear: their ability to use and commercialize their traditional knowledge and herbal medicines and the protection of their culture and society under the Treaty of Waitangi is not mentioned in the TTTGA proposals.

In the USA, each state has responsibility for legislation regarding CAM practitioners and there are regulatory controls that cover licensing, scope of practice, malpractice, professional discipline and third-party reimbursement. Federal laws, particularly the food and drug laws, control the use of herbal medicines. The unlicensed practice of medicine is a crime and non-licensed practitioners of CAM, such as herbalists and homeopaths, as well as licensed CAM practitioners such as chiropractors, risk prosecution if they exceed their legislative power. In most states the practice of any kind of medicine including CAM is limited to licensed physicians. Osteopaths and chiropractors are recognized in all states and osteopaths are fully licensed physicians regarded as part of mainstream medicine. Chiropractors are regulated in all states but are not licensed physicians and are not recognized as being part of the mainstream. The situation as regards the other CAM professions is complex but in most states the practice of medicine is limited to licensed physicians and CAM practitioners face legal risks. Some states have developed regulatory or licensing arrangements for CAM practitioners; for example New York State passed the Alternative Medical Practice Act in 1994 which recognizes all CAMs and supports consumer choice in health care. The states of Arizona, Connecticut and Nevada have specific licensing boards for homeopathic physicians. The White House Commission on Complementary and Alternative Medicine Policy recommends that government agencies should explore ways in which to integrate CAM into their health care systems, that states should evaluate and review their regulation of CAM practitioners and ensure their accountability to the public. It also recommends that the federal government provide assistance to the states to improve CAM practitioner regulation. Herbal medicines are regulated under the Dietary Supplement Health and Education Act 1994 which is less rigorous than the regulations that control drugs. Traditional native North American medicine in the USA is regulated under the Self-Determination Act. In Canada the situation is somewhat similar with each province responsible for the regulation of health professionals. The Federation of Medical Licensing Authorities provides a set of criteria for developing regulations for CAM practitioners that are intended to promote consistency between provinces. In effect, the situation for many CAM practitioners is uncertain and they remain outside the scope of specific regulation and are subject to practice under the 'laws of general application'.

It seems likely that as the move towards legislation to regulate CAM professions develops there will be increasingly an integration of CAM with the national health provisions of most western countries with perhaps CAM and allopathic medicine being practised side by side. China provides perhaps the best model for this kind of health care system. Traditionally China depended upon Traditional Chinese Medicine (TCM) which is a complete diagnostic and treatment system based upon acupuncture and herbal medicine that was developed over thousands of years. With the introduction of western allopathic medicine, TCM started to become displaced by the end of the 19th century. The Communist party further tried to eradicate the practice of TCM but the latter found a champion in the form of Chairman Mao who was in favour of integrating the old with the new. A universal health system was developed integrating western allopathic medicine and TCM following the First National Conference in 1955. The majority of general hospitals in China now have TCM departments. TCM practitioners are regulated by the State Administration of Traditional Chinese Medicine. TCM physicians are required to hold an appropriate degree qualification. It is common in China for physicians to be trained in both TCM and western allopathic medicine. This is less likely to happen in the UK where there have traditionally been few allopathic physicians trained in CAM compared to Europe and other developed countries and it is more likely that CAM practitioners will continue to be separately trained but work as specialist practitioners alongside medical physicians. With the arrival of statutory regulation of CAM, the future safety and position within the mainstream of health care for CAM therapies is now assured.

References

Broughton, A. and Denham, A. (2000) Hypericum and drug interactions. *The European Journal of Herbal Medicine* 5: 19–25.

Department of Health (2001) *Government Response to the House of Lords Select Committee on Science and Technology's Report on Complementary and Alternative Medicine* (London: Department of Health).

Department of Health (2004) *Regulation of Herbal Medicine and Acupuncture Proposals for Statutory Regulation* (London: Department of Health).

Department of Health (2005) *Statutory Regulation of Herbal Medicine and Acupuncture – Report on the Consultation* (London: Department of Health).

House of Lords Select Committee on Science and Technology, 6th Report 1999–2000: *Complementary and Alternative Medicine* (London: Department of Health).

Juckett, G. (2004) Herbal medicine. In Craig, C. R. and Stitzel, R. E. (eds), *Modern Pharmacology with Clinical Applications*, 6th edn (London: Williams, Wilkin, Lippincott).

MHRA (2005a) *Consultation on Proposed Herbal Medicines Advisory Committee, MLX318*.

MHRA (2005b) *Proposals for the Reform of the Regulation of Unlicensed Herbal Remedies in the United Kingdom Made up to Meet the Needs of Individual Patients: Summary of Responses to Consultation Document, MLX299*.

The Prince of Wales Foundation (1997) *Integrated Health Care: A Way Forward for the Next Five Years?* (London: Prince of Wales Trust).

The Prince of Wales' Foundation for Integrated Health on Behalf of the Herbal Medicine Regulatory Working Group (2003) *Recommendations on the Regulation of Herbal Practitioners in the UK* (London: Prince of Wales Trust).

The Prince of Wales' Foundation for Integrated Health on Behalf of the Acupuncture Regulatory Working Group (2003) *The Statutory Regulation of the Acupuncture Profession.*

WHO (1998) *Regulatory Situation of Herbal Medicines: A Worldwide Review* (Geneva: WHO).

WHO (2001) *Legal Status of Traditional Medicine and Complementary/Alternative Medicine: A Worldwide Review* (Geneva: WHO).

Wicke, R. (2004) Herb–herb and herb–drug interactions: modes of interaction. In *Herbal Review* 3, http://www.rmhiherbal.org/review/2004-3 htm

Part II

Research Supporting Health Professionals

Introduction

Using qualitative research techniques in health care

This section introduces some recent studies of health care environments, health professionals and patients in a number of health care situations. It begins with a critical discussion relating to the principles and practice of qualitative research and goes on to depict the problems, pitfalls and successes when using various models and, in some cases, health policies that inform the studies as well as the techniques used. Some reflections upon the processes are also offered with the aim of assisting other researchers who wish to embark upon enquiry in the health field.

Qualitative means of gathering data are defined either in their process, the conditions of operation or the message they convey. For example, Faltermeir sees it as:

> research ... concentrating more on the whole person in his/her 'life world', relying more on subjective reports and experiences, giving more room for meaning in life, allowing for more openness for unanticipated meanings and connections that all the data have to be interpreted, analyzing data and generalizing from understanding the single cases in a more inductive and controlled way and aiming more at the formation of concepts and theories. (Faltermeir 1997: 357)

Sandelowski, on the other hand, describes it as '... an array of techniques that operationalize a view of reality ... as socially constructed and a desire to observe phenomena in a manner as here of artifice as any human project will allow' (Sandelowski 1996: 359–60). The conditions for conducting such investigations are emphasized by Bowling as 'a method of naturalistic enquiry which is usually less obtrusive than quantitative investigations and does not manipulate a research setting. It aims to study people in their natural social settings and to collect naturally occurring data' (Bowling 1997: 311–12).

Qualitative methods of gathering information for the purposes of study have a long established tradition in the field of anthropology (Malinowski 1922; Evans-Pritchard 1976). This was extended by the Chicago school of sociologists before the Second World War and has gained increasing prominence in the field of health studies over the years, especially in relation to lay perspectives associated with health and illness (Thomas and Znaniecki

1977; Williams and Calnan 1996). It has been predominantly overridden by critics due to its lack of objectivity and scientific rigour (Davis 1991) in favour of quantitative techniques partially accounting for its secondary status during the late 1980s. However, notwithstanding such criticisms, qualitative research in the health field is coming into its own. Indeed the combination of both qualitative and quantitative approaches has been extremely beneficial in not only providing richer sources of data, but increased accuracy in capturing a view of reality.

Gathering data through unstructured interviews, case studies and observations has its benefits as some researchers have proven. Storytelling provides rich data where there is little pre-existing knowledge or where issues are sensitive or complex. For example, Bott et al. in their study of experiences of smokers attempting to give up, stated that 'despite the vast literature on smoking cessation, no study actually describes the experience from the perspective of the subject' (Bott et al. 1997:258). Pearlin et al. (1981) also made use of qualitative techniques to identify the complex processes that develop into stress-related illness as it becomes manifest in the individual. Such description would not be possible in a technique that yielded pure numerical analysis, as it would state nothing about human experience.

Generally speaking, qualitative techniques employed in research are able to capture the subjectivity of human experience in terms of language, dialogue and interaction, unlike quantitative methods where evidence is often only partial and, for the most part, inflexible. Bendelow's open interview technique revealed some sensitive and interesting accounts of pain and misfortune such as when one of her interviewees stated: 'Most nights if I'm honest I spend watching TV and drinking enough to blot it out ...' (Bendelow 1996:176). Questionnaires would rarely yield such a stark account of the reality of human suffering or means of coping.

Another strength in the qualitative method is the range of application. Early examples have been afforded by Goffman (1961) in his work in the field of mental illness. More recently, the individual's role in the prevention of health problems and illness has uncovered other means of interpreting health behaviour. This has emerged through descriptions of family life, observation of doctor–patient interaction and analysis of patients' means of communicating their experiences of illness (Martin 1989; Silverman 1996).

Qualitative research has the advantage of being able to exercise curiosity about cause-and-effect relationships in the phenomena observed. The researcher is able to make close observation and obtain a great deal of in-depth information that can be tested in subsequent quantitative studies if necessary and appropriate. Mackenzie (1995) discovered that the process of the in-depth qualitative interview was the best way to identify the components of culture in the NHS trust hospitals during her investigation. She discovered 'the key values within the organisation ... the use of heroes, rituals, and ceremonials to reinforce core values ... the use of rewards and punishments and attitudes of deviants' (Mackenzie 1995:73). This was one approach which assisted in the unmasking of aspects of the organization's culture. From this rich source of information, she was able to develop a questionnaire for a larger scale study within the trust.

In the process of conducting research, the qualitative methods sometimes present an opportunity for the researcher to adapt to the situation, so offering greater flexibility, as Orr demonstrated: 'when possible I took notes ... I did not want the research to intrude or detract from the group experience' (Orr 1993, p. 31). Gatter (1995) made use of discussions around posters and then held in-depth interviews to verify perceptions identified about HIV in a clinical setting.

Qualitative research, like other methods of enquiry, is bound by a number of principles that strive to give credence to the field of academic research. The principles range from the development of understanding to the formulation of theory. However, these principles attract strong criticism.

As identified earlier, the researcher uses techniques categorized as 'qualitative' to make sense of human behaviour and institutions by getting to know the persons involved, their values, beliefs, traditions and emotions. Faltermeir (1997) observed that this process is not yet employed on a grand scale in the assessment of treatment outcomes. The testing of causal hypotheses takes place in epidemiological studies that equate with the traditional positivist views of science. In other words, the scientific method is applied where standard and repeatable methods are employed to gain understanding of phenomena. Single case or biographical studies have found little credence in studies of a population, for example (Stake 1995).

Case studies have, however, in recent years emerged as a heuristic device for generating knowledge and for testing accuracy, relevance and utility (Eisenhardt 1989; Feilding 1994). They are now considered the best way to optimize understanding of a single phenomenon or, as Simons (1980) calls it , the development of the 'science of the singular'. They have been known to permit naturalistic and idiopathic generalizations to be made from and about cases and are favoured in the fields of nursing, psychoanalysis, law and ethics.

Kuhn stated: 'what we see depends on what we look at and what previous visual conceptual experiences have taught us to see' (Kuhn 1970, p. 103). He signals a note of caution in that the researcher will undoubtedly make assumptions and develop theories from their own individual value base, which itself has grown from their own unique experiences. Thus, the awareness in analysing research information is regarded as an important principle. Foster (1990) found this to be problematic when reporting his research findings and was accused by his critics of being blind to racial discrimination in the school where his investigation took place.

Like scientists, qualitative researchers attempt to meet the principles of value freedom and objectivity in their work. This is now regarded as a little naive (Bowling 1997) as most research in the social sciences is value-laden (Frankfort–Nachmias and Nachmias 1992). Throughout the entire process, from the conception of the idea to analysis and consideration of funding bodies to publication, the values of the broader spectrum may be communicated and hence assimilated either wittingly or unwittingly. Indeed, some researchers like Stacey (1986) feel there seems little point in disguising the fact. Also Scavenius and Orland, in their study of health workers on multiple sites, also confessed that 'in our preliminary formulation of the research problem, our attention was focused in a rather traditional way. On meeting the demands of the methodological constraint, in the process we neglected the content-related constraints' (Scavenius and Orland 1996: 511).

Another underlying principle of qualitatative research is the extension of knowledge. Popper (1959) argues that scientific hypotheses can never be more than informed estimates about the universe since they cannot be proven to be totally correct. He argues that scientists should operate within a particular framework where predictions can be made and then construct their investigations in an attempt to disprove their hypothesis. So he implies that knowledge can only be developed through falsification, that is, by setting up testable theories that can be potentially disproved by a process of deduction. This can be problematic for researchers using less conventional techniques for data collection and is attested to in the works of Glaser, Strauss and others in the years invested in the development and use of grounded theory where there is no initial hypothesis (Glaser and Strauss 1967; Kools et al. 1996).

Brown's (1977) theories gained credence through other means. He argued that the refutation of hypotheses is not a certain process, as it is dependent on observations that may not be accurate. Owing to the problem of measurement, deductions may provide predictions from hypotheses, but there is no logical method for the comparison of predictions with observations from which new hypotheses emerge. To follow Brown's reasoning, one may begin with a topic and allow what is relevant to that topic to emerge from analyses as in grounded theory.

Merton (1968) also refuted Popper's claims on the falsification of theory. Research observation, according to Merton, must precede theory because it initiates, formulates, deflects and clarifies theory. In the philosophy of phenomenology, for example, Merton and his followers place emphasis on social facts that are characterized by their meaningfulness to members in the social world. The interactionist notion, as communicated by Merton, sees reality as socially constructed through a multiplicity of interaction. Individuals use symbols to interpret each other and assign meanings to perceptions and experience. These are not imposed by external forces. Thus Merton underlines the point that to use the tools of natural science as emphasized by Popper is to distort the view of reality and reduce, even fragment, the lived experience.

Participant observation is a method of enquiry that can be used by the researcher to develop a view of social reality. It is justifiable on the grounds that it makes possible the study of inaccessible groups or groups that do not reveal to outsiders certain aspects of their lives. It has been criticized for a number of reasons. First, the researcher may disturb the setting. As Erikson notes, 'a stranger who pretends to do something else can disturb others by failing to understand the conditions of intimacy that prevail in the group' (Erikson 1967: 368). This underlines the importance of using gatekeepers when entering new territory to guide the researcher. Evans-Pritchard (1976) was able to make use of gatekeepers in his study of the Azande people, but he had difficulty in accepting that he was regarded as different to the group. This gave a slightly different emphasis to his study (Wilkinson and Kitzinger 2000; Merriam 2002).

A second criticism rests with the decision about what to observe. This is noted in situations where the researcher is unable to evoke responses and behaviour without raising suspicion. This was noted in the study by Holm and Smidt (1997) in their observations of children's dietary needs in a clinical setting. Although their study severely criticized staff behaviour, they were not able to elicit direct information from children through questioning as this would have implications for their results and would not be based on observation. Finally, critics argue that the reporting of observations or taking notes is considered impossible on the spot. Time lags in writing up observations may introduce selective bias. This appeared to be the case in the study conducted by Kools et al. in a clinical setting where there were nurses and confused elderly patients. They found that the information had to be supported by the use of interview material and verification reports from members of the research team (Kools et al. 1996), thus emphasizing the importance of triangulation in qualitative approaches to investigation.

Ethnography is a form of qualitative investigation that is directed towards producing what are referred to as 'theoretical', 'analytical' or 'thick' descriptions. Ethnographers, it is claimed, test theories by the process of using them (Geertz 1973). These may be of societies, small communities, organizations, spatial locations or social worlds. Theory develops from the data collected. However, it is claimed that the ability to formulate theories is problematic as there needs to be a distinction between theory and description. What is developed is largely intuitive because one cannot be certain that what has emerged through observation has been correctly interpreted and that it represents universal scientific principles (Hammersley 1989).

Hammersley's argument is a strong plea for scientific credibility. However, he does not capture the spirit of the approach, that is, the development of meaning or assigning of meaning to social phenomena. As Kermode, attempting to make sense of descriptions and theories, stated 'texts always have their secrets' (Kermode 1983, p. 136). This is strongly supported by Iser who states that it is up to the researcher or reader to make sense of their own inferences 'to bring into play our own faculty for establishing connections – for filling the gaps left by the text itself' (Iser 1980, p. 125). Ayres and Poirer (1986) support the view that the interpretive process occurs in the mind of the researcher and it is therefore essential to the realization of meaning; without interpretation, the text is without meaning. Iser and Kermode, along with Stacey (1986), agree that the bringing of the values of the researcher to the investigation and interpretation of the meaning of a text arises from the interaction of the mind, which includes the personal history of the researcher, with the respondent, both formulating the initial meaning or the 'virtual' text from which analysis flows and flourishes. Perhaps, therefore, Hammersley implies that what emerges is a theory that is partial, but not pure. He can take heart from the position that one may never uncover truth in its purest sense because theories and social situations are not static but are constantly altering. But it is the duty of the researcher to attempt to make sense of what is happening in the situations they observe. Research, after all, is a process of discovery.

The principles and practice of qualitative research outlined in this discussion are largely supportive of their value to social scientific enquiry. However, there are reservations in the sense that the social environment needs to be a consideration in the collection and interpretation of data. The social environment, for the author, also impinges on the values, beliefs, behaviour and traditions of the participants, as well as shaping the unique experiences of those negotiating that social space. This is particularly important in health care settings as users of the service, 'actors' within the service and visitors to the settings will contribute to altering the setting. At the same time, the social environment and the negotiators of that environment in qualitative research are difficult to separate, and it may be the case that separation would distort the findings.

References

Ayres, L. and Poirer, S. (1996) Virtual text and the growth of meaning in qualitative analysis. *Research in Nursing and Health* **19**: 163–9.

Bendelow, G. A. (1996) 'Failure' of modern medicine? Lay perspectives on a pain relief clinic. In S. J. Williams and M. Calnan (eds), *Modern Medicine: Lay Perspectives and Experiences* (London: UCL Press).

Bott, M. J., Kuckleman-Cobb, A., Schelbermeir, M. S. and O'Connell, K. A. (1997) Quitting: smokers relate their experiences. *Qualitative Health Research* **7** (2): 255–69.

Bowling, A. (1997) *Research Methods in Health: Investigating Health and Health Services* (Buckinghamshire: Open University Press).

Brown, H. J. (1977) *Perception, Theory and Commitment: The New Philosophy of Science* (Chicago: Chicago University Press).

Davis, D. S. (1991) Rich cases: the ethics of thick description. *Hastings Centre Report* **21** (4): 12–17.

Eisenhardt, K. M. (1989) Building theories from case study research. *Academy of Management Review* **14**: 532–50.

Erikson, K. T. (1967) A comment on disguised observation in sociology. *Social Problems* **12**: 368–70.

Evans-Pritchard, E. E. (1976) *Witchcraft, Oracles and Magic Among the Azande* (Oxford: Oxford University Press).

Faltermeir, T. (1997) Why public health research needs qualitative approaches. *European Journal of Public Health* **7** (4): 357–63.

Feilding, S. I. (1994) Case studies: a case of egalitarianism. *Qualitative Sociology* **17**: 423–31.

Foster, P. (1990) Case not proven: an evaluation of two studies of teacher racism. *British Educational Research Journal* **16** (4): 335–48.

Frankfort-Nachmias, C. and Achaia, D. (1992) *Research Methods in the Social Sciences*, 4th edn (London: Edward Arnold).

Gatter, P. N. (1995) Anthropology, HIV and contingent identities. *Social Science and Medicine* **41** (11): 1523–33.

Geertz, C. (1973) *The Interpretation of Cultures* (New York: Basic Books).

Glaser, B. G. and Strauss, A. I. (1967) *The Discovery of Grounded Theory: Strategies for Qualitative Research* (New York: Aldine Publishing).

Goffman, E. (1961) *Assylums: Essays on the Social Situations of Mental Patients and Other Inmates* (New York: Doubleday Anchor).

Hammersley, M. (1989) *The Dilemma of Qualitative Method: Herbert Bulmer and The Chicago Tradition* (London: Routledge).

Holm I. and Smidt, S. (1997) Uncovering social structures of and status differences in health systems. *European Journal Public Health* **7**: 373–8.

Iser, W. (1980) The reading process: a phenomenological approach. In J. Tompkins (ed.) *Reader Response Criticism* (Baltimore: Johns Hopkins University Press).

Kermode, F. (1983) *The Art of Telling: Essays in Fiction* (New York: Oxford University Press).

Kools, S., McCarthy, M., Durham B. and Robrecht, I. (1996) Dimensional analysis: broadening the conception of grounded theory. *Qualitative Health Research* **6** (3): 312–30.

Kuhn, T. S. (1970) The structure of scientific revolution, 2nd edn (Chicago: Chicago University Press).

Mackenzie, S. (1995) Surveying the organisational culture in an NHS trust. *Journal of Management in Medicine* **9** (8): 69–77.

Malinowski, B. (1972) *Argonauts of the Western Pacific* (London: Routledge).

Martin, E. (1989) *The Woman in the Body: A Cultural Analysis of Reproduction* (Buckingham: Open University Press).

Merriam, S. et al. (2002) *Qualitative Research in Practice* (San Francisco: Jossey-Bass).

Merton, R. K. (1968) *Social Theory and Social Structure* (New York: Free Press of Glencoe).

Orr, J. (1993) Working with women's health groups: the community health movement. In P. Abbott and R. Sapsford (eds), *Research into Practice: A Reader for Nurses and the Caring Professions* (Milton Keynes: Open Univesity Press).

Pearlin, I. J., Lieberman, M. A., Menagan, E.G. and Mullan, J. F. (1981) The sleep process. *Journal of Health and Social Behaviour* **22**: 337–56.

Popper, K. R. (1959) *The Logic of Scientific Discovery* (London: Hutchinson).

Sandelowski, M. (1996) Using qualitative methods in intervention studies. *Research in Nursing and Health* **19**: 359–64.

Scavenius, M. and Orland, J. (1996) Theoretical constraints in the first phase of a multi site case study of health services. *Qualitative Health Research* **6** (4): 506–25.

Silverman, D. (1996) *Discourses of Counselling: HIV Counselling as Social Interaction* (London: Sage).

Simons, H. (1980) *Towards a Science of the Singular: Essays about Case Study in Educational Research and Evaluation* (University of East Anglia: Centre for Applied Research in Education).

Stacey, M. (1986) Concepts of health and illness and the division of labour in health care. In C. Curren and M. Stacey (eds) *Concepts of Health, Illness and Disease: A Comparative Perspective* (Oxford: Berg Publishers).

Stake, R. F. (1995) *The Art of Case Study Research* (London: Sage).

Thomas, W. and Znaniecki, F. (1977) *The Polish Peasant in Europe and America* (New York: Alfred A. Knopf).

Williams, S. J. and Calnan, M. (1996) *Modern Medicine: Lay Perspectives and Experiences* (London: UCL Press).

CHAPTER 8

Studying Organizational Health Culture in a Hospital Setting: Some Reflections on the Process

CAROL WILKINSON

Introduction

This pilot study took place over a period of three months in a combined hospital and community health trust in central England. It was intended to clarify the questions for a larger research project and to ascertain whether the method of data collection selected was suitable for the purposes of the project. In order to arrive at some accommodation, it is intended to:

1. describe the location and provide some relevant background detail about the trust and its relationship with the local environs;
2. discuss the actual material collected and reasons for doing so;
3. provide some reflections on the methods, the questions posed, the approach taken and some initial insights into the main issue of the culture of workplace health.

The study was undertaken at a time when New Labour policy, relating to *Saving Lives: Our Healthier Nation* (DoH 1998), had been introduced into the trust after eighteen months.

The NHS trust hospital is located in central England not far from Netherbridge council estate (fictitious name) and is in close proximity to the community trust buildings. Altogether there are 3,500 staff who provide a health service for the local community. The trust has an extremely busy Accident and Emergency Department, and its main specialty within the region is the prevention and treatment of cancers.

During the period of the study, local hospital trust reports for that year indicated that the trust had exceeded its contractual obligations by 5.9%.

It dealt with 20,014 inpatients, 7,446 day case procedures and 131,404 outpatients. This was a considerable increase on the previous year. Like all trusts across the country, the hospital and community trust was undergoing change in terms of organization and structure as a result of new government policy. This caused considerable stress, particularly in managerial and administrative circles, in terms of anticipation and uncertainty of tenure. Other stressors related to increasing discontent with the nurse training programme that had been introduced within the sector and poor levels of staffing in some areas of the trust. Portering, domestic and catering services were all undertaken on a contractual basis, sometimes making working relationships difficult in times of dispute.

The trust had experienced a winter where pressure on the acute sector meant making provisions with the local community hospital and one in the neighbouring town for extra beds. Additional staff were employed in the A&E Assessment Unit that was open daily from 11 am to 11 pm.

The attitude towards health promotion had an established history and had been highly commended within the region. Some five years earlier, the Human Resources Department had set up an employee assistance programme that provided advice and counselling for employees experiencing stress-related problems. Its success in reducing sickness absence was recorded in *The Best of Health – Good Practice in the NHS, No. 2*, the following year. The programme was then taken over by the Occupational Health Department, becoming less high profile with a reduced budget and staffing input (staff had to pay for the service originally, a flat fee of £20 per person), although awareness-raising information about stress management issues was disseminated through staff induction programmes and updates.

At the time of the study, the trust had an active Health for All Committee. This group included the health authority, the local community health council, the hospital and community NHS trust, the Council for Voluntary Organizations, the local Race Equality Council and the Local Agenda 21 representatives. They operated within the World Health Organisation (WHO) framework with its underpinning principles of equity, community participation and intersectoral collaboration. A series of priorities and actions had been set out in a strategy document up to the year 2004. Their achievements as a collective included a seminar on good practice for the maintenance of health and well-being for the local black and ethnic minority population, as well as a single regeneration budget project with two local council estates. Their 'Take a Break' community café received a Bronze Food Award from the health minister that year. Areas that remained of some concern included poverty, racism and service provision and access for the poor. They were working in partnership with the local county council to develop projects that would assist in reducing these problems.

The annual budget held by the health authority for health promotion projects across the entire community was a meagre £7,500. Hence projects were limited and undertaken on a priority basis. The fund did not include support for the range of hospital and community-based health care employees. There was no budget for health promotion projects undertaken by the Occupational Health Department within the trust. The planning of a health event for staff, discussed in this study, was being funded through external sponsorship and the good will of local service providers.

A health festival for employees of the trust was the idea of staff located in the Occupational Health Department. It was created with a view to promoting well-being among the workforce and showcasing the often hidden work remit of the department in terms of health promotion (as many staff equated it only with health and safety), as well as an annual health check. This staff health promotion initiative initially met with suspicion and hostility as well as a lack of commitment from the managerial hierarchy. It took months of careful negotiation with interested parties, including the person who acted as the researcher's gatekeeper, to gain the support and permission to go ahead with the scheme. The planning committee had to ensure that positive publicity was provided for the trust.

Aims of the study

These were:

- to identify the culture of workplace health promotion within the service sector;
- to utilize research findings to inform policy and practice of health improvement at work.

Research objectives

To unmask the culture of workplace health promotion, it was intended to observe the connection between the service (incorporating elements of health promotion, disease prevention and health protection, that is, the traditional work of an occupational health department in a large teaching hospital) and the maintenance of health and well-being. Interventions and support structures for the workforce and whether workers participated in the process of maintaining health and well-being at work was seen as an important objective. In order to underline this point, a series of questions were drawn up, linking what makes people ill at work and the mechanisms that enable people to develop health awareness in the workplace. However, there was also a need to uncover the peculiarity of the organization in terms of the nature and commitment to health matters for workers alongside the interactions of individuals at the workplace. Hence the following questions were posed:

1. To what extent do employees participate in the whole process of health maintenance and improvement at work and what is the main driving force behind their participation/non-participation?
2. The ideological framework for workplace health promotion (WHP) evades the needs of workers by seeing them as a discrete group rather than different groups with differing needs. How can the missing elements of gender and 'race' be expressed?
3. What is the relationship of the elements in (1) and (2) to the culture of the workplace?

These questions were tentative for the purposes of a pilot study, the intention being to further develop them after initial findings.

Establishing a position for investigation

Health at work

There are many definitions of health but, for the purposes of the project, the issue of health is derived from a position of the negotiation of social situations. In stating this, it is acknowledged that ill health arises from social circumstances of deprivation and exploitation (Gerhardt 1989). In the workplace, a number of theoretical perspectives have underlined this phenomenon. For example, Gardell's work demonstrates that lack of control over work tasks, reduction in interaction with others and a reduced ability to plan work tasks as a result of work fragmentation have a marked impact on the mental well-being of workers in a range of manufacturing and service industries (for examples, see Gardell 1971, 1976). Marmot and Theorell (1987, 1988) and Johnson (1986) have identified issues such as lack of control over individual workloads in relation to the organizational hierarchy and the predisposition to cardiovascular disease amongst workers. Boredom of workers due to inappropriate levels of work, lack of skill discretion and lack of employment security have an impact on blood pressure, weight gain and stress (Knox 1985; Alfredsson et al. 1985; Marmot and Theorell 1988; Frankenhauser 1991).

The gendered position of workers places greater emotional burden on those who work in service industries, predominantly women, especially when linked to the variable of control (Hall 1991). Women also do more deep and surface acting than men because of their often subordinate position; this maintains their unequal status in the workplace (Duncombe and Marsden 1995). The issues of class, emotions and inequalities in the workplace are inextricably linked (Williams 1995; Hochschild 1983) and were identified as areas requiring further investigation.

With specific reference to the service sector, it has been recognized that emotional labour is a feature of face-to-face service contact work (Fineman 1993; Hosking and Fineman 1990). Service workers are trained to be 'caring', 'benign', 'objective' and 'scientific', although Finemen recognizes that nurses, doctors and social workers are paid for their skill in emotion management, as there are costs if the mask slips. Emotion labour and its link to health at work results in reduced spontaneity of human interaction, and this can have negative consequences for the employee in working relationships (Fineman 1993). Burn-out and emotional numbness are also distinct features of emotion labour (Van Maanen and Kunda 1989).

Investigating the private–public divide of home and work demonstrates that relaxing after work is a male privilege when childcare and domestic household chores are taken into consideration; hence the stress experienced by working women in these situations is prolonged (Frankenhauser 1991). This is recognizable in symptoms such as blood pressure, heart rate and others self-reporting in daily activity. The new forms of work organization of the recent past, such as flattened management structures and altered labour processes and employment patterns, were intended to encourage flexibility in working arrangements and solidarity between citizens (European Commission 1997). This however has not prevented poor practice in the workplace from impacting on the lives of those on the receiving end. However, family-friendly policies have been introduced into the National Health Service. How this has affected the self-reported total workload for men and women is an area that requires some consideration as it is very much connected to issues of stress and control in the service sector, particularly for women (Hall 1991).

Global developments in workplace health promotion

The current literature on workplace health issues in Britain presents a picture of neglect in terms of developments in policy and strategic direction for worker health improvement. For example, although workplace health has been discussed in a number of policy documents over the years, there has been no national strategy (see, for example, Waldron 1996). The Health and Safety Executive and various health promotion bodies in England, Scotland, Wales and Northern Ireland have developed local policies based on local community matters, which has led to fragmentation of workplace health issues. There is also evidence at grassroots level that health promotion experts have tremendous difficulty entering, negotiating and developing a health-promoting ethos within an organization (Wilkinson 1999), despite the fact that the World Health Organisation's mandate established a position to encourage such activity (WHO 1988).

Workplace health promotion (WHP) is an evolving concept and relatively underdeveloped from a European perspective, although since the 1970s it has been welcomed and is flourishing in the United States and Canada. The differences between the geographical locations are mainly economic. The American attitude to workplace health promotion, although largely associated with lifestyle and behavioural change, arose out of three distinct issues. First, there was the concern to contain costs. As a key issue of corporate health policy, managers envisaged that if companies could reduce their medical insurance and disability claims costs, this would lead to lower health care costs and sickness benefits, thus reducing operational costs. Also, as employee productivity was seen as crucial within a competitive market, keeping workers healthy meant greater productivity (Wilkinson 1997).

Secondly, there is the issue of risk as associated with lifestyie. The medical profession emphasizes that there is scientific justification for implementing strategies to improve employee health. Medicine regards individual lifestyle and behaviour in terms of risk factors that are central to the development of chronic disease. This approach has, however, been heavily criticized on the grounds of victim-blaming and often provides a self-serving justification for medical services and medical research (Conrad 1987).

Finally, health interests in the US have been promoted by cultural and social values rather than scientific advances. Workplace encouragement in the late 1980s saw over 60 million people between the ages of 20 and 50 years participate in jogging. These were largely the professional middle-classes who also stimulated the sales of health foodstuffs, participated in exercise classes at work and accounted for increased attendance at health and fitness clubs (Wilkinson 1997).

The European dimension of WHP is a developing phenomenon. In 1988 the WHO produced a pamphlet entitled *Health Promotion for Working Populations* in which WHA 40.20 resolved to 'pay due attention to workers' health programmes and to develop guidelines on health promotion in the workplace'. In almost two decades, very little work has been undertaken that has made any impact on Britain and Europe in achieving these aims. Findings of a European project highlighted that little work was being undertaken outside the occupational health and safety requirements of the individual countries (Wynne and Clarkin 1992). The few exceptions were located in Germany and Wales.

In Britain, workplace health improvement preceded the Ottawa Charter that was introduced after the successful 'Look after Yourself' programmes in the days of the Health Education Council. Some years later, a further step was taken by the Health of the Nation Taskforce which provided training for interested parties in health improvement in the workplace. However, the medical model continued to prevail with an emphasis on care, safety and treatment as opposed to health promotion. Some work undertaken by health promotion experts has involved the introduction of award schemes, for instance, Corporate Health – Corporate Action and Health at Work in the NHS. Individual incentives undertaken by private companies have also been notable. However, for the most part, the work has been poorly evaluated (Springett and Dugdill 1995).

The momentum in WHP has gathered pace in recent years. Government policy in Britain, *Saving Lives: Our Healthier Nation* (DoH 1988) has encouraged reform to include more active health promotion in workplaces, hospitals and schools. Allied to this, other European activity in WHP has been prompted through Framework Directive 89/391/EC on safety and health at work. The Framework has prepared the ground for the reorientation of traditional occupational health and safety legislation and practice and the increasing profile of the workplace as a public health setting (Breucker 1998). The psychosocial health problems born out of a recognized lack of control, including exploitation and emotion labour, mentioned above, have become part of the broader picture at work which the Framework has addressed.

With these developments in policy, workplace health promotion has now been defined within the European context as 'the combined efforts of employers, employees and society to improve the health and well being of people at work. This can be achieved through a combination of improving the work organisation, and the working environment, promoting active participation, and encouraging personal development' (Luxembourg Declaration of Workplace Health Promotion 1997). This is a departure from the American policy that advocated lifestyle and behaviour change issues and was born out of a practical problem-solving approach to health improvement in the workplace. For example, the 'Live for Life Project' from the Johnson and Johnson corporation advocated a business planning approach with strategies for health improvement along with training in cardiopulmonary resuscitation (Fielding and Breslow 1983; Kizer 1987).

Although the European definition is a positive step towards a policy agenda for health improvement at work, it is based on a total quality management model that largely suggests management focus and hence should be management driven. Although that is not a bad place to be in terms of initiatives for resource allocation and driving change, the employee's perspective could be made more explicit in the process of development. The perspective of those specializing in health promotion in the workplace is also crucial to any work of this nature that is to be undertaken in future. The European definition does fall short, though, in the consideration of the social dimensions of workplace health.

The social relations of the workplace: organizational culture

Harrison (1972) was the first to develop a basic taxonomy of organizational culture. This was later popularized by Handy (1985) and comprised elements associated with power, role, task and person. It is acknowledged that there is more than one culture operating in any given environment. This gives rise to tensions and conflicts amongst competing ideologies and interests. Such challenges will at certain points rise up and become dominant at the cost of subordinating another set of values. The process is cumulative and dispersive yet, at the same time, never quite sheds all of its core features.

Deal and Kennedy (1983) argue that behaviour is shaped by shared values, beliefs and assumptions about the way an organization should operate, how rewards should be distributed, the conduct of meetings, even how people should dress. They do not consider whether behaviour within organizations is a result of reaction to intrinsic and extrinsic motivators. They state that the organizational culture relates to its success. Sathe (1983) argues that culture guides the actions of an organisation's members without the need for detailed instructions or long meetings that discuss how to approach particular issues or problems; it also reduces the level of ambiguity and misunderstanding between functions and departments. In effect, culture shapes the purpose and context of the organization. Indeed, Barratt develops this, stating that 'values, beliefs and attitudes are learnt, can be managed and changed and are potentially manipulable by management' (Barratt 1990: 23). So managers have an important influence on the culture of an organization (Schein 1985).

There are a number of definitions of organizational culture. Silverman (1970) contends that organizations are societies in miniature and can therefore be expected to demonstrate aspects of their own cultural characteristics. This may be the case in that there is the implication that, within these societies, there exists conflict, consensus and interactions that lead to behavioural change and that the rules for living are reflected within the organization as in wider society. It follows then that culture defines how those within the organization should behave in a given set of circumstances. It has been observed that cultural systems contain elements which prescribe forms of behaviour or allow behaviour to be judged acceptable or not (Turner 1971).

The fundamental elements of organizational culture are observed and monitored in many ways. Beckhard (1969) identified what was meant by a healthy organization. Positive correlations have also been found between culture and organizational effectiveness (Ouchi 1981; Deal and Kennedy 1982; Denison 1984). Information-sharing, delegating, results-oriented, developmental, egalitarian, employee-centred cultures are believed to enhance adaptiveness, productivity, innovation and performance (Kanter 1983; Denison 1984; Walton 1985). The strength of cultures within organizations is also seen as important. It is suggested that strong cultures (clan mechanisms) may enhance organizational efficiency only under conditions where there is uncertainty and ambiguity (Wilkins and Ouchi 1983; Wilson 1992).

Others see organizational culture as a system of shared values, beliefs, norms and routines that becomes evident through anecdote and myth, all of which serve to communicate and reinforce those shared values (Peters and Waterman 1982). This is further developed by others who see organizational culture as a basic set of assumptions that a given group has created, discerned or developed over a period of time through a process of learning to cope with the issues or problems that arise within an organization. It is a process of adaptation to the environment. Such means of adapting are usually taught to new members of the organization and determine the behaviour of its members through visible artefacts such as office layout, architecture, dress codes, behavioural patterns and speech (Schein 1985).

Taking the elements discussed by Schein (1985) as a practical way of understanding the culture of organizations, a model was developed for gathering data. The stages of exploration are outlined briefly in Figure 8.1 below. Schein's model was selected originally because it provided some insight into ways in which material could be collected that would inform the researcher about the structure, functions and behaviours within an organization. This was important because it presented the potential for gaining insight into the levels at which culture operates within an organization. To understand issues that relate to workplace health, taking into consideration the environment, its people, its policies and actions which impinge upon health, it was important to gain as full a picture as possible. The pilot study was intended to test some of the elements of Schein's model in terms of feasibility for data collection.

Gaining access

Gaining access to the trust came about through initial contact with the Occupational Health Department based in the large teaching hospital. They were hosting a Health Festival at the hospital in March that year. It came as a surprise to be invited to meet with the Occupational Health Coordinator (ML: she became my gatekeeper) who subsequently secured an invitation to meet the planning committee members. Although invited to a series of meetings, it was not until two days prior to the event that I was granted permission to interview participants as well. This was linked with the proviso that an evaluation of the event be provided at a later date to the planning committee.

Actual material collected

Prior to the event, details concerning the organization were requested and obtained from the human resources department relating to policy for health promotion and health improvement, past and current initiatives undertaken by the organization to improve health (for example, they had introduced a no-smoking policy some twenty months prior to my study) and other material and services to support staff to give up smoking. The health authority headquarters provided further statistical details, as well as information about services, business plans and strategies for the trust. Specific details concerning the work of the occupational health department were obtained through discussion and semi-structured interviews with my gatekeeper.

Notes were also made concerning my impressions of the organization, its décor, activity, structure and functions in areas where I had access. It was incredibly useful to sit in the hospital reception area simply observing activity and exchanges between people. The event outlined a major aspect of health promotion material that I needed but, allied to this, unearthing perspectives on health at work was a feature of my research, so it was important to observe, take notes and speak to people about this. As culture is an important aspect of the study, a combination of approaches was required for collecting the data. It was intended to be qualitative research, as it was my view that the observation of social interaction of participants in the study was important, and questionnaires would not necessarily yield the richness of data that, say, an interview or recording activity would present. I was also of the view that any information collected would only provide a partial account of phenomena, hence a triangulated approach to data collection was necessary for the purposes of checking and forming links between actions and events. In the study, it was possible to record details in a diary; notes were taken of observations and a series of interviews was also undertaken. This was indeed a lot of work, and yielded a great deal of data for a pilot study, but as most researchers are aware, nothing is ever wasted and links between the data can be made in a variety of ways.

The diaries recorded a series of thoughts, observations and discussion with interested parties about initial meetings leading up to and beyond the event.

The event itself was observed including interaction between participants. Observations were made by participating in the event as an employee. As the only other person aware that I was conducting research was ML, I was free to capture aspects of activity at the event as I saw them and speak to participants. Some volunteers gave me their contact details for a follow-up interview. All exhibitors were spoken to regarding their main role. The best way to do this was to try out some of the materials and treatments on offer or stand alongside some of the attendees and listen to exchanges. This proved a valuable source of information.

The organizer was interviewed before and after the event, and other staff involved in the planning committee after the event only. Some members of the workforce volunteered to participate in interviews a few days after the event. Negotiating this was not particularly difficult; many more could have been interviewed, but I was conscious that this was only a pilot study.

Background details: the event

The event was planned by ML together with LW (manager of the Occupational Health Service across the trust) from the Occupational Health Department. It was based on an idea LW had developed as a result of observing events undertaken at a neighbouring health authority. Both were armed with the knowledge that a five-day event was not feasible as it discouraged attendance and so settled on one day instead. Each member of staff at the hospital and community health trust, many of whom work a shift system, was granted permission by their managers to take an additional hour in their break to attend the event. Others attended on their day off duty. The event was attended by at least 600 people. A range of exhibitors was available, providing an opportunity to sample goods and services. These included acupuncture, aromatherapy massage, beauty and skin care for men and women, juggling, travel health, tai chi, meditation, reflexology and Indian head massage amongst many other things. Prizes were donated by hospital friends and major exhibitors.

Utilizing Schein's model

Schein's (1985) model has been interpreted as shown in Figure 8.1.

As stated above, an adaptation of Schein's (1985) model was utilized in this study to gather data that would provide some insight into aspects of the culture within the organization. Extracts of the data are presented below using a sample of the ten stages of action model, although it must be stated that, for reasons of brevity, not all ten stages are discussed here.

Stage One – beginnings: gaining entry/initial impressions

7th January

Arrive at 11.05 a.m. for my meeting with ML. I am ten minutes early but am greeted by the receptionist. She plainly thinks that I am a patient and directs me to the patients' waiting room. The room is small but brightly coloured and cluttered with chairs, a table on which a few plastic bricks from a children's toy box are scattered. Beside a few glossy magazines, I also notice a woman sat opposite clutching her bandaged wrist. On one wall are a series of photographs of the team members of the OH Department, all suited and tidy, mainly women, with one male, the consultant. All caucasian. Just spotted the one of ML so at least I know who to expect. The other walls are filled with posters and leaflets about the OH service and health matters.

Soon I am called by the receptionist and am taken through the hall and down the corridor into an office where I am warmly greeted by ML. She is a woman of medium height and slight features. Her non-verbal communication displays much animation. I think she is pleased to see me and immediately recalls that she last spoke to me when I had a rather awful dose of flu – we chatted and laughed about that for a while.

ML then launched into discussion about the work she was involved in – obviously excited and busy with the arrangements for the event, she is anxious to tell me absolutely everything that she has done so far ... this goes on for about fifteen minutes; then she remembered I was here to do some research and so promptly asked me to tell her about myself and what I do ... I did contemplate which 'me' she wanted to know about, but then talked about my interest in health

Stages of exploration	Comments
1 Entry -- focus on surprises	Systematic observation of organization; surprises encountered; initial expectations of outsider.
2 Systematic observation and checking	Note repeated experiences to verify surprises
3 Locating a motivated insider	The outsider must find someone inside the culture who is capable of deciphering what is going on.
	Participating in a project with an individual may be a useful way of doing this.
4 Revealing surprises	Relationship established.
	Hunches can be discussed with 'insider' who often sets the scene by asking what outsider thinks after 'induction'.
	Stick to own observations and question on the basis of own needing to know.
5 Joint exploration	Communication between parties and observation can assist in categorizing and confirming assumptions -- theorizing.
6 Forming assumptions	Hunches about the culture are formed.
	Data obtainable in operational values.
7 Systematic checking and consolidation	New evidence is obtained through interviews or observations.
	Systematic interviewing of informants, content analysis of documents and other artefacts; other means of data collection may be mobilized here.
8 Pushing the levels of assumptions	Need to move beyond articulated values and attempt to understand deeper layer of assumptions.
	Knowing when one's behaviour fits the culture and when it is counter to it.
9 Perpetual recalibration	As new data surface, the outsider, now better acquainted, can modify model and construct test with insiders.
10 Formal written description	Write down assumptions and explain how they relate to each other in a meaningful way.

Figure 8.1 Schein's model (1985)

promotion and why I wanted to do research with the Trust. Her eyes lit up when I started to talk about workplace health promotion and I could feel her drawing in every bit of information; then she tested my knowledge on occupational health matters that were current and I think I passed, judging by her enthusiasm towards me. We arrived at the conclusion that we could work together. She then outlined issues of clearance and the structure of the planning committee and invited me to attend all the meetings leading up to the event.

Later I was provided with paper information about the event and introduced to LW, her manager, and taken on a tour of the hospital and the site where the event will be taking place.   (Diary entry)

This introduction to the organization was amiable and I was left with a good impression of the keenness of my gatekeeper to support the work I was there to do. Generally it had been an informative and frenzied first meeting but seemed promising. I then thought I should find out more detail about the organization and so made my way back to the main reception area of the hospital:

Staff were milling through in rather an efficient manner. My arrival in the main reception area prompted a chat with the male receptionist. I asked if he had a brochure for the hospital; his reply 'Not at the moment' was accompanied by groping for a leaflet under the counter. He handed it over and said they should have brochures in a few days – they had just been updated. He was very friendly and courteous.   (Diary entry)

Stage Two – systematic observation and checking

Schein observes that notes should be scrutinized to identify any examples of duplicated experiences that serve to confirm unexpected results:

17th January

On my approach to the main hospital reception area, I see a couple of uniformed hospital porters standing chatting and smoking. The ground area near them appears to be littered with cigarette ends and discarded 'roll-up' papers.   (Diary entry)

and

8th February

Arrive at the hospital at 1 p.m. On my approach to the main entrance, an assortment of people, staff, patients' relatives and a couple of what seem to be patients, as they are in dressing gowns, standing outside the doors smoking and chatting. This may be indicative of the policy of the hospital (I need to check). The entrance is marked by cigarette butt ends and is not actually a very inviting sight to behold.   (Diary entry)

The links between these entries provide an indication that there may be no designated smoking area in the hospital. I did check later and discovered that the hospital had indeed introduced a no-smoking policy, hence the sight outside the main entrance of the hospital that somewhat contradicted the image the trust was trying to present.

Stage Three – Locating a Motivated Insider

Schein notes that the researcher should locate someone inside the culture who is capable of deciphering what is going on. This can be achieved by participating in a project. One of the planning meetings for the health festival was ideal for doing just this:

29th January

Arrived a few minutes late for the meeting, having spent the last ten minutes trying to find somewhere to park! I enter the room located in the Post-Graduate Medical Centre in the hospital grounds, and am warmly greeted by ML. Immediately, KB, the Non-Executive Director of the trust, introduces herself and her colleagues in turn, announcing their job titles and their specific interest in the event. ML provides me with a copy of the agenda for the meeting and the discussions begin. (Diary entry)

[...]

The business flows with some useful interjections by KB who provides me with a running commentary of the 'politics' of the situation in terms of presentation of the Trust, delicate negotiations with the in-house nursery team, who as yet have no formal nursery, and the juggler who is apparently being funded by them. This is currently in conflict with the normal duties as the hospital are lobbying for nursery facilities for staff with children on site. The nearest local authority nursery, at Netherbridge, is finding difficulty filling its places, whereas the hospital has an oversubscribed waiting list for potential places. KB is herself heavily involved in this lobbying as ML let slip that KB has an eighteen-month-old son who would benefit from nursery facilities on site. ... KB's motivation is driven by her need to return to full-time work. She is a former police officer who gave up work in the service on health grounds but has been involved in the NHS in some capacity for a number of years. She appears to be a staunch ally of ML who is keen to drive several initiatives of this kind forward. (Observation notes)

Reflections on the organization and its people

Recording observations on a notepad and using a dictaphone were the best ways of registering my impressions of the work setting and its people. Sometimes after parking my car in the hospital grounds I would walk to the main hospital entrance and observe and listen to people as they sat or stood outside the sliding doors, smoking, talking to friends and relatives, waiting for transport. On other occasions, I would sit in the reception area and observe the work of the receptionist and others involved in exchanges in the hairdresser and in the shop adjacent to the reception desk. On other days I would wander along the corridor, observing the décor as I approached the Occupational Health Department or visit the employees' restaurant. Nobody seemed to mind that I was there, or at least there were no questions asked.

Reflections on method

Leading up to and including the event, I felt very comfortable observing activity and gathering subjects for interview, although I was initially apprehensive as the number of people at the event itself was overwhelming. Where to begin? Exhibitors? Workers or participants? On the whole, I found a ready acceptance at the planning committee over the weeks that I attended. They were plainly highly motivated and willing to provide material so long as it focused on the event itself. Frankly, I felt the urge to explore further in terms of procedures and policies but the group would have become suspicious of my motives – unmasking aspects of the culture of the organization rather than capturing the spirit of the event. Staff readily gave permission to be interviewed on tape. People were also prepared to chat 'off record' about their views of the organization and the event as well. Many expressed their views about health matters at work as well.

In terms of observation, there was much to take in and I was alerted to the need to retreat on occasions so as to avoid being overwhelmed by the extent of new avenues for exploration. For example, at one point I spoke to the UNISON representative about his non-attendance of the event. Plainly he had not received any information and was disappointed as other staff on his ward whom I interviewed clearly had. Also a couple of porters, who were peering through the entrance door to the staff restaurant where the event was being held, wanted to go in and sample it but felt inhibited, despite encouragement to participate. They considered it was 'not for them'. The men they saw attending the event were doctors and managers or, as one put it, 'the suits', who were not like them at all.

Reflections upon the research questions

Participation. It was plain that the extent of participation was dependent on knowledge, motivation and employee concerns about health issues. One of the planning committee interviewed felt that her fellow health visitors did their own thing. She thought (rather guiltily) that her team tended to operate in a fragmented way and had no true sense of team-working or solidarity except at a national level. They considered their health work was more important for their patients than themselves, and that, frankly, they knew it all, and tended to deal with their own health matters themselves, it being considered a personal thing. To be seen to be failing to deal with matters of stress was seen as not coping, despite their knowledge of mechanisms available to them within the health authority. The issue of individualism and privacy was important to her team, many of whom did not attend the health festival as there was a 'them' and 'us' attitude (which she explained had a long history) between the community and hospital workers. The issue of participation was a common theme in the observation material collected and in interviews, despite the image portrayed in written documentation. The extent of participation by domestic and portering staff, frequently mentioned, was limited because they did not feel a part of the hospital team, despite the vital tasks they performed on a daily basis in the workplace. They were curious and expressed their curiosity by talking to ML and LW as well as myself, but were still afraid to take any further step towards active participation. It was pointed out that participation would cost them nothing but they remained unconvinced.

Gender and 'Race'. 'Race' is an issue discussed in the broader context of the community and its documentation in relation to health strategy. A few black women (mainly nurses and health care assistants) attended the event and were willing to sample some of the materials/products available. LW commented that a couple of the women complained that there was nothing for them in terms of skin care range. On investigation, this was discovered not to be the case as Max Factor and Chanel beauticians both sell products for black skin (although admittedly, one had to ask). What these women were probably referring to were familiar brand names that they could readily relate to, e.g., 'Iman', 'Fashion Fair' and so on, so it could be argued that they had a point. Also it was apparent that there were no ethnic foodstuffs on display. In terms of the presence of role models, there were a couple of exhibitors, one demonstrating Indian head massage and the other products for the prevention of osteoporosis. In terms of worker relations issues, again some matters arose during interview but they require further exploration.

Relaxation was an issue of importance to both men and women. Both groups expressed interest in complementary therapies and took away useful information from the event. Double shifts and the inability to unwind were concerns that were expressed during interview, particularly by nurses with young families who were finding combining shift work with motherhood stressful. Women tended to reveal this if issues of children and social life were brought into the discussion. One staff nurse confessed after a while that she had no time for a social life with her four children. It was a matter of organizing them by doing domestic chores before and after work. In fact she came to work for a rest!

Needs of Workers. The event was organized by people with a professional stake in the organization. Canvassing opinion of the entire organization was not undertaken by the planning team, which I felt was problematic in terms of generating interest, ideas and cooperation, but also for potential participation in the event itself.

It was through listening to, observing and interviewing staff that I was able to uncover their needs and attitudes to health matters at work. More interviews with staff over a longer period of time would have been beneficial and will be a consideration for the study itself. It was interesting that catering staff saw themselves mainly as onlookers in the planning and participation of the Festival. One group questioned the weekend after the event mentioned that healthy eating issues were discussed to the point of boredom in the work they do and the courses they have taken but they would have liked some other activities such as tai chi or reiki. One of their colleagues had such an appointment the following week, as apparently the tai chi workshops were arranged to operate fortnightly after the Festival as part of the move by the trust to manage staff stress.

Emergent themes from the pilot study

Thematic analysis was undertaken of the material that was collected. Emergent themes from the observations and interviews were as follows:

- the desire to publicize the hospital as a health promoter/nice place to work;
- managers interested in reputation only:

  'They were initially hostile to any interventions that were not initiated by them.' (Respondent 2)

  'The Chief Executive shook my hand and asked "Are you from the press?" When she discovered that I was not, she breathed a huge sigh of relief, and chatted about the wonderful display in the foyer instead.' (Observation note – the event)

- staff interest in health promotion issues in some spheres but time an issue. Others see health promotion in terms of their patients rather than for themselves. Health was seen as a private matter for the individual and to be kept so.
- ambivalence of the role of the organization, care-oriented.

  'They were prevention oriented and needs of staff was largely piecemeal, not at the heart of the organization.' (Respondent 3)

- operation within political and financial constraints.

  'They were awaiting the publication of the White Paper on Public Health and how the organization should comply rather than taking a pro-active stance.' (Observation notes of Planning Meeting No. 2)

Reflections upon my approach to data collection

Focusing on what to explore in the beginning was difficult as gaining a sense of the organization through impressions of its activity was more important in the early days. Making discoveries and allowing situations to present themselves was something I quickly learned to do as I became used to the environment, and referring to my field notes initially to make sense of the environment was extremely beneficial. It was only after several observations and much note-taking and ordering, did something more cohesive begin to emerge, enabling me to plan future observations, and prepare questions to ask during interview situations. For example, this would include observing the reactions and responses of others in a meeting to the gatekeeper, noting who was actually in charge, who were the motivators on the committee and so on.

There were many influences, such as group dynamics, that made for a more flexible approach to data collection. Adopting a rigid focus would have meant overlooking crucial factors such as the politics of the planning committee, their views on their managers, health and people generally. Their personalities began to emerge as time moved on. It was also interesting to find out about some of the 'life' of the organization. It was apparent that a lot of information documented in my diary reflected upon meetings and the event itself. The use of semi-structured interviews provided much more focus and control for me as interviewer as I knew the issues I wanted to explore further but this was only achieved some time after scrutinizing observation and diary data, so in a sense the process of data collection flowed from one to another, although it must be stated that keeping the main research question in view is something I had to maintain, otherwise it would have been easy to drift into other areas of interest, which is why so many qualitative researchers end up with superfluous data that require a good deal of editing.

I also felt that observation of the event was useful in terms of gaining access to the true views of people in the organization. The process of triangulation in the study was extremely useful in a methodological sense because I was able to combine aspects of the analysed data to obtain a distinct impression of the organisation's attitude to workplace health issues. Theoretical triangulation provided the focus for adapting ideas about culture and workplace health improvement.

I decided that this would require further development in the main study and found the Schein model useful, but I felt the need to develop my own based on further reading and my developed understanding of hospitals as a setting in which to undertake research of this nature. I did find a better way of making distinctions between structure, function and interaction within the organization and related health issues.

References

Alfredsson, L., Spetz, C. L. and Theorell, T. (1985) Type of occupation and near future hospitalization for myocardial infarction and some other diagnoses. *International Journal of Epidemiology*, **14**: 378–8.

Barratt, E. S. (1990) Human resources management: organisational culture. *Management Update* **2** (1): 21–32.

Beckhard, R. (1969) *Organisational Development: Strategies and Models* (Reading: Addison-Wesley).

Breucker, G. (1998) *Success Factors of Workplace Health Promotion* (BKK, Germany: Bundesverband).

Conrad, P. (1987) Wellness in the workplace: potentials and pitfalls of worksite health promotion. *Milbank Quarterly* **65**: 255–75.

Deal, T. E. and Kennedy, A. A. (1982) *Corporate Culture: The Rites and Rituals of Corporate Life* (Reading: Addison-Wesley).

Deal, T. E. and Kennedy, A. A. (1983) Culture: A new look through old lenses. *Journal of Applied Behavioural Sciences*, **19** (4): 497–507.

Denison, D. R. (1984) Bringing corporate culture to the bottom line. *Organizational Dynamics*, **13** (2): 5–22.

Department of Health (1993) *Taskforce, Health of the Nation* (London: Department of Health).

Department of Health (1998) *Saving Lives: Our Healthier Nation* (London: Department of Health).

Duncombe, J. and Marsden, D. (1995) Can men love? 'Reading', 'staging' and 'resisting' the romance. In L. Pearce and J. Stacy (eds), *Romance Revisited* (London: Lawrence and Wishart), pp. 238–50.

European Commission (1997) Green Paper. Partnership for a New Organisation of Work. European Commission, Belgium.

Fielding, J. and Breslow, L. (1983) Health promotion programs sponsored by Californian employers. *American Journal of Public Health* **73**: 538–42.

Fineman, S. (1988) Dominant discourse, professional language and legal change in child custody decision-making. *Harvard Law Review*, **101**: 727.

Fineman, S. (1993) *Emotions in Organizations* (London: Sage).

Frankenhauser, M. (1991) *A Biopsychosocial Approach to Work-Life Issues* (New York: Baywood Publishing).

Frankfort-Nachmias, C. and Nachmias, D. (1992) *Research Methods in the Social Sciences* (London: Edward Arnold).

Gardell, B. (1971) Alienation and mental health in the modern industrial environment. In L. Levi (ed.), *Society, Stress and Disease*, vol. 1 (Oxford: Oxford University Press).

Gardell, B. (1976) *Job Content and Quality of Life* (Stockholm: Prisma).

Gardell, B. (1979) Technology, alienation and mental health. *Acta Sociologica*, **19** (1): 83–93.

Gerhardt, U. (1989) *Ideas About Illness: An Intellectual and Political History of Medical Sociology* (Basingstoke: Macmillan).

Green, G. M. and Baker, F. (1991) *Work, Health and Productivity* (New York: Oxford University Press).

Hall, E. (1991) *Gender, Work Control and Stress: A Theoretical Discussion and Empirical Test* (New York: Baywood Publishing).

House of Commons Select Committee on Science and Technology (1983), *Occupational Health and Hygiene Services*, 2nd report, vol. 2 (London: HMSO).

Handy, C. (1985) *Understanding Organisations* (Harmondsworth: Penguin).

Harrison, R. (1972) Understanding your organisation's character. *Harvard Business Review* **3**: 119–28.

Hochschild, A. (1983) *The Managed Heart: The Commercialisation of Human Feeling* (Berkeley, CA: University of California Press).

Hoskin, D. and Fineman, S. (1990) Organizing processes. *Journal of Management Studies* **27** (6): 583–604.

Kizer, W. M. (1987) *The Healthy Workplace: A Blueprint for Corporate Action* (Canada: John Wiley and Sons).

Knox, S. (1985) The relation of social support and working environment to medical variables associated with elevated blood pressure in young males: a structural model. *Social Science and Medicine*, **21**: 525–31.

Marmot, M. (1984) *Immigrant Mortality in England and Wales 1970: Causes of Death by Country of Birth* (London: HMSO).

Marmot, M. and Theorell, T. (1987) Look after your heart: stress and cardiovascular disease – a studiable case? *Health Trends*, **19** (3): 21–5.

Marmot, M. and Theorell, T. (1988) Social class and cardiovascular disease: the contribution of work. *International Journal of Health Services*, **18** (4): 659–74.

Ministry of Health (1964) *Health Education Report of a Joint Committee of Central Scottish Health Services Councils (The Cohen Report)* (London: HMSO).

Merriam, S. et al. (2002) *Qualitative Research in Practice* (San Francisco: Jossey-Bass).

Ouchi, W. G. (1981) *Theory Z* (Reading, MA: Addison-Wesley).

Peters, T. J. and Waterman, R. H. (1982) *In Search of Excellence* (New York: Harper and Row).

Van Maanen, J. and Kunda, G. (1989) 'Real feelings': emotional expression and organizational culture. In M. M. Staw and L. L. Cummings (eds), *Research in Organisational Behaviour*, vol. 11 (London: JAI Press), pp. 43–103.

Sathe, V. (1983) *Managerial Action and Corporate Culture* (Homewood: Irwin).

Schein, E. (1982) The role of the founder in creating organisational culture. *Organisational Dynamics* (Summer: 13–63.

Schein, E. (1985) *Organisational Culture and Leadership* (San Francisco: Jossey Bass).

Silverman, D. (1970) *The Theory of Organisations* (London: Heinemann).

Springett, J. and Dugdill, L. (1995) Workplace health promotion programmes: towards a framework for evaluation. *Health Education Journal* **54**: 88–98.

Waldron, H. A. (1996) Occupational health during the Second World War: Hope deferred or hope abandoned? *Medical History*, **41**: 197–212.

Walton, R. (1985) The management of interdependent conflict: a model and review. *Administrative Science Quarterly*, **14**: 73–84.

Wilkins, A. L. and Ouchi, W. G. (1983) Efficient cultures: exploring the relationship between culture and organisational performance. *Administration Science Quarterly* **28**: 468–81.

Wilkinson, C. (1997) *Managing Health at Work* (London: E. F. Spon/Chapman and Hall).

Wilkinson, C. (1999) Managers, the workplace and health promotion: fantasy or reality? *Health Education Journal* **1**: 54–65.

Wilkinson, S. and Kitzinger, C. (2000) Thinking differently about thinking positive: a discursive approach to cancer patients' talk. *Social Science and Medicine*, **50** (6): 797–811.

Williams, S. J. (1995) Theorizing class, health and lifestyles: can Bourdieu help us? *Sociology of Health and Illness*, **17** (5): 577–604.

Wilson, B. (1992) Staff nurses' perception of job empowerment and organisational committment: a test of Kanter's theory of structural power in organisations. *Journal of Nursing Administration*, **24** (4): 39–47.

World Health Organisation (1988) *Health Promotion for Working Populations. Technical Report Series 765* (Geneva: WHO).

Wynne, R. and Clarkin, N. (1992) *Under Construction: Building Health in the EC Workplace* (Dublin: European Foundation for the Improvement of Living and Working Conditions).

CHAPTER 9

Integrating Herbal Medicine into the National Health Service: Perspectives of General Practitioners

ANNE PARKIN AND CAROL WILKINSON

Herbal medicine has been used for thousands of years – according to recent knowledge, it was the ancient Egyptians who discovered medicine (Menzies-Trull 2003). Virtually all evidence of this ancient herbal knowledge was found written on six papyri; the medical papyrus is held in the British Museum (No. 10059) (Menzies-Trull 2003). Dating back to 1500 BC there are more than 700 herbal remedies described on the Egyptian Ebers Papyrus (DoH 2003a).

The philosophy of herbal medicine is the holistic principle that looks upon the body as a complete system, with all its parts being mutually dependent. Disease disturbs the homeostasis of the body, so the cure must not just treat the symptoms of the condition but the person as a whole. It is claimed that general practice is holistic (Allsop 1995), but this point can be argued as conventional medicine still focuses treatment on symptoms, although some preventative medicine does take place. GPs as generalists need to know something about everything, including having a working knowledge of complementary medicine, but they would not be expected to become practising herbalists per se.

Herbs are the foundation of therapeutic systems in many countries throughout the world. Eighty per cent of people in Africa use traditional herbal medicine as their main, if not their only, source of primary health care (World Health Organization 2003). Today where pollution, pesticides, hormone-fattened animals and so-called wonder drugs (Hedley and Shaw 2002) are commonplace, people have begun to look for safer alternatives, particularly in health care. An estimated 30 per cent of British people have tried herbal medicine and approximately £31 million is spent on herbal remedies and treatments annually (Ernst 2004).

Literature review

Looking at the available literature in reports, journal articles and books, there seems to be an increasing interest in complementary and alternative medicine (CAM) but with no reported information on the possibility of seeing a herbalist at a local GP's surgery, or in fact being referred to a herbalist by a doctor. The National Health Service (NHS) ought to look at this matter seriously as it is argued that it could reduce its sizeable drug budget considerably with relatively low cost herbal medicines (Ernst 2004).

The large pharmaceutical companies would probably not look favourably upon herbal medicines, unless they could see a way into the market themselves. If pharmaceutical companies became involved, millions of pounds could be generated for research that may ultimately be beneficial to western herbal medicine, unless they closed ranks and tried to squeeze herbalism out of the picture completely. A survey in 1996 indicated that a mere 0.08% of the NHS research budget in the UK and only 0.05% of the medical charities budget was allocated to CAM research (House of Lords 2000).

There is some information on the integration of various medical therapies, but none on GPs' reactions to this possibility. The review of literature puts forward the theory that most people would like to see an integrated NHS that puts all forms of treatment within reach of the public at large – should they so wish – and not just those who can afford to pay for alternative treatments. If the latter were the case, it would accentuate a two-tier system, allowing the wealthy but not the poor a choice of treatments (Weil 2003) unless it was available on the NHS or was sponsored. 'We consider that without a shift of resources to the less well off, both in and out of work, little will be accomplished in terms of a reduction of health inequalities by interventions addressing particular "downstream" influences' (Shaw et al. 1999, p. 209).

According to Allsop (1995), there is evidence of more widespread use of alternative medicine, including self-help remedies. In an ideal scenario, to complement existing GP services, health centres could employ acupuncturists, herbalists and other therapists as appropriate all under one roof, funded by the NHS or medical aid schemes, thereby empowering the patient to take charge of their health under complete medical supervision (Weil 2003).

The national 'health policy' is largely restricted to the policies of reigning governments, which refers to the 'intent about action which relates to the maintenance of good health in individuals and populations; the cure of disease and illness; and the care of the vulnerable and frail' (Allsop 1995, p. 4).

The health policy has three main approaches:

1. to focus on an individual and their health care;
2. to achieve a more equal distribution of health services;
3. to follow a structuralist approach – to seek wider-ranging social improvements beyond a conventional health service (Allsop 1984).

The table of health service priorities, referred to by Bowling (1993), that showed the mean priority rankings of the public and doctors indicated that complementary and alternative medicines were rated extremely low by GPs, consultants, public health doctors and the public in general. The lowest priorities were given to complementary medicine, low-birth weight babies, infertility treatment and cosmetic surgery. Seeing how the latter three have gained respect and have become acceptable, perhaps CAM as a whole and herbal medicine in particular will be perceived differently now. Since the research was conducted, there has been a renaissance in complementary medicine over the last decade. Consequently, if the same opinions were canvassed today there might be a different outcome.

Looking at recent research in Israel, a survey conducted by Mizrachi et al. (2004) shows that there is increasing use of alternative therapies in the population generally. Up to a quarter of the adult population in western European countries and almost half of the population in the United States have used some form of alternative therapy (Mizrachi et al. 2004). There have been many reasons for this swing to CAM, namely:

> the growing disillusionment with the technology and bureaucracy of biomedicine and increased questioning of its excessive invasiveness; heightened consumer awareness of iatrogenic effects of modern medicine and growth in expectations for quality service including structural changes in the physician–patient relationship as well as widespread demystification which have led to considerable erosion of confidence in Big Science as a means of solving problems. (Mizrachi et al. 2004, pp. 24–5)

In research conducted in Bath in the 1990s, the public indicated that the community should be more involved with, and have a say in, the purchasing intentions of health authorities (Bowling 1993). One of the problems highlighted was that there was a limited amount of information available regarding cost-effectiveness and the outcome of treatments (Bowling 1993). This lends itself to the argument that herbal treatments could work out less expensive than pharmaceutical drugs, and their outcomes could, on the whole, be positive as there are relatively few side effects compared with many conventional treatments.

Bowling (1993) also noted that that 52 per cent of people interviewed strongly agreed that preventing illness was at least as important as curing it, and 44 per cent indicated that they strongly agreed that financial cost should not be considered when deciding whether to provide treatment or not. This demonstrates that the cost of herbal medicine should not be the deciding factor in determining whether or not it should be offered as a treatment of choice for patients in GPs' surgeries. Again, if this research was conducted today the results might be even more favourable as there has been such a huge upswing in the interest in CAM since 1993.

Back in December 2001, an article in the *Sunday Times* reported that the government had said it would be prepared to offer patients alternative treatments on the NHS if (and this could be the 'get-out' clause for the government, as there has been very little research conducted) the government regulators confirmed their effectiveness (Carr-Brown 2001). Alan Milburn, who was Secretary of State for Health at the time, indicated that he wanted complementary medicine practitioners to be licensed to work under contract to the NHS, using medicines and treatments that would be approved (Carr-Brown 2001). Alan Milburn's spokesman admitted receiving thousands of letters each year from patients who receive complementary treatments, and he felt CAM did have a place in the NHS (Carr-Brown 2001). Yet Alan Milburn was also reported as saying that he believed that the NHS should be spending more on drugs (ABPI 2003); this could have something to do with the fact that the 2000 Labour Party Conference was financed by various drug companies (Rattigan 2003).

The CAM market has reached figures in excess of one billion pounds per annum. With figures like these and five million people reportedly paying for such treatments (Carr-Brown 2001), something should be done to incorporate CAM into primary care. GPs would be able to set up contracts with approved complementary therapists (Carr-Brown 2001); this practice could also be extended into secondary care. Herbal medicine is valuable in primary care due to the fact that it treats the patient holistically. 'Western herbalism is characterised by a person-centred approach where the patient rather than the disease is the focus of the practitioner's attention' (DoH 2003, p. 30).

Doctors in general practice usually have ten-minute consultations, which do not allow time to treat the person holistically; there is only time to treat the symptoms. In herbal medicine, treatment is supported by advising patients on lifestyle choices and nutrition, with many practitioners today supporting a combination of both traditional and scientific values (DoH 2003b).

Practice-based commissioning is a new development that is indicative of the way in which both primary care and the NHS are changing. Health care professionals will see their responsibilities expand as new partnerships are formed with GPs to deliver GMS and PMS (DoH 2005a). The Rt Hon John Hutton, in a speech to GPs on 9 March 2005, said: 'If there is an alternative that is better for the patient and better for the NHS, they will have the freedom to change the way services are delivered. It gives the initiative to primary care professionals to the lead the debate about how essential services are reformed' (DoH 2005a).

Prince Charles, His Royal Highness the Prince of Wales, has always maintained that alternative forms of medication should be freely available on the NHS for all patients and he has been outspoken about his approval of CAM, although many people criticize his philosophy on life in general. What he says makes sense. He spoke to NHS managers about CAM availability for all patients, and although the managers did not agree with what he was saying, 75 per cent of the UK population would like to see complementary medicines freely available on the NHS (*Medical News Today* 2004). Most people still want to have conventional medicine freely available to them, but many would prefer to use complementary treatments for everyday minor illnesses (Ranshaw 2003). Dr Gill Morgan, from the NHS Confederation, stated that the NHS can only use therapies that have been shown to work, basically that are tried and tested, and evidence-based which, given the nature of CAM, means that many forms of practice would presumably be eliminated (*Medical News Today* 2004). There are numerous conflicting ideas as to what is best practice for the NHS, but by incorporating complementary therapies, e.g., western herbal medicine, into mainstream medicine, patients would be encouraged to take some responsibility for their own treatment, by emphasizing and encouraging preventative medicine (*Medical News Today* 2004).

The National Institute for Clinical Excellence (NICE) in the United Kingdom is the body that advises the NHS on the best treatments and therapies available. It has guardedly welcomed treatments such as reflexology and t'ai chi, for example, for the treatment of multiple sclerosis, because they are known to relieve the symptoms (*Medical News Today* 2004).

Since the inauguration of the NHS in 1948, the Royal Homeopathic Hospital in London has been part of the system. There has been no further integration of complementary and alternative medicines into the NHS. In the late 1970s, the government in Britain started to look more positively at movements that placed greater emphasis on preventative medicine and community care (Turner 1996). Prince Charles has been involved with the current government's decision to launch a five-year programme of research into complementary medicine. The research was programmed to start at the latter end of 2003, with funding of approximately £7.5 million. Some complementary therapies may be found to be ineffective from a scientific basis and there are bound to be some negative conclusions, but these results are important too, as the research should bring together all forms of medicine, creating an integrated health care system (*Medical News Today* 2004).

Many GPs would agree that there are significant gaps in the ability of conventional medicine to treat a wide range of chronic diseases, such as arthritis, anxiety, mild depression, irritable bowel disease and psychosomatic diseases (Ranshaw 2003), and they would be happy for these patients to be treated, for example, with herbal medicine. It seems logical therefore that the NHS should be able to offer both conventional and complementary medicine as part of an integrated approach to health care (Ranshaw 2003). Patients may feel more confident if their GP is part of an integrated team, who is able to refer the patient to a CAM practitioner within the practice. It has to be better and safer than the current system, where many patients seek complementary therapies without their GP's knowledge (Ranshaw 2003).

Modernizing the NHS could be said to be courageous and ground-breaking. Many GPs and their patients would like to see an NHS that provides integrated health care services with greater choice for patients (Illich 1995). If building a truly patient-centred, modern NHS – that offers both conventional and complementary medicine as the norm – is considered worthwhile, what is the government waiting for? Moving towards a patient-centred health service might be beneficial in more than one area; it may also take the pressure off the current financially fragile NHS by substantially reducing the nation's drug budget (Ranshaw 2003). 'The White Paper *The New NHS – Modern and Dependable*, which was published in 1997, claimed that Health Action Zones would "blaze the trail" for modernising the NHS' (Shaw et al. 1999, p. 175).

To date, there have been no new or innovative developments in primary care, apart from doctor appraisal and the abolition of fund-holding, which was government policy. There is the scope to incorporate many types of medicine into mainstream practice. The number of complementary practitioners available would hopefully reduce the workload of overstretched GPs, whilst offering a valuable service to patients. The government has said that it will look favourably on alternative medicine, but has failed thus far to deliver its proposals.

Inequalities in health, discussed by Frank Dobson, Secretary of State at the time, in 1998 (Shaw et al. 1999) have not changed over the last six or seven years. People who are financially secure have a choice of medical treatment, whereas the people who are the worst off have no option whatsoever. In the same paper, Dobson suggested that without waiting for changes in the law, local area small-scale research/surveys could be conducted to gather information and indicate what could be achieved (Shaw et al. 1999). What evidence is there that any small-scale surveys have been conducted? It is just such research that may prove beneficial and worthwhile for future medical practice.

Considering that £1.6 billion was spent on the rocketing complementary medicine business last year, it is a worrying realization that less than 8p of every £100 that the NHS spends on medical research funds was actually spent on complementary treatments (*HealthMall*, n.d.). The Lords Science and Technology Committee (2000) reported, after conducting a fifteen-month inquiry, that there should be stricter regulations regarding the complementary medicine business to protect consumers (Mills 2001). It indicated that patients were being put at risk due to lack of research and the dependence on self-regulation throughout the alternative medicine field. One positive aspect of the report suggested that therapies with a proven track record of research (acupuncture, herbal medicine, homeopathy and osteopathy) should be made available on the NHS (Mills 2001). This is good news for all concerned should it ever become a reality. However, Saks (1992) reported these same findings in the early 1990s.

According to research conducted in north-east Scotland in 1999, 65 per cent of patients using CAM had consulted their GP previously for the same complaint, which seems to indicate that the lack of improvement resulted in patients seeking alternative medication (Emslie et al. 2002). Of these patients, 37.5 per cent said that their GP knew that they were using alternative medicines, 9 per cent of them receiving CAM treatment from their GP (Emslie et al. 2002).

When looking at the relatively small amount of information that is available, CAM professionals should expect to be accredited independently, and this ought to be standardized across the board (Mills 2001). If CAM professionals have undertaken a three- to five-year degree course, in addition to having to fulfil a minimum of 500 hours of clinical experience, they should be suitably qualified to work in primary care. GPs should also endeavour to become more familiar with CAM (Mills 2001), especially as its popularity has grown over the last decade or so. It would be an ideal scenario to have patients treated by a qualified herbalist, working in conjunction with a GP, rather than patients self-medicating and their doctors being unaware of any alternative medication that their patients are ingesting. A recent report stated that those people working in the best regulated CAM professions (herbal medicine and acupuncture ought to be in this group) should work towards integration with conventional medicine (Mills 2001).

One report stated that German GPs readily referred their patients for CAM treatments, with herbal medicine being one such treatment (Schmidt et al. 2002). The same report claims that both Germany and the United Kingdom have a positive approach to, and a high interest in, CAM. This interest would be investigated in the proposed research for this project, albeit a small research assignment in respect of national figures. When questioned, many members of the public expressed concern about taking conventional medication, describing it as 'artificial, chemical and unnatural' because pharmaceutical drugs are manufactured rather than naturally occurring (Britten 1996).

Like the United Kingdom, the United States of America is having a CAM boom. In 1999 a study was carried out on practitioners, both mainstream and complementary, who met to discover whether 'integrative medicine' could be practised. They had to work together to examine, diagnose and prescribe for a patient with a particular problem (Anderson 1999). One finding was that they could all relate to and discuss the problem, but terminology was limited to scientific biomedical language (Anderson 1999). Such coordination could easily become a reality in this country, if the General Medical Council (GMC) and the European Herbal Practitioners Association (EHPA) boards could liaise with the NHS and the Prince of Wales' Foundation for Integrated Health (PWFIH) over the future of CAM.

After qualifying, education and reflective practice should continue in all fields of medicine. The role of the medical practitioner will constantly be re-shaped in years to come by the reorganization and rationalization of medical care (Schön 2003). This can already be seen in the acceptance of nurse-practitioners and nurse-prescribers as part of the medical team. With a little foresight and restructuring, western herbal medicine could be usefully incorporated into the realms of clinical practice.

Looking at research conducted by Shuval and Mizrachi (2004), the boundary between conventional medicine and complementary medicine can be seen to have moved over the last few years. The findings show an integration by complementary practitioners into fields that have traditionally been the domain of biomedicine (Shuval and Mizrachi 2004). Due to the very different styles of practice followed by CAM and conventional medicine, the smooth transition of CAM into integrated medicine will probably meet with some antagonism, particularly from the biomedical side. Conventional practice 'focuses on the principles of the natural sciences, especially biology and biochemistry, in terms of irreducible cellular and molecular processes and is guided by assumptions of objectivism, determinism, and positivism' (Shuval and Mizrachi 2004, p. 2).

The National Centre of Complementary and Alternative Medicine (NCCAM) describes alternative medicine as 'a group of diverse medical and health care systems, practices and products that are not presently considered to be part of orthodox medicine' (Shuval and Mizrachi 2004, p. 2).

In herbal medicine, there have been very few controlled, evidence-based trials; therefore many doctors doubt its efficacy, even though it is effective for many people, and has been used successfully for thousands of years. As conventional therapeutics have relied heavily on evidence-based medicine recently, 'whole categories of intervention, such as complementary therapies, may be relatively neglected, owing to a combination of therapist suspicion of trial methodology and the absence of funding. This results in an absence of evidence for potentially useful treatments, about which guidelines therefore have to remain silent' (Goodman et al. 2000, p. 55).

Currently there are large areas of medicine where there is very little evidence-based, clinical data available, but that 'lack of evidence must not be mistaken for lack of effort, or for that area's unworthiness' (Goodman et al. 2000, p. 39). By encouraging doctors to practise up-to-date medicine through adopting evidence-based practice protocols and submitting to strategies that have been proven in previous random clinical trials, herbal medicine is also under threat of having to undergo scientific, double-blind trials and further research: 'The practice of evidence-based medicine means integrating individual clinical expertise with the best available external clinical evidence from systematic research' (Sackett et al. 1997, p. 3).

CAM embraces so many different forms of medicine and health-related therapies that it is unfortunate, in some respects, that herbal medicine has been grouped with the likes of crystal therapy and aromatherapy. Herbal medicine adheres to a holistic approach as its hypothesis in health care, where the patient will be able to heal himself or herself bodily by using the energetic qualities of herbs.

In Israel, as in the United Kingdom, complementary medicine is not financed by the state but patients can purchase extra cover from their medical aid or sick funds to include this service. In 2000, 45 per cent of the Israeli population purchased these supplementary insurance policies (Shuval and Mizrachi 2004). The number of practising CAM practitioners in Israel has increased from 5,500 part- and full-time practitioners in 1998 to 8,800 in

2003 (Shuval and Mizrachi 2004). This rising number demonstrates that there is a demand for this form of medicine, indicating the way in which demand is going. Many people in the United Kingdom would like a choice of health care to suit their needs. Herbal medicine could prove to be a viable form of complementary medicine available to all NHS patients in the future.

For the medical profession in Israel to retain its status, power and control, the changing direction of large sectors of the medical fraternity needs to be seen against the growing demand for CAM practitioners by the general public (Shuval and Mizrachi 2004). In the United Kingdom, if herbal medicine were to be phased into general practice gradually, there would be no threat to either set of practitioner (conventional or herbal) because treating patients is not a competition and neither speciality can claim exclusively that their method of practice is better than any other. The overall benefit to patients, however, would be invaluable.

At least 66 per cent of all medical schools in the USA offer CAM information in their core curriculum (NCCAM and the Royal College of Physicians 2001) but it stands to reason that a practitioner, who has specialized in phytotherapy, training for three to five years to degree level, will have more expertise in herbalism than a GP who has studied herbal medicine as a small part of his or her wide-ranging curriculum.

With CAM degrees being offered at approximately five universities in the United Kingdom, the knowledge of western herbal medicine will increase, as will the number of practitioners who therefore may be available to work in general practice when state registration occurs. Statutory Regulation of Herbal Medicine and Acupuncture is currently also being considered (DoH 2005a): 'It is anticipated that the statutory self-regulation of herbalists and modernisation of the medicines legislation will bring about a number of much needed improvements that will ensure the safety and quality of herbal practice and medicines' (DoH 2003a, p. 33).

The proposal for the regulation of herbal practitioners in the United Kingdom is outlined in the Department of Health document, which also includes a recommendation for the reform of section 12(1) of the Medicines Act 1968 (DoH 2003b). There are 45,000 CAM practitioners in the UK alone (Saks 1999) with 1,300 being herbal practitioners who are members of voluntary registers, with half of them practising western herbal medicine (DoH 2003b). One option for regulation has been to have a shared council, the Complementary and Alternative Medicine Council (CAM Council), for both herbal medicine and acupuncture. Such a council would be advantageous in that there would be a greater number of practitioners, which in turn would prove more cost effective. 'A larger council would have a greater degree of influence and would be better equipped to protect both the interests of patients and practitioners' (DoH 2003a, p. 16).

With herbal degree courses now being available, the so-called 'quacks' could be prevented from working in the medical world. Unfortunately, some excellent herbalists, who are self-taught or have undertaken short courses and have been practising successfully for many years, would possibly be prevented from working with doctors in a primary care setting because they are not graduates. This may be unfair as many herbalists provide a high quality service. From a biomedical slant, the degree courses offer an excellent grounding in anatomy and physiology, important not only for diagnoses and physical examinations but also for enabling herbalists to converse confidently with GPs, from a medical point of view, when discussing patients.

Looking at the available literature, there appears to be no information on herbalists working in general practice as most work privately. As there is a gap in the literature on the subject of whether GPs would consider working together in practice with western medical herbalists, and the research, albeit on a small scale, conducted for this project, there is still scope to discover whether or not it would be beneficial to pursue this idea. There is a significant amount of literature available regarding CAM and conventional medicine, but little evidence of GPs' thoughts on the matter of working with and referring to western medical herbalists.

Method of investigation

Background information to study

Currently most herbalists work in private practice but within the new general practice framework, it could be in the interests of the NHS to diversify and employ herbalists as there is a shortfall in doctors entering general practice, and many practices are understaffed. The extent of the shortage is evidenced by the number of foreign doctors being brought in to fill these positions (*Source Correspondent* 2003).

Having spoken to a number of GPs socially over the past year, there seems to be a mixed attitude towards herbal medicine. Many GPs do not have any understanding of what it entails, most relating it to homoeopathy or Chinese herbal medicine. Surprisingly, however, some GPs are totally in favour of complementary medicine and demonstrate an interest in herbal medicine. Those GPs (and a number of consultants) who are opposed to herbal medicine are very often the ones who believe it is restricted to homoeopathy, which is probably due to a lack of knowledge. Given the huge costs that burden the National Health Service, herbal treatment could prove to be a relatively safe and less expensive option for some chronic disease management (Ranshaw 2003).

Research objectives

This study uses the qualitative approach of phenomenology which quite simply means 'the study or description of phenomena' (Hammond et al.

1991, p. 1), originating from the Greek words 'phainomenon' meaning an appearance, and 'logos', denoting a reason or a word, therefore it is a 'reasoned enquiry' (Stewart and Mickunas 1974, p. 3). The phenomenon is 'anything that appears or presents itself to someone' (Hammond et al. 1991, p. 1) and anything which appears to 'consciousness is a justifiable area of philosophic exploration' (Stewart and Mickunas 1974, p. 3). It 'aims to make sense of, or interpret, phenomena in terms of the meanings people bring to them' (Greenhalgh and Taylor 1997). Information must be obtained without any prejudice or preconceived ideas on the part of the researcher. In this study, the researcher will attempt to discover GPs' beliefs regarding integrated medicine and whether they would consider working alongside western medical herbalists in primary care.

The process of investigation enabled data to be collected from taped interviews with GPs that was transcribed at a later date, allowing for observation of the respondents in conjunction with listening to their replies to questions (Locke et al. 2000). Although the interview questions were pre-set, they were open-ended questions allowing for freedom of discussion and unbiased responses – which is also referred to as naturalistic research (Locke et al. 2000). This approach is both sensitive and humanistic as there was a two-way interaction between interviewer and interviewee, allowing for non-verbal communication to also be accessed.

The design

For this qualitative study, it was appropriate to interview GPs rather than send out questionnaires. Initially five GPs were interviewed for a pilot study, testing reliability, where results are produced consistently, and validity, addressing the same issue concerning the degree of confidence (Bowling 1997) in the questions. This number was ideal for purposive sampling (Locke et al. 2000). Purposive sampling was used because the researcher selected participants who were both willing and able to provide the best information to accomplish the objectives of the project (Kumar 1999). This means of selection was advantageous due to the time constraints on this research project. The pilot study determined whether the questions in the interview schedule were correctly structured, or whether they needed altering or omitting entirely. With regard to the interview questions, it was felt that specific answers might be given during previous questions which could stilt the flow of the interview; therefore a semi-structured interview, allowing for flexibility of questioning, was required (Saunders et al. 2003).

Once the pilot study of five interviews had proved to be of value and reliable, meetings with another five GPs were arranged. Information letters and consent forms were sent to a number of GPs. The GPs who agreed to the research were interviewed, using the revised questions from the interview schedule. Interviews were conducted at a mutually agreeable time and place.

Taking into consideration that GPs have severe time constraints, the aim was to be able to conduct each of these interviews within thirty minutes, taping the dialogue for transcription at a later stage.

Interviewing was the method of data collection that helped to collate valid and reliable information which was pertinent to the research questions and objectives (Saunders et al. 2003); whereas the interview schedule was the research tool used to collect information (Kumar 1999). Although the questions were predetermined and were the same for each interviewee, the semi-structured interview sanctioned further development, allowing the researcher to ask supplementary questions that gave scope for individual expansion. Questionnaires would not have been an ideal format as numerous open-ended questions were asked (Saunders et al. 2003).

It was important to elicit information that was unbiased and correct from the data, and that was not clouded by the researcher's own thoughts, ideals and desired outcomes. According to Bowling (1997), qualitative research is not as intrusive as quantitative investigation in that it does not influence the research setting, despite the fact that the researcher is attempting to examine people in their usual environment whilst collecting naturally occurring data.

Interviewing was advantageous due to its flexibility, allowing an interviewee to answer questions freely and to digress if necessary. This method also allowed the interviewer the freedom of pursuing lines of investigation if required (Melia 1987). The interviewer could observe the interviewee's reactions because verbal and non-verbal communication were witnessed first hand.

The phenomenological approach was best suited to this research because it is 'the analysis of everyday life' and allows the researcher 'to establish its underlying assumptions' (Turner 1996, p. 4). It is a 'lived experience', and offers information derived from this knowledge.

This research, although on a small scale, is neither minor nor trivial as it could, in the future, be beneficial to patients, GPs, herbalists and the NHS alike. If adopting a phenomenological approach, various phenomena sanctioned by the respondents need to be understood, resulting in a detailed set of data being collated (Saunders et al. 2003). Interpretism 'clarifies and extends meanings of interviewee's statements, but without imposing meaning on them' (Bryman 2004, p. 325). In essence, it is interpreting the data collected verbatim and transcribing the information without changing the fundamental essence of the replies.

Data collection procedure

The method of data collection was justified, as the time allocated to complete the project was only six months. For this study ten GPs in total were interviewed, five in the pilot and five in the main study.

After receiving approval for the research from the Lincolnshire Local Research Ethics Committee (LREC), the interviews were conducted over a period of seven weeks. The pilot interviews helped to collate relevant data that was applicable to the research questions and objectives (Saunders et al. 2003). The respondents were given the option of being interviewed at their respective surgeries, or at a suitable place, and time, convenient to them. Seven opted for their surgeries, two their homes and one interview was conducted in a supermarket coffee shop!

Ethical considerations

Considering the ethical aspects of any research is paramount. This does not only relate to the respondents and materials used in the research process, but also to the appropriateness of the interviewer's behaviour in relation to the rights of those who become the subject of the investigation (Saunders et al. 2003). Informed consent was sought from the GPs taking part in this research, and strict confidentiality regarding the interviews was adhered to. According to Kumar, 'seeking informed consent is probably the most common method of data collection used in medical and social research' (Kumar 1999, p. 192).

Data protection is important and all materials used in the research process would be kept safely locked away until completion of the project (a period of six months), after which any research material would be erased or destroyed to comply with local ethics requirements. This ensured that anonymity and confidentiality were adhered to. Quotes from interviews would also be used anonymously. The Data Protection Act of 1998 implements the EC Directive 95/46/EC, one of the primary purposes of which is to protect an individual's fundamental rights (DoH 2000). In January 2005 the Freedom of Information Act was fully implemented, when the General Right of Access to recorded information for all public authorities, including the NHS, came into force (Information Commissioner 2000). As a result of this legal requirement, total anonymity was upheld. Bias is another form of unethical behaviour; the researcher should neither hide what has been discovered in the study nor emphasize data inexplicably (Kumar 1999).

On completion of the research proposal, a copy was submitted to the academic supervisor for verification, prior to it being sent to the University of Lincoln's Ethics Committee. A further copy of the proposal was sent, in electronic form, to LREC for their approval. As the research was to be based in the local vicinity, LREC was approached as the committee to approve this project. Concurrently permission had to be sought from the local NHS Primary Care Trust (PCT) (in this case West Lincolnshire PCT) in order that GPs could be interviewed. Once the proposal had been approved and an honorary contract with the NHS was granted, research could commence.

Plans for analysis

When editing data obtained from the interviews, the information was scrutinized to reduce 'errors, incompleteness, misclassification and gaps in the information obtained from the respondents' (Kumar 1999, p. 200). Problems could occur, after interviews, when trying to recall information that had not been classified, as doing this could introduce mistakes into the data (Kumar 1999). Telephoning a respondent to clarify information could be a way of correcting mistakes, but could be time-consuming when time had been allocated in the first place for the interview. However, with taped interviews, apart from being unable to decipher muffled words, the need to clarify information should not arise.

Coding of data was possibly the most difficult part of this research, second to the analysis thereof. Attitudes towards an issue can be measured on an interval or ratio scale. Coding depends both on the way in which the measurement scale is used in the measurement of a variable and on how the questions are structured, whether they are open-ended or closed (Kumar 1999).

To code qualitative questions the content analysis must be adhered to. Although it was important to have specific categories identifying common areas, the variety of answers given by the respondents was vital too. Usually in qualitative research, the responses are used verbatim or are structured under specific themes and the actual responses are provided to validate them (Kumar 1999).

All the relevant data from audio tapes was transcribed. Devising a coding system required data to be batched according to the set criteria. This could be done numerically and/or alphabetically, according to the findings being analysed. The coding for these results was developed by taking specific language, common to several interviews, into account and each theme was coded with different coloured dots. Repetition of language, particular themes and styles, would be observed and noted too. Each piece of information was deciphered, ready for analysis at a later stage. This process was refined as coding progressed. 'Analysis of qualitative data can and should be done using explicit, systematic and reproducible methods' (Greenhalgh and Taylor 1997, p. 740).

In qualitative research the desired result is to collect information from individuals to gain a full understanding of the experience of those people (Greenhalgh and Taylor 1997). It is also important to realize that it is difficult to eliminate totally the researcher's bias in qualitative research (Greenhalgh and Taylor 1997). This is evident when 'participant observation is used, but it is also relevant for other forms of data collection and of data analysis' (Greenhalgh and Taylor 1997).

Once the information had been obtained, transcribed and coded, arbitrary authentication of the process was instigated until all variables for discrepancies had been isolated (Kumar 1999) and the coding was proven accurate. The researcher analysed the data systematically, looking for cases that challenged or disputed the theories derived from the majority of instances (Greenhalgh and Taylor 1997).

The researcher hoped that the research conducted would prove interesting as this could be the way forward for the integration of general practice with western herbal medicine. It would also provide an alternative for those patients who have tried conventional practice with little satisfaction. GPs would be the first to admit that there are just such patients in every practice. In the long run, the National Health Service should also benefit from this integrated system of medical practice, particularly as it has been highlighted in the *WHO Traditional Medicine Strategies 2002–2005* (WHO 2002).

Reflection

Downloading and completing the NHS Research Ethics Committee Application Form online proved to be quite a challenge. The form was extremely repetitive and took far too long to complete. On reflection it would have been easier to have had a hard copy to complete but, in the age of the internet, it is probably deemed easier for committees to access the completed application forms from source. The process of telephoning to have the form 'unlocked' online to alter two numerals, and then to have it relocked before reprinting the 57-page document seemed futile and a waste of paper!

LREC invited the researcher and supervisor to attend their monthly meeting on Wednesday, 17 November 2004, in Sleaford, Lincolnshire. The purpose of the researcher attending the meeting was to clarify anything that the committee was unsure of. It was quite daunting to sit in front of a panel of twelve members who questioned the researcher on various aspects of the study.

A week after the meeting, the researcher received a letter outlining changes that had to be made to the proposal before permission could be granted. This information had to be altered and highlighted, and resubmitted to the chairman of the committee via the administrator of LREC. A letter confirming a favourable ethical opinion was issued by LREC.

Concurrently, permission had to be obtained from the relevant primary care trusts to interview NHS GPs. This permission was approved, and two of the three trusts approached granted permission to interview GPs, i.e., West Lincolnshire PCT and Lincolnshire South-West PCT. East Lincolnshire PCT expressed a few concerns with the study and therefore was unable to approve the research. An honorary contract was issued to the researcher for the duration of the research by the Human Resources Department of the West Lincolnshire PCT NHS. This presumably was necessary for interviewing GPs at NHS premises and during hours where GPs were employed by the NHS. The research could then commence, some three months after initially submitting the research proposal to the university ethics board for approval. Hence only three months remained to conduct the research, analyse the data and have the project bound.

Pilot study

Beginning a pilot study can be quite daunting; in this case, the interview schedule had to be tested in an environment with professional people. Telephone calls were made to receptionists, secretaries or practice managers of surgeries that had been selected randomly. There was some difficulty making appointments initially; one reason perhaps could have been that GPs receive frequent calls from people requesting interviews for research, or from pharmaceutical companies trying to promote products, therefore time becomes an issue. Another reason was possibly a lack of interest. Perhaps if the research were to ultimately affect them, they would have been more approachable and amenable. The first interview of the pilot study was conducted with some trepidation, but the researcher felt quite comfortable asking the questions and expanding on anything that was misunderstood by the GP. It proved to be invaluable, as it made the interviewer realize how some questions could be answered in a single sentence. The respondent appeared relaxed during the interview and as the discussion developed. This interview proved interesting in that some of the questions asked later in the interview had already been answered in previous responses. LREC had advised that Question 14 be rephrased to read 'What are the implications of conventional medical treatment when considering a range of complementary medicines available to the public?' In the pilot study, GPs asked for this revised question to be repeated, as they were unsure what it was actually asking, which was the researcher's sentiment too! The original question was reinserted to read: 'What do you think the future holds for medicine, in light of the range of treatments available, both conventional and complementary?' In other words, how do GPs see all forms of medicine advancing in years to come?

The questions were answered briefly, considering they were open-ended. The interview lasted approximately twenty minutes. The outcome of the pilot study was reasonable given that these questions were being tested. Modification of one question was necessary plus, after the fourth interview, Question 8 was inserted after Question 5, a logical sequence which improved the interview flow. The interview schedule was satisfactory for the research being conducted. When conducting future interviews the researcher would endeavour to elicit more information from GPs, resulting in questions being answered more fully. The researcher was aware that Question 9 could appear as though future employment was being sought, so made light of the question, whilst still obtaining the information required. However, it could be advantageous for a practice to be the first to appoint a herbalist as a member of staff, especially as Beacon Practices seem to be the innovative practice in PCTs who provided leadership with new ideas and good standards of practice. This would be progress indeed in the integration of all forms of medicine.

Results and analysis

The transcribed data were analysed and common patterns and themes discovered (Saunders et al. 2003). These themes were partially determined by the interview questions and partly by common subject matter derived from the interviews. Responses obtained from the interviews have been arranged according to the order in which they appeared, probably led by the interview questions. Various quotes were used to substantiate GPs' thoughts and beliefs. GPs' names and the names of their practices have been omitted, ensuring confidentiality and anonymity, with each being assigned a respondent number for cohesion of replies. Some of these responses are quite lengthy, but the researcher deemed it necessary to include more of the content of the quotations in order that the essence of the replies would not be lost. Including interviewee's quotes in qualitative research is the equivalent of tables and graphs in quantitative research (Saunders et al. 2003). The purpose of this chapter is to present the facts obtained during the interview process.

Main themes emerging from analysis

As the eleven interviews with GPs progressed, key themes emerged from the content analysis. These themes can be related to the initial research question and are as follows:

1. Medical specialism
2. Connection with complementary medicine in terms of:
   (a) interest/lack of interest
   (b) training
3. GPs' definition of herbal medicine
4. Use of herbal medicine:
   (a) general use
   (b) patients admitting to using herbal medicine
   (c) GPs recommending herbal medicine to patients
5. Employment of a complementary therapist
6. Consumer information about complementary medicine
7. Economic factors in relation to complementary medicine on the NHS
8. Use of complementary medicine as a referral
9. The future of complementary medicine

10. The values of the use of complementary medicine
    (a) value to the patient
    (b) personal value to the GP
11. Responsibility for the patient

1. Medical specialism

All GPs are experts in their field of general practice, yet many have additional interests and specialities, which they use within their own practices. These range from:

'Dermatology is my main interest' *(Respondent 1)*

'Dermatology, physical medicine and orthopaedics' *(Respondent 4)*

'I do training and I'm involved with clinical governance' *(Respondent 2)*

'My main interest is psychiatry' *(Respondent 3)*

'I do all the minor surgery in the practice and some for the PCT' *(Respondent 5)*

'Minor surgery and orthopaedics, but that is all – no herbal stuff' *(Respondent 9)*

Others had a particular interest in women's health or paediatrics and one had an interest in complementary medicine, albeit not herbal medicine.

'I am interested in family planning' *(Respondent 7)*

'Women's health, obstetrics and gynae, psychiatry and I am just starting to do diabetes' *(Respondent 8)*

'Quite a lot of women's medicine, so gynaecology, I like paediatrics and I do a fair bit of family planning' *(Respondent 10)*

'Homoeopathy' *(Respondent 6)*

2. Connection with herbal medicine

(a) *Interest/lack of interest.* Many doctors admitted to not having any particular interest in complementary medicine:

'Don't dismiss it out of hand, but no particular interest in it' *(Respondent 1)*

'Not really, because we are so evidence-based now that we don't have the luxury to try things that haven't got a load of clinical trials behind them to say that this is justified prescribing' *(Respondent 3)*

'Not usually. I do sometimes advise people who are struggling to go for, you know, osteopath, chiropractor or something like that. I know very little about it' *(Respondent 9)*

'Not in terms of actively pursuing it, but certainly I think people are asking about it more and more. I've got lots of ladies asking about alternatives to HRT. I think people are often looking for alternatives, aren't they?' *(Respondent 10)*

Then there are the doctors who appeared to be more open-minded about other forms of medical treatment.

'Yes, I do. I suppose I am flexible in that I don't believe there is anything wrong in having complementary medicine and I will often recommend people for homoeopathy, acupuncture, etc., but I don't know very much about herbalism, although I have used some herbal products or recommended them occasionally' *(Respondent 4)*

'I am open-minded about complementary medicine. I don't discourage people from trying complementary treatments' *(Respondent 6)*

Doctors who have trained or worked overseas seem to have a better understanding and are more accepting of CAM:

'I do. I used to work with a GP in Australia, and he did complementary medicine' *(Respondent 8)*

'I am open-minded. I think herbal medicine is a bit more favourable in Ireland' *(Respondent 9)*

(b) *Training.* There has been very little in the way of CAM education, at medical school or elsewhere, and many doctors mentioned the shortened medical degrees.

'No, there was one lecture on it, an evening talk. You are looking at shorter courses for medical students to try and cut the cost of training so how you are going to get another thing is difficult' *(Respondent 1)*

'Not at medical school. We've had various sessions within the practice and through the vocational training scheme, e.g. homoeopaths, chiropracs, reflexologists and acupuncturists to talk about it. No herbalists. I think people should know, because we know a huge proportion of patients are using alternative practitioners, so we ought to really have knowledge of what sort of assessment they are getting, how the treatments work and what they are like really' *(Respondent 2)*

'No, but as part of the VTS we had a session with homoeopathy with Dr J' *(Respondent 7)*

Others, on the other hand, although they think it would be beneficial, would not want to see it taking the place of conventional medical training, which has been shortened recently:

'I think the training is tight enough. As far as I am aware there is not enough slack in the undergraduate training system so I suppose some exposure to it is probably helpful, but I wouldn't want to see it taking the place of some of the conventional training' (*Respondent 5*)

'I think inclusion in terms of familiarization. Times have changed and things have gained respectability, and certainly doctors couldn't know all the complementary therapies available, but whether it could be included, given some kind of working knowledge of it, but as it is – medicine is spread so thinly these days' (*Respondent 6*)

'We did have a little bit, yes, we did have like a section on Complementary medicine where they just went through the different types and explained what they were. I'd like to understand more, about all the alternative medicines, because it impacts on the drugs you give and we want to give the best management for the patient whether that's using alternatives practitioners. The outcome has got to be the best possible' (*Respondent 8*)

'I think there is a vogue for them so that we are not totally in the dark and if we had even one hour lecture on each of the different specialties of Complementary Medicine – it would be useful' (*Respondent 9*)

'I don't think there is any choice. I think it has to be included because it is being used more and more, and if you are starting to give advice about other things that you can buy, we need to know what we are talking about really. And as I say I am often recommending different things for women with menopause and people coming in having taking St Johns Wort. We are talking to people already about it, but in an unqualified way really, so I don't think there is any choice but to include it really' (*Respondent 10*)

Instead of querying whether the GP has had any training in CAM, doctors could query a herbalist's training:

'I suspect they wouldn't have the confidence to refer to a herbalist, because again a herbalist is somebody we don't really know. We don't know what the training has been; we don't know what happens with consultations' (*Respondent 6*)

3. GPs' definition of herbal medicine

Many GPs have very little understanding of herbalism and what it entails, and how a patient, seeking this form of complementary medicine, would be treated by a western medical herbalist:

'This is where I have to express a fair bit of ignorance. I don't know what actually happens in the herbalist's consultation with the patient' (*Respondent 2*)

'I have only come across herbal medicine in Hong Kong when I did my elective and there it was the bane of the doctor's life, because Chinese Herbal Medicine often contains steroids' *(Respondent 3)*

This indicates that Chinese Herbal Medicine and western herbal medicine have been grouped together as one and the same thing, which they are not. Chinese herbal formulations could contain herbal, animal and mineral ingredients whereas western herbal medicine contains plants materials only:

'To be truthful, I don't really know. I think it is modelled on taking extracted plant materials. I am not certain how a herbalist goes about diagnosis. The problem is that it doesn't have a scientific base' *(Respondent 6)*

'I know absolutely nothing about it, or very little about it to be honest. I know it is plant extracts. Our big problem is (a) Not knowing anything about it and (b) not knowing how it interacts with what we can prescribe' *(Respondent 9)*

Some doctors seemed to have a clearer understanding of what herbal medicine entails:

'I always understood it was the use of natural plants basically to produce a remedy for whatever you are treating' *(Respondent 1)*

'Herbal medicine I see as a complementary medicine, and hopefully one without as many side effects as conventional medicine. I would have thought that you would have taken a history and probably examined the patients, made a diagnosis and given them an appropriate herbal medication' *(Respondent 4)*

'I presume the medicines are derived from herbs, plants. I presume there is some activity within the herbs to treat various things' *(Respondent 5)*

'It is someone who just uses herbs like St John's Wort or Chamomile – I think that they can use it for a variety of problems. And like your herbalist, a lot of them make up, like, a tonic or whatever that you drink or eat. But I am not sure whether herbalists do inhalations of herbs and things as well, or whether it's more that they make up something that they take internally' *(Respondent 8)*

'I presume that they would have some parallels to what we do in terms of they'd take a history. I don't know what they would do or anything in terms of examination. They'd bring it together and try and formulate something as we would, that they feel would help the individual. There are lots of parallels with standard medicine really as we see it' *(Respondent 10)*

4. Use of herbal medicine

This refers to the general use of herbal medicine with patients who admit to using it and possibly ask their GPs for advice on various herbal remedies. It is surprising to discover that some GPs are recommending over-the-counter forms of herbal medicine, even though they cannot specifically refer a patient to a herbalist at this stage.

(a) General use

'People come up and ask me about it, but I have very little experience so I just say I don't know. There are a lot of people with chronic conditions who don't find satisfactory remedy from standard medicine. If herbal medicine was available they would obviously try that and if it was successful they would carry on with it. Normally it would be for arthritis, depression, stress, all of that; skin conditions and that sort of thing. There are lots of things you'd use it for' *(Respondent 1)*

'The only problem is learning about it and having an evidence-base for it, so it isn't very widely available. I think I'll have to admit to a fair degree of ignorance about how effective it is for whatever, because we don't get any teaching in it. I think we would see some difficulties in not knowing what you were recommending, and dealing with the responsibility if you had recommended the treatment. It's alright if the patients are doing things off their own bat' *(Respondent 2)*

Some doctors went as far as admitting that not all conventional treatments were particularly successful, especially in light of some of the reported side effects, therefore it was thought that herbal medicine might offer some benefit.

'I don't know enough to know which ones would be benefited, but my guess is that things like arthritis would be benefited, because we don't treat arthritis particularly well and it's a bit hit and miss with anti-inflammatories and they have their whole list of side effects that go with them and chronic pain, because it is so subjective' *(Respondent 3)*

'I think if we had the evidence that herbalism works, and if there was evidence that it was as effective as conventional medicine – yes. I think it will grow from the point of view of lack of side effects' *(Respondent 4)*

'Our problem is that we don't know about interaction with herbal medicines. I think it is inevitable and if it was worked out properly it could be okay' *(Respondent 5)*

'Well, I see it working. I think every time we have a scare like we have had with vioxin and celebrex, then people will turn to herbal medicine' *(Respondent 6)*

'There are things that have been around for a long time that some people swear by, like St John's Wort. It's first line on the continent for mild depressive symptoms. Everything that we can't treat' ... [relating to what herbal medicine can treat] 'I think there are certain conditions that it probably does benefit, maybe it is the placebo effect, mind over matter, that sort of thing' *(Respondent 9)*

'Yes, I think it would be beneficial and as I say for people looking for alternatives to standard medicine quite often, so I'd particularly like to see it doing lots of ladies stuff and I think a lot more about HRT and alternatives to HRT. There are often alternatives that work for things like depression, and again conventional anti-depressants in general have had quite a slating' *(Respondent 10)*

(b) Patients admitting to using herbal medicine. Four GPs stated that some of their patients admitted to using herbal medicine for specific complaints

'I've had patients who have come back and said "I've seen a herbalist and it helped"' *(Respondent 8)*

Others are quoted as saying:

'I suspect there are a lot more people taking alternative medication' *(Respondent 5)*.

(c) GPs Recommending herbal medicine to patients. GPs have been giving advice regarding complementary treatments for some time. However, many feel that their hands are tied as there is no referral strategy in place, due to herbalists not being state-registered at this stage.

'I have suggested the alternative of feverfew at times for migraine, if other things have failed and St John's Wort for some people who don't tolerate anti-depressants' *(Respondent 2)*

'I refer people for acupuncture, because the physio that works in the practice is trained in acupuncture' *(Respondent 3)*

'I know a pharmacist who has an interest in herbalism and I refer them to his pharmacy but, other than that, no' *(Respondent 4)*

Some doctors are sceptical about herbal medicine, yet often pharmaceutical drugs produce more side effects than the publicized incidents regarding drug–herb interactions:

'I don't discourage people from trying things assuming that they are fed up with their conventional drugs, but I think their lives will be difficult, because most doctors wouldn't recommend complementary medicine or herbal medicine because of the potential interactions with hypertensives, etc' *(Respondent 6)*.

Women are the main users of complementary medicines and many are concerned about the menopause and breast related problems. GPs are finding it difficult to suggest alternatives, e.g. for HRT, that could be a direct result of the 'Million Woman Study':

'I don't know because it is not usually something I recommend [talking about herbal medicine]. Well, no, that's not true at all. I do suggest black cohosh. The main problem is since all this stuff about HRT, the problem has been finding alternatives' *(Respondent 7)*

'I advise my patients to take over-the-counter herbs; anyway, ones that I know have shown to be useful. But things like evening primrose oil they have taken off the NHS, because they said the studies show it was no better than a placebo, but that's not what you find with patients who have breast pain: it's useful' (*Respondent 8*)

'I say, well, you can try black cohosh, something that has got plant derived oestrogens in. I would like to see clearer advice as ladies are looking for alternatives for menopausal type symptoms' (*Respondent 10*)

5. Employment of a complementary therapist

When discussing the employment of a complementary therapist, most GPs thought that, if they were in a position to appoint one, an acupuncturist would be useful. This could be because it is a complementary treatment for most conditions, whereas herbal medicine could, as Respondent 4 suggested, be 'complementary, in addition or in place of' conventional medicine.

'An acupuncturist' (*Respondents 2, 4, 5, 6, 7* and *8*) 'but because of our ignorance of herbalism really' (*Respondent 4*).

Yet Respondent 7 said:

'I think it would be useful to have someone who knew about herbal medications, things like black cohosh and all that kind of thing would be helpful.'

When discussing employing a herbalist Respondent 3 replied:

'Given all the criteria – yes. The branch surgery that I work in – there are a lot of elderly patients with chronic problems who would maybe benefit' (*Respondent 3*)

Quite a few suggested that a therapist would have to be state-registered, or registered with a governing body before employment could be considered.

'I suppose the complementary therapist would have to be registered with a governing body. Any professional body has got to have its own self-governing qualification and redress' (*Respondent 3*)

'I'm not sure what line the NHS would take on an actual herbal practitioner. I don't think it would be allowed "to do that" until it was regulated and gone through standard systems. Yes, I do, yes' [reply to: "Do you think that it would be beneficial having a herbal practitioner in your practice?"]' (*Respondent 10*)

6. Consumer information about complementary medicine

This refers to information readily available regarding any form of complementary medicine:

'You've got to be very careful; we get some people [patients] come into us and know everything ...' [referring to information on the internet]   (*Respondent 1*)

'Where would you go now for information? You can't go to a pharmacist; you can't say, well, here is my script, can you tell me about it? In the health shop, if they don't have the interest, then who can advise them?'   (*Respondent 6*)

A few doctors suggested that some form of herbal formulary, similar to the BNF, was required:

'If we had something with the drug-herb interactions on-line or in the BNF it would help, we would then know what we were up against'   (*Respondent 5*)

'It's that we haven't got a BNF for herbal medication'   (*Respondent 7*)

'The problem is we haven't got a formulary for it like we have for standard medicine, so also, because we are NHS practitioners, you can only advise to take over-the-counter products'   (*Respondent 10*)

7. Economic factors in relation to complementary medicine on the NHS

The cost from the patient's perspective was discussed.

'If it was on the NHS they would use it, but if it is not they won't pay for it. The trouble is I can't see the NHS funding it on a large scale because there is such a backlog of conditions to treat, so it is going to be quite difficult to get herbal medicine funded on the NHS nationwide'   (*Respondent 1*)

'It is interesting in Southern Ireland where you pay for your medication, people are much happier to go to an alternative practitioner than to see their doctor. Often they would go for reiki, physiotherapy, acupuncture, homoeopathy without actually seeing their doctors. It is a cultural thing'   (*Respondent 4*)

'In other countries where people do pay for things a lot more, it is probably appreciated a lot more. As long as it is free of charge' [Discussion about herbal medicine being available on the NHS]   (*Respondent 10*)

Economically, the cost-effectiveness of herbal medicine and also the financial gain with regards to pharmaceutical companies was mentioned by most of the interviewed GPs:

'Drug companies aren't going to make any money out of it – because they can't patent it'   (*Respondent 2*)

'The drug companies are the ones with the money and they need to have a financially viable product at the end to market, which then will take it out of your hands because of licensing'   (*Respondent 3*)

'Possibly the cost as well – being cost effective – and I think people would be less frightened of it and, if it was available over-the-counter, they would just go and have it recommended' (*Respondent 4*)

'If herbal medicine was recognized, I think it would be a much cheaper option' (*Respondent 6*)

8. Use of complementary medicine as a referral

All the GPs interviewed said that they would be more than happy to receive communication from a herbalist regarding a patient, whether it be a referral back to the GP or merely a letter discussing medication.

'If somebody else has just spent an hour with the patient, got the history out and put it in a typed letter, so if somebody has already gone through that – thank you very much!' (*Respondent 3*)

'I would be open to it if you were a qualified herbalist – yes, certainly. You know us doctors don't like being told what to do – but from an equal professional – yes, that's fine, and we receive referrals from physiotherapists and acupuncturists and all sorts of people. We're open to that, yes' (*Respondent 4*)

'I think communication is the ultimate. It is happening more and more, from chiropractors, osteopaths, herbalists – we are getting more information back, and that is helpful' (*Respondent 9*)

Some mentioned the need for protocols on methods of referral to be put in place if state registration occurs. Others made it quite clear that it would be more of a worry if herbalists did not refer patients back to their GP if there was a problem that the herbalist could not deal with:

'I don't think we'd have a problem with that. It would be more of a worry if they didn't refer patients back, if there was a problem. They should know their limitations' (*Respondent 2*)

'If you do one day come under the NHS umbrella, then we've got to have some sort of protocol on methods of referral. I wouldn't see a problem with it. If you saw one of our patients with a problem, I would be more worried if you didn't refer them back to me if you couldn't deal with the problem' (*Respondent 5*)

'I think we'd be generally happy with it if we knew the person or if we knew their qualifications. The problem is at the moment, I am sure other people have said this to you, if you know nothing about a clinic and nothing about the person's qualifications or if they have got qualifications or what they mean. Whereas a referral from another colleague in Lincoln and you know what they are like and know their standard of practise, you'd accept it happily. But I think because it is so up and coming, it would take a while for us to get used to what the qualification means' (*Respondent 10*)

A few GPs saw it as a positive step because they would then know that either the patient required another form of medical treatment or that possibly the herbalist had highlighted a problem with the patient:

> 'I think that would be good, because then at least I'd know that the patient wanted something alternative and then I could look at the medication, and discuss possible interactions with them, and I could see what sort of things they wanted to try. I would see that as good, rather than them doing it and taking herbal medication and normal medication and not being aware of what they were taking' (*Respondent 7*)

> 'I think that's good. I've had patients do that. Whether it was from a herbalist or any other alternative, they'll come in and say there is something wrong with my thyroid or whatever, which is a good thing – to work together' (*Respondent 8*)

One GP indicated that under the present system there would be some hesitation referring to a herbalist:

> 'I think that interchanging information has got to be beneficial. I would hesitate in this present system to refer to a herbalist; I think if someone came and said, 'Can I do this?'', I would say, "Well, these are the problems", for example, but I wouldn't actually refer to a herbalist. But if a herbalist wanted to write back to me and say that they have seen this patient and to discuss the patient, I couldn't comment on what they were having, but I would appreciate the feedback on what was happening' (*Respondent 6*)

9. The future of complementary medicine

Bearing in mind the general public's understanding of different forms of medicine, GPs were quoted as saying the following regarding the future of CAM:

> 'If herbal medicine was offered, the demand would expand, but I don't see it reducing the workload. I think that there may be a bigger input, yes. If it was funded and the government supported it, yes' (*Respondent 1*)

> 'I'm sure it would, yes. Most people would like to try alternative treatment because the conventional treatments just don't work for a lot of people. I think it is possible to work in a complementary way, when I think of the Patrick Patromi Health Centre with complementary practitioners working alongside, and that is encouraged. I think it is possible. I think there will probably be increasing public pressure to include some of the alternative treatments in the NHS' (*Respondent 2*)

Consideration ought to be given to the likely changes that may occur in the future that could benefit patients and may make it more acceptable for both GPs and herbalists alike to work alongside each other:

'I think with Prince Charles's sort of thrust for complementary medicine and organic food, we see that there is a gradual acceptance and I think, yes, it's going to grow. And I think it is going to grow quite big. With the over-the-counter vitamins and minerals sale actually booming, I think if herbalism is sold in the right way that will do the same' (*Respondent 4*)

'It is inevitable that it is there. I'm sure complementary medicine will continue to grow. I would say there will be dramatic changes in the legislation' (*Respondent 5*)

'There are lots of things happening in conventional medicine, you know, cost of drugs, etc. – there are lots of things happening, and there would be the same parallel with complementary and herbal' (*Respondent 9*)

Some GPs did not see herbal medicine as the forefront of medical progress and others were not quite sure where it would all lead:

'I think that complementary medicine will always lag behind in the sense that it is an issue and is likely to remain an issue' (*Respondent 6*)

'I don't know. I'm not sure. Conventional medicine will continue and people will always want an alternative, like herbal medication. I think it would be better if the herbal medication was regulated and that we knew they had just as much side effects as well. It doesn't mean that they are necessarily safer than conventional medicine. I think it would make people aware that it is not just a harmless herb. If it was regulated, at least you'd know then that people weren't being ripped off' (*Respondent 7*)

10. The value of using complementary medicine

(*a*) *Value to the patient.* This respondent had some mixed views regarding value, emphasizing that evidence is necessary regarding the effectiveness of herbal medicine:

'If someone is not practising safely, there is someone who knows about it that will be able to look and say you shouldn't be doing this and we'll strike you off our list. Partly because you have the luxury of time, if you spend an hour with people, then they feel understood. And then you have the time to follow them up, and you can say, well, come back in a week, rather than wait a month. And people will feel then that they have been heard' (*Respondent 3*)

(*b*) *Personal values to the GP.* For this respondent the issue of spirituality was important:

'That is another side of complementary medicine that I am very wary of, because quite often there's a spiritual element that is opening up channels and I do believe that there is good spiritual, but then there is also bad spiritual. The first premise has always got to be – do no harm' (*Respondent 3*)

11. *Responsibility for the patient*

Many of the GPs voiced concern about responsibility:

'If you recommend something, then you have to carry some of the responsibility for the consequences. I think it is hard to see who would have prime responsibility for the patient, how you would define the working practices and division of responsibility. One has got to look at that. If you refer someone to a complementary therapist working alongside, where does your responsibility begin and end? What is the communication going to be?' (*Respondent 2*)

'I think we would see some difficulties in not knowing what you were recommending, and dealing with the responsibility if you had recommended the treatment. It's alright if the patients are doing things off their own bat' (*Respondent 2*)

'The problem will come with responsibility, that you will have to be responsible for what you do, and the resistance will come if it keeps coming back, "Well, ask your GP" and they make another appointment to say "Well, can I take this with what I have already?" and that will really wind doctors up' (*Respondent 3*)

Issues of regulation and litigation were mentioned:

'There are so many interactions. The main problem is that it is not regulated' (*Respondent 7*)

'And how much concern is there that there is the potential that patients may sue you?' (*Respondent 6*)

'If we do it, we can be brought in, if there is an adverse event we can be brought in, and we take the rap. If we went to see the lawyer he'd say who did refer her? Who takes the responsibility – the herbalist or do we do it, because we have referred? It's a grey area and is high risk' (*Respondent 9*)

Discussion

From the interview data, eleven themes emerged which were relevant to the research question. These themes will be discussed and compared to the available literature to identify any evident gaps pertaining to this study.

After scrutinizing the literature, the researcher was unable to find any available information on herbalists working in a GP's surgery, or patients being referred to a herbalist by their doctor. This could be because herbalists have not yet become state registered. A couple of decades ago, the General Medical Council (GMC) deemed it unethical for doctors to refer patients to be treated by herbalists, acupuncturists and homoeopaths, thus forcefully prohibiting the practice of those practitioners without justifiable medical qualifications (Saks 1995).

Only one GP, of the ten interviewed, had a definite interest in complementary medicine, although not in herbalism. The GP was open-minded regarding CAM, but then so were many of the others who were interviewed. They were aware that CAM had more to offer in terms of longer consultation times and a more holistic approach. Many GPs (and their patients) would like to have an integrated health care system in place and logically it should be supported by the NHS. The DoH (2003a) and Ranshaw (2003) reinforced these two notions respectively.

It could be argued that, as some GPs suggested, the popularity of CAM has increased immensely over the last decade, as substantiated by Carr-Brown (2001). This could be the beginning of a two-tiered health system, with only those who are able to afford to see a herbalist privately benefiting. Shaw et al. (1999) highlighted these inequalities in health.

With so many people self-medicating or seeing complementary practitioners, GPs need to be offered some training in the subject and, according to Mills (2001), they should attempt to become more familiar with CAM, which would lead to an understanding of drug–herb interactions. Familiarization with CAM ought to be offered as part of the medical school curriculum in the UK. As reported by NCCAM (2001), 66 per cent of all medical schools in the USA offer CAM instruction as part of their core curriculum.

Integrated medicine should be available to everyone, and should include complementary practitioners such as herbalists and acupuncturists, according to Mills (2001). As Schmidt et al. (2002) claim, the UK has a positive approach to, and a high interest in, CAM, as was evident from the information that emerged during the interviews. More than half the doctors would favour the inclusion of CAM, as long as the practitioner was registered and accountable, as was highlighted in the Department of Health's (2003b) *Statutory Regulation of Herbal Medicine and Acupuncture*. The respondents admitted that some patients, who were dissatisfied with conventional treatments, sought alternative forms of medicine. This theory is supported in the literature by Emslie et al. (2002).

According to Turner (1996), the government has been trying over the last thirty years to place a greater emphasis on preventative medicine and community care and more recently on integrated medicine which is supported by both the DoH (2003a) and *Medical News Today* (2004). If, as is planned, statutory regulation is granted, GPs would feel more confident in referring patients to herbalists because, as the DOH (2003b) claims, it will bring about a number of necessary improvements that will certify the safety and quality of herbal practice and medicines.

Many GPs see the shape of medicine changing in the future, with conventional medicine still moving forward, but with a place for CAM in a new and integrated system. This altering of boundaries between the various types of medicine is reflected by Shuval and Mizrachi (2004) in their research. Due to the fact that medicine today is very much evidence-based, as mentioned by a few of the respondents, Goodman et al. (2000) argued that herbal medicine should not be discredited just becasue of a lack of scientific validation.

Analysis of the data showed that GPs were struggling to suggest alternatives, for example to HRT, for their menopausal patients. This is probably a direct result of two studies conducted over the last decade: the 'Million Woman Study' in Britain and the 'Women's Health Initiative' (WHI) in the United States. In these circumstances, concerned patients will very likely seek out natural alternatives to alleviate their symptoms. If this is the case, herbal medicine will become a more acceptable alternative when dealing with such issues.

A comparison of the methods of therapeutic treatments in various countries indicates that, where there is a national health care system in place, patients tend to select the option that is free at the point of service whereas, in countries where health care is funded by the individual, there is more often a tendency to choose an alternative practitioner. Respondent 1 believed that if herbal medicine was offered, demand would expand but this GP did not see it reducing doctors' workloads. Yet it can be argued that many chronic cases could be treated with herbal medicine, which would then prevent patients returning time and time again for allopathic medicines.

The method of interviewing was appropriate for this study. Using a phenomenological approach allowed the respondents' experiences to be evaluated. Interviewing is particularly useful if it relates to the interviewees' particular work; in this case it may not be relevant at the moment but, within the next few years, the face of medicine could be quite different in this country.

Novelty

The novelty value of such research is that GPs probably have not thought much about herbal medicine in the past, except where there have been reported cases of drug–herb interactions. With more information appearing fairly regularly in medical journals, e.g., the recent article regarding St John's Wort (*British Medical Journal*, 4 March 2005), and an eleven-week series in *The Doctor* magazine, 'Alternative medicine: the facts' by Professor Ernst, more awareness is being generated about CAM, probably from necessity rather than personal interest.

One common theme that recurred during the interview process was a genuine concern about the lack of a worthwhile alternative to HRT after the recent scares. With so many patients looking for alternatives for menopausal treatment, GPs are recommending herbs like black cohosh. One respondent, who claimed to be dubious about herbal medicine but was extremely concerned about menopausal patients had within a week of the interview informed a patient at the university's polyclinic about herbal medicine. As a result the patient was delighted to find a herbal alternative. This was a direct result of the interview conducted during the research. If a suggestion that a patient try herbal medicine has been made by one GP already, only time will tell whether other GPs would consider it a helpful alternative to conventional drugs. If this was the case it could be argued that it would be beneficial for patients to be referred within their own practice to a herbalist who perhaps specializes in the menopause.

Relating directly to the research into whether GPs would consider working together in practice with western medical herbalists, a few of the doctors considered that it would be beneficial to have a herbalist with whom they could discuss drug–herb interactions and treatments for diseases and illnesses where conventional medicine is failing, or where patients have tried everything and there seems to be no further option. In this situation, GPs would be able to discuss patients on-site and would be able to monitor progress too, if they so chose.

Most GPs were unaware of what herbal medicine entailed. Some thought that it had a place, but would prefer it to be state registered. A few GPs also said that they would like guidelines to be issued regarding the referral process and concern was expressed regarding responsibility for the patient. Would the doctor who referred the patient be responsible or would the medical herbalist be accountable?

This area of discussion was probably as a result of GPs' concerns about litigation. With conventional medicine being evidence-based, many GPs cannot accept that herbal treatments, used over thousands of years, could be used alongside their medicine when there is no scientific basis. A few doctors suggested that a herbal equivalence to the BNF is what they require so that they can establish what herbs are used for and what drug–herb interactions there are, if any. Yet ironically many are already suggesting that their patients use St. John's Wort (*Hypericum perforatum*) and black cohosh (*Cimicifuga*) for depression and menopause respectively. In herbal medicine the whole person has to be taken into account; therefore a herbal practitioner's prescription for a menopausal patient could contain between seven and thirteen herbs, and black cohosh may or may not be included within the formulation. So by taking black cohosh as a supplement the symptoms of menopause may not be alleviated.

GPs' acceptance of acupuncture, as a complementary medicine, within the general practice framework was surprising, because herbal medicine was not mentioned specifically. This could be due to the fact that many physiotherapists and NHS pain control clinics already practise acupuncture, although they are not state registered. In many cases, herbal medicine could be used as the only method of therapeutic treatment so in effect it could be said to be in direct competition with general practice, although it could also be used complementarily to conventional medicine.

Because there has been a huge increase in complementary medicine use over the last decade, the need to regulate this practice has become necessary. With many more people asking their GPs about CAM, there has to be provision for some education at medical school. If statutory regulation, there is a possibility that herbal practitioners and acupuncturists could be employed directly by the NHS within the next couple of years.

Now that most people have access to the internet, patients are able to investigate many illnesses and diseases and their treatment strategies and medication. Articles and reports about drugs and their side effects are available for scrutiny via the internet, as are herbal medicine and drug–herb interactions. Today people are better informed than ever before, and as a consequence of the 'rights' that it demands, the general public has more information available to it regarding its health. Given the cost of herbal medicine, to employ a herbal practitioner in primary care and stock a wide range of herbs in a dispensary may be costly to set up initially but this would be no more expensive than purchasing drugs for patients. In the long run, herbal medicine could work out to be by far the cheaper option.

Limitations

The difficulty of obtaining an appointment with a GP was a valid concern. Under the new appointment system in place in most surgeries, one receptionist even suggested phoning 'on the day' for an emergency appointment, something the researcher declined as this would have been an abuse of the emergency appointment scheme! GPs are hard pressed for time so few wanted to commit twenty minutes to an interview. Two methods were used to try and gain access to GPs. First, a few surgeries were telephoned, informing them of the research, and the call was followed up with information letters and consent forms (Appendix 1 and 2 respectively). Alternatively letters were posted initially to GPs and were then followed up with telephone calls. The response rate was very poor for either system.

There was only one GP who agreed to interview without a personal request because the letter had in fact been addressed to another member of the practice. It was probably thought that someone with an interest in CAM, such as the GP in question, might be better qualified to do the interview but this was not the case from the interviewer's point of view, as both positive and negative feedback was sought. The researcher was known to a few of the GPs approached; some obliged and some did not even reply. The researcher had hoped to interview GPs from ten different practices, but due to the difficulty in finding willing GPs, seven practices were utilized in the end. This still gives a clear indication of feelings in the area.

Gaining ethical permission from LREC to conduct GP interviews was probably one of the most difficult parts of the whole research process. It took approximately three months from completing the forms, attending the LREC meeting and changing the required alterations to finally gaining a favourable ethical opinion and being awarded an honorary contract with the NHS, all of which were required before research could commence. This long process at the time seemed unreasonable for the type of research being conducted, as there were no 'vulnerable participants' to be interviewed. Future researchers should consider whether their study is worth the extra work that going through the LREC process entails. In this particular case, the researcher was pleased to have had such an opportunity.

One disadvantage with taped interviews was that the quality of the sound was not absolutely clear in one fifth of the interviews. This was not identified until the pilot study had been completed. The researcher would ensure that future research interviews would be conducted with the tape recorder situated as close to the respondent as possible, or use a microphone extension. Another disadvantage is that each interview took approximately four hours to transcribe. Possibly a foot-operated transcription machine might speed up the process (Bryman 2004). In this case, however, the advantages of conducting taped, semi-structured interviews most certainly outweighed the disadvantages.

The researcher felt that for any future qualitative research, Kath Melia's (2000) interview advice might be useful: 'less from the interviewer is more'. On transcribing the tapes it was found that the interviewer had sometimes replied to a question at the same time as the respondent spoke, which resulted in neither comment being clear.

In conclusion, taking into account that this was a relatively small-scale study, the researcher was moderately satisfied with the outcome. Given that complementary medicine is being used more frequently, it is inevitable that it is here to stay and everyone should work towards the common goal of an integrated medical system. With both herbalists and acupuncturists undergoing statutory regulation at the moment, it is possible that within two years this may become a reality.

Upon statutory regulation a regulatory body will be formed, possibly known as the Herbal Council or CAM Council, and this body will have responsibility for establishing and maintaining a Register of Practitioners who are deemed competent to prescribe and use herbal products as medicines (DoH 2003a). The DoH (2003a) outlined three competencies required by herbal practitioners:

1. professional values and behaviour;
2. knowledge;
3. specific skills.

As with the medical profession, herbal practitioners would be expected to maintain and increase their competency through continuing professional development, and compulsory arrangements will be put into place a year after the establishment of a statutory council (DoH 2003b). The EHPA demands certain minimum course requirements as part of the process of accreditation, ensuring competent, safe and effective practitioners (DoH 2003b).

Granted, there are real concerns emerging relating to the evidence-base of herbal medicine, but it can be argued that this form of medicine has survived thousands of years, so what is required in the way of evidence? There have not been many research projects conducted because there is insufficient funding available for research into CAM. Possibly after state registration, programmes may be set up for further research, as many treatments have worked successfully but there is little or no evidence to substantiate their efficacy.

At the beginning of most interviews, GPs appeared bemused by the fact that the researcher was asking questions regarding their thoughts on herbal medicine's integration into mainstream medicine. The outcome was that more than half had already been recommending various herbal remedies for their patients, in the form of over-the-counter supplements, which is slightly different from the way in which herbal medicine is practiced. Even the doctors who initially sounded sceptical admitted to recommending it in one form or another. In this situation, would it not be preferable to have someone within a practice to prescribe herbal formulations for patients? If not, GPs could cross-reference with correspondence with a herbalist.

The research identified the need for GPs to receive up to date information on herbal medicine, preferably a herbal equivalent of the BNF, or inclusion within the BNF. Drug–herb interactions was a subject most GPs mentioned, so again relevant information should be readily available to them. The researcher was under the impression that if this information could be accessed online in a computer-based formulary, time-constrained GPs would be quite satisfied. Otherwise a disc containing all the relevant information could be made available to them. The common area where GPs would like to see some advice, and would consider using herbal medicine, is as a substitute for HRT. It was evident from the study that over half of the GPs would consider working with a herbalist, but certain aspects would need to be clarified initially, e.g. state registration (or a member of a recognized body), referral procedures and the important issue of responsibility.

Doctors clearly do not understand CAM sufficiently at the moment and they are not up to date with much of the available evidence. The value of this study has highlighted the need for further education on this subject for health professionals as practising GPs and in other parts of the NHS. Some knew about the relatively small number of cases where herbs have interacted with drugs, which have been sensationalized by the media or been included in articles in the *British Medical Journal* for example.

As a novice researcher, the process of obtaining LREC and NHS approval for the study was far more time consuming and frustrating than had been anticipated. The researcher felt that some GPs were cynical initially, probably because complementary medicine is one area that most do not know anything about, which is understandable. From a normal position of authority, the doctors were trying to discuss something which they did not understand, especially as it is something which is neither scientific nor evidence-based. Given the same opportunity again the researcher would prefer to have the full six months to conduct the research and have more time to consolidate ideas.

However the researcher felt the study was successful and could lead, in the future, to further investigations.

Ideas for further investigations

1. Herbal medicine used in the treatment of the menopause in general practice.
2. To focus on the employment of herbalists after statutory regulation.
3. The costs of herbal medicine as opposed to drugs for a specific illness.
4. The cost of setting up a medical herbal practitioner in primary care.
5. Employing a herbal practitioner in a 'super surgery'.
6. Whether practices would need a herbal dispensary, as pharmacists may not want to stock herbal medicines given the large number of herbs that would be required.

References

Allsop, J. (1984) *Health Policy and the National Health Service* (New York: Longman).

Allsop, J. (1995) *Health Policy and the NHS: Towards 2000*, 2nd edn (New York: Longman).

American Cancer Society (ACS) News Center (2003) Another blow for hormone therapy [online]. Available from: *http://www.cancer.org/docroot/NWS/content/ NWS_1_1x_Another_Blow_for_Hormone_Therapy.asp* [accessed 03.04.05].

Anderson, R. (1999) A case study in integrative medicine: alternative theories and the language of biomedicine. *Journal of Alternative and Complementary Medicine* 5 (2): 165–73.

Association of the British Pharmaceutical Industry (ABPI) (2003) British pharmaceutical industry: medicines for a healthy future [online]. Available from: *http:// www.abpi.org.uk/publications/publication_details/annualReview2003/ar2003_04- highlights.asp* [accessed 09.05.04].

Bowling, A. (1993) *What People Say about Prioritising Health Services* (London: King's Fund Centre).

Bowling, A. (1997) *Measuring Health: A Review of Quality of Life Measurement Scales*, 2nd edn (Buckingham: Open University Press).

Britten, N. (1996) Lay views of drugs and medicines: conventional and unconventional. In S. J. Williams and M. Calnan (eds) *Modern Medicine: Lay Perspectives and Experiences* (London: UCL Press), pp. 48–73.

Bryman, A. (2004) *Social Research Methods*, 2nd edn (Oxford: Oxford University Press).

Carr-Brown, J. (2001) Ministers call for herbal cures on NHS, *Sunday Times*, 30 December.

Department of Health (2000) *Data Protection Act 1998* [online]. Available from: http://www.dh.gov.uk/PolicyAndGuidance/OrganisationPolicy/RecordsManagement/Data ProtectionAct1998Article/fs/en?CONTENT_ID=4000489&chk=VrXoGe [accessed 04.03.05].

Department of Health (2003a) *Recommendations on the Regulation of Herbal Practitioners in the UK* (London: Herbal Medicine Regulatory Working Group).

Department of Health (2003b) *Prescriptions Dispensed in the Community: Statistics for 1992 to 2002: England* [online]. Available from: http://www.dh.gov.uk/ assetRoot/04/03/58/54/04035854.pdf [accessed 08.09.04].

Department of Health (2005a) Speech by Rt Hon John Hutton, Minister of State (Health), 9 March 2005: Practice Based Commissioning [online]. Available from: http://www.dh.gov.uk/NewsHome/Speeches/SpeechesList/SpeechesArticle/fs/en? CONTENT_ID=4106433&chk=DBCAAS [accessed 02.04.05].

Department of Health (2005b) *Statutory Regulation of Herbal Medicine and Acupuncture: Report on the Consultation* (London: Department of Health).

Department of Health and Human Services: National Institutes of Health (NIH), National Heart, Lung and Blood Institute (NHLBI) (2005) 'Women's Health Initiative' [online]. Available from: http://www.nhlbi.nih.gov/whi/factsht.htm [accessed 03.04.05].

Emslie, M. J., Campbell, M. K. and Walker, K. A. (2002) Changes in public awareness of, attitudes to, and use of complimentary therapy in North East Scotland: surveys in 1993 and 1999. *Complementary Therapies in Medicine* 10 (3): 148–53.

Ernst, E. (2004) Herbal medicines put into context, *Student British Medical Journal* 12 [online]. Available from: http://www.studentbmj.com/back_issues/0104/editorials/ 2.html [accessed 09.10.04].

Goodman, N. W., Miles, A., Hampton, J. R. and Hurwitz, B. (eds) (2000) NICE and the new command structure: with what competence and with what authority will evidence be selected and interpreted for local clinical practice? In NICE, *CHI and the NHS Reforms: Enabling Excellence or Imposing Control?* (London: Aesculapius Medical Press).

Greenhalgh, T. and Taylor, R. (1997) How to read a paper: Papers that go beyond numbers (qualitative research), *British Medical Journal* 7110: 740–3.

Hammond, M., Howarth, J. and Keat, R. (1991) *Understanding Phenomenology* (Oxford: Blackwell).

HealthMall (no date) 'Prince Charles Calls for Research into Alternative Medicine': Alternative Medicine Newsletter [online]. Available from: http://www.chiro. org/alt_med_abstracts/FULL/Prince_Charles_Calls_for_Research.html [accessed 14.05.04].

Hedley, C. and Shaw, N. (2002) *Herbal Remedies* (Bath: Paragon Books).

House of Lords (2000) Science and Technology – Sixth Report Appendix 3 [online]. Available from: http://www.chiro.org/alt_med_abstracts/FULL/House_of_Lords/ APPENDIX_3.html [accessed 16.03.05].

Illich, I. (1995) *Limits to Medicine: Medical Nemesis: The Expropriation of Health* (London: Marion Boyers Publishers).

Information Commissioner (2000) *Health Data Protection* (London: HMSO), 108: 9–10.

Kumar, R. (1999) *Research methods: A Step-by-Step Guide for Beginners* (London: Sage Publications).

Locke, L. F., Spirduso, W. W. and Silverman, S. J. (2000) *Proposals That Work: A Guide for Planning Dissertations and Grant Proposals*, 4th edn (London: Sage Publications).

Medical News Today (2004) Prince Charles is wrong about complementary medicines, say NHS managers [online]. Available from: http://www.medicalnewstoday.com/ index.php?newsid=6239 [accessed 01.05.04].

Melia, K. (2000) Conducting an interview, *Nurse Researcher*, 7(4): 75–89.

Menzies-Trull, C. (2003) *Herbal Medicine: Keys to Physiomedicalism including Pharmacopoeia*, 1st edn (Newcastle: Faculty of Physiomedical Herbal Medicine [FPHM]).

Melia, K. (1987) *Learning and Working: The Occupational Socialization of Nurses* (London: Tavistock Publications).

Mills, S. Y. (2001) The House of Lords Report on Complementary Medicine: a summary. *Complementary Therapies in Medicine*, 1 Mar 2001; 9 (1): 34–9.

Mizrachi, N., Shuval, J. T. and Gross, S. (2004) Alternative medicine in biomedical settings. *Sociology of Health and Illness* 27 (1): 20–43.

National Center for Complementary and Alternative Medicine (NCCAM) and the Royal College of Physicians (sponsors) (2001) *Can Alternative Medicine be Integrated into Mainstream Care?* [online]. Available from: http://nccam.nih.gov/news/pastmeetings/012301/ [accessed 27.11.04].

Ranshaw, K. (2003) 'The Importance of Integrated Health' Prince Charles Online [online]. Available from: http://pco.teamhighgrove.com/ihart.htm [accessed 10.05.04].

Rattigan, P. (2003) *Disease Gridlock National Health: Towards Gridlock* [online]. Available from: http://patrattigan.mysite.wanadoo-members.co.uk/page6.html [accessed 09.10.04].

Sackett, D., Richardson, W. S., Rosenberg, W. and Haynes, R. W. (1997) *Evidence-based Medicine: How to Practice and Teach EBM* (New York: Churchill Livingstone).

Saks, M. (1992) *Alternative Medicine in Britain* (Oxford: Oxford University Press).

Saks, M. (1995) *Professions and the Public Interest: Medical Power, Altruism and Alternative Medicine* (London: Routledge).

Saks, M. (1999) The wheel turns? Professionalisation and alternative medicine in Britain. *Journal of Interprofessional Care* 13 (2): 129–38.

Saunders, M., Lewis, P. and Thornhill, A. (2003) *Research Methods for Business Students*, 3rd edn (Harlow: Pearson Educational).

Schmidt, K., Jacobs, P. A. and Barton, A. (2002) 'Cross-cultural differences in GPs' attitudes towards complementary and alternative medicine: A survey comparing regions of the UK and Germany'. *Complementary Therapies in Medicine*, 10 (3): 141–7.

Schön, D. A. (2003) *The Reflective Practitioner: How Professionals Think in Action* (Aldershot: Ashgate Publishing).

Shaw, M., Dorling, D., Gordon, D. and Davey Smith, G. (1999) *The Widening Gap: Health Inequalities and Policy in Britain* (Bristol: The Policy Press).

Shuval, J. T. and Mizrachi, N. (2004) Changing boundaries: modes of coexistence of alternative and biomedicine, *Qualitative Health Research* 14 (5): 1–16.

Source Correspondent (13/05/2003) Recruiting Foreign Doctors. *Public Management Journal* [online]. Available from: http://www.sourceuk.net/indexf.html?03330 [accessed 12.10.04].

Stewart, D. and Mickunas, A. (1974) *Exploring Phenomenology: A Guide to the Field and its Literature* (Chicago: American Library Association).

The United Kingdom Parliament (2005) The Government's Public Health White Paper (CM6374) [online]. Available from: http://www.publications.parliament.uk/pa/cm200405/cmselect/cmhealth/uc358-i/uc35802.htm [accessed 23.03.05].

Turner, B. S. (1996) *Medical Power and Social Knowledge*, 2nd edn (London: Sage Publications).

Weil, A. (2003) Frontline [online] Available from: http://www.pbs.org/wgbh/pages/frontline/shows/altmed/interviews/weil.html [accessed 09.10.04].

World Health Organization (2002) WHO Traditional Medicine Strategy 2002–2005 [online]. Available from: http://www.who.int/medicines/library/trm/trm_strat_eng. pdf [accessed 09.10.04] pp. 44–5.

World Health Organization (2003) Traditional Medicine Fact Sheet No 134. [online]. Available from: http://www.who.int/mediacentre/factsheets/fs134/en/ [accessed 03.03.05].

CHAPTER 10

The Therapeutic Relationship in the Dental Setting

LIANNE AQUILINA AND CAROL WILKINSON

The perception and behaviour of dental nurses and dentists can do much to influence patient satisfaction. The link between care and treatment of patients, and maintaining their well-being, generated the researcher's interest in the testing and application of a therapeutic intervention model, often used in the field of complementary medicine.

Complementary medicine involves the patients' active participation and the opportunity for therapeutic intervention using the principles underlying Chinese medicine. These are 'looking', 'hearing' and 'asking' (Maciocia 1997). Traditional Chinese medicine associates not only the symptoms and signs but also many other 'manifestations', to form the representation of a particular person, observing a patient emotionally as well as clinically, and then responding accordingly. These factors are applicable to the dental setting. A patient's emotional and behavioural disposition resulting from a dental intervention ought to be managed accordingly, with patients supported and efforts made to ensure a therapeutic alliance. Complementary medicine places great emphasis on the therapeutic relationship as well as its physical counterpart. However, the opportunity to correlate and apply data directly to a dental setting has previously been overlooked. Therapeutic techniques facilitate positive outcomes and have a powerful impact on those who experience them. A therapeutic intervention provides an opportunity for dental surgeons to convey mutuality, trust and care. Research also supports the quality of the relationship with the patient in terms of rapport and empathy and establishes this as the key factor in modifying attitudes and changing behaviour (Burke and Freeman 1994).

Therapeutic intervention in a dental setting

The therapeutic process of mutuality → trust → care → challenge → performance, then returning to mutuality, permits warmth, empathy, genuineness,

Table 10.1　The therapeutic relationship in a dental setting

Therapeutic consultation task	Therapeutic skills
1　Mutuality Adult-to-adult interaction (transactional analysis)	Opening phase – layout of surgery
	Discuss patients' views and provide them with an opportunity to consider before committing to treatment.
Clothes protector: 'Would you like me to put it on for you or would you like to put it on.'	'So today we are going to do (*brief description*) to ensure (*brief description*). What are you thoughts on this?'
2　Treatment – trust Reduce patients' anxiety (CBT model – how thoughts, feelings and behaviours are linked).	Show your patients you can tolerate and accept their feelings.
Support patients during clinical activities	Acknowledge how vulnerable a patient maybe – responding accordingly and helpfully.
Increase verbal interaction – 'This will not take too long'	'I sense that you're anxious – but try not to worry. It is quite natural to feel like this. We always manage to make this as easy as possible for our clients.'
'If you would like a break, please raise your left hand and I'll stop for a few seconds.' 'You can do this anytime you like throughout the treatment.'	'You are doing really well you know'
3　Care Transactional analysis	Take into account your own potential biases and preconceptions
To avoid 'cross' transactions. Maintenance of complementary transactions preferably adult ego state.	Self-awareness Active listening and monitoring of verbal and non-verbal cues.
4　Challenge To provide psychological safety for clients	Respect and behave courteously to all members of staff at all times.
	Inter-personal skill: 'Thank you'; 'Great'; 'That is a good mix'
5　Performance and end – return to mutuality Summarizing follow up	Give the patient credit for any positive outcomes.
	Alternatively, if they are maintaining oral health sufficiently.
Dental after-care: advise fillings/dentures/extractions Positive reinforcement	'The treatment went really well. Thank you for your collaboration. We shall see you at your next appointment. I would like to see you again in six months/next check up.'

Source:　Burke and Freeman (1994); Maciocia (1997); Mitchell and Cormack (1998); Cole and Bird (2000).

authority, respect and collaboration amongst the parties involved (Mitchell and Cormack 1998) – see Table 10.1. The therapeutic relationship disregards an individual's rationale through the generation of a connection between health professional and patient. A relationship may be shaped and outcomes influenced.

The therapeutic relationship (Mitchell and Cormack 1998) in a dental setting gives support to the vulnerable and offers a working alliance that is based on mutual respect, positive expectations and shared understanding. It offers a means for trust, provides boundaries and establishes safety for the dental patient. The therapeutic relationship permits care as a patient may relate to it; emphasis is focused upon the dental patient and a concern for dental patients' feelings are ascertained and responded to, and managed appropriately. A dental patient, the dental surgeon and the dental nurse are able to acknowledge their contribution within the encounter. These processes in a therapeutic relationship suggest the potential to improve an experience within the dental setting.

The need for a therapeutic relationship within a dental setting

Increasingly, it has been recognized that the interpersonal aspects of health care, particularly the practitioner–patient relationship, are essential to the good treatment of patients and their health problems (Locker 1989).

Nuttall et al. (2001) report that only 43 per cent of the UK population attended regularly for a dental examination in 1998: 14 per cent had an occasional check-up and 43 per cent only went to a dentist when they had problems with their teeth or gums. There was only a slight increase (43 per cent to 59 per cent) between 1978 and 1989 in the population attending regular dental check-ups and it is adults over 55-years-old who were the most likely to say they attended regularly. Almost half (48 per cent) of younger adults (16–24 years) visited the dentist less often than five years previously. It is reported that in dental anxiety, mutual participation and an estimate of the cost of treatment remain problems for many dental patients. The effective treatment of physical and oral conditions are said to always depend upon the patient's initiative in seeking diagnosis and treatment (Locker 1989). It is acknowledged that it is not only understanding treatment-seeking and utilization behaviour, but also responding to it, that are necessary for the promotion of effective and efficient dental care.

The dentist

In dental education, most emphasis has been placed upon clinical and technical skills. Less significance has been attached to the development of scientific skills and to the ability to develop a satisfactory relationship with patients, manage patient behaviour and provide for the social and psychological needs of patients (Locker 1989). These lapses may be easily identified and correlated with the overall anxiety felt by dental patients, utilization of the dental setting and patient satisfaction. Patients and the dental team are able to observe the existence of dental anxiety. It may be suggested that, like other health professionals, the dental team must develop a variety of communication skills and therapeutic techniques in order to provide safe and effective patient care and that this is particularly important for the dentists themselves, due to their interventions, which directly affect patients.

The patient

Locker (1989) asserts that patients judge dentists on their personal qualities rather than their technical competence and are more satisfied with those dentists who are successful at relieving anxiety. It is suggested that this ability depends on the quality of the interaction between dentist and patient. In addition, Veldhuis and Schouten (2003) found that dentists need to pay attention to their personal communication style.

Further research that explores the effects of the therapeutic relationship is essential as studies have demonstrated that limited verbal interaction between dentist and patient leads to less anxiety reduction, less positive attitudes and lower levels of satisfaction (Gale et al. 1984). Moreover, positive and negative communication has been found to influence patients' dental anxiety (Rouse 1990). A willingness to listen, to explain and to deal with the patients' concerns are taken as an indication of a general interest in patients and their welfare and these qualities are most appreciated by patients (Locker 1989).

Improving communication in the dental setting remains the dentists' responsibility (Kankin 1985) but the goal of consultation is not simply that of arriving at diagnosis and formulating a treatment plan. Patients also need to be offered the means to make sense of and develop a sense of control over their illness and its course (Locker 1989).

The dentist–patient relationship

Freidson (1970) believed that the doctor–patient relationship is characterized by conflict rather than harmony. This conflict (which rarely surfaces during the actual consultation) originates in the different perspectives of doctor and patient. The doctor views the patient's condition in a detached, scientific manner and evaluates its severity and significance according to the clinical criteria. The patient, however, is more personally involved with the illness and assesses its significance in terms of its social and psychological impact and its implications for his or her life as a whole. Freidson acknowledged in his work that 'a physician should at least act like a member of the therapeutic team' (1970, p. 134).

Locker (1989) discusses the activity–passivity model, which occurs in many dental consultations, the patient lying passively in the dental chair while the dentist undertakes some restorative or other procedure. Another type of relationship is the guidance–cooperation model in which the dentist instructs the patient on what needs to be done about the presenting complaint; the patient then cooperates by following this advice. Locker (1989) suggests that mutual participation is becoming more common, due to the increased prevalence of chronic disease and the need for preventive health behaviours. A good example is said to be found in dental health education, where a dentist provides the patient with the necessary knowledge and skills, the patient then takes the responsibility for improving and maintaining their oral hygiene. In this model, the professional helps the patients to help themselves. However, with the fast-growing need for dental hygienists, this particular 'opportunity' for mutual participation is being delegated to other health professionals. Dental patients have distinct preferences in relation to treatment decision-making. Further studies have established that these may not always be met during consultation with the dentist. Chapple et al. (2003) found a high preference for mutual participation, especially where the patient and dentist share equal responsibility for decision-making.

Locker (1989) explains that encounters between dentists and patients are constrained by the patients' conditions and the nature of the treatment offered, and that the relationship between them is highly variable. This is due to the change over the course of a patient's treatment or during the single course of the patient's consultation. However, it has been established that the practitioner is generally in control of the consultation, as it is his or her preferences and perceptions of the patient which will ultimately determine its form.

The absence of a therapeutic relationship

Locker (1989) establishes that it is not unreasonable to suppose that health professionals offer less information to those whom they assume do not share their values with respect to oral health. Corah (1986) claims that dentists' views are influenced primarily by those patient characteristics which are manifested during treatment.

Locker (1989) discusses cognitive processes as having their origins in failure, comprehension, interpretation and memory, suggesting that, even when professionals make special efforts to communicate more effectively, many patients remain dissatisfied. It is suggested that this may be due to certain features of the patient–practitioner relationship by inhibiting patients' understanding and retention of information. Patients are understandably not familiar with the technical language of dentistry and may not understand messages that are presented in this technical vocabulary. Patients also find consultations with doctors and, especially, dentists anxiety-provoking and anxiety has a negative effect on memory. Corah et al. (1988) discuss whether an approach to anxiety-reducing behaviours needs to be studied.

Gale et al. (1984) establish that it takes no more time for dentists to interact with patients than it does not to interact and 'busyness' does not hinder information-sharing. However, the dentist's practising style plays a role. As Lahti et al. (1995) note, there is a clear gap in communication between dentists and patients. They find that patients would like more interaction and wanted to be encouraged during the dental treatment. Schouten and Vinkestijn (2002) also note that communication problems between dentist and patient play an important role in complaints and it is important that dentists provide comprehensible information to their patients. Schouten et al. (2003) discuss dentists' communicative skills in informing patients adequately, so that patients can reach a well-informed decision about treatment, in relation to 'informed consent'. Lahti et al. (1996a) found that expectations of patients concerning 'mutual communication' and 'fair support' were not met. However, Ley and Spelman (1988) discuss findings on patient satisfaction with the amount of information received during a consultation and its association with compliance, acknowledging that simply informing patients is, in itself, not enough.

Benefits of a therapeutic relationship in a dental setting

Communication is now more than ever regarded by health professionals and social scientists as a key process in health care provision. 'Effective' communication provides the foundation for diagnosis and treatment. Communication is important to the patient, as it allows the patient to understand, manage and feel at ease with their health problems. However, despite the significance attached to communication, it remains a major area of patient dissatisfaction (Locker 1989).

Research highlights that behaviour such as empathy, friendliness and support is closely associated with patient satisfaction (Corah 1988) and patients are sensitive to dentist behaviours (Kankin and Harris 1985). Locker (1989) suggests that poor communication is attributed to differences in class and status between patients and their professional health care providers. It is suggested that such differences lead to diffidence on the part of patients and reluctance to make demands on the professional's time. Middle-class patients were more likely to ask for information than working-class ones. A number of general practice studies support the observation that people similar to doctors and dentists in terms of social class are more able to communicate effectively with them. Working-class patients are likely to say less than middle-class patients about their problems; they ask fewer questions, get less information and are offered fewer explanations, despite the fact that they wish to know as much as possible about their health. It is suggested that doctors and dentists may also contribute to these class differences in communication because of the perceptions and assumptions they make about their patients (Locker 1989).

Recent research promotes the view that dentists who have a far more accurate understanding of patients' perceptions will leave the patient feeling better understood, less vulnerable and more cared for (Chapman and Kirby-Turner 2002). Gale et al. (1984) believe that it is possible that dentists will give more satisfaction to their patients as they increase their interaction but Sondell and Soderfeldt (1997) note that any theory of 'communication' is lacking in the dental context. There is a necessity in the dental setting to identify and incorporate opportunities for therapeutic relationships and determine their effects.

Current educational standards

The Dentists Act (1984) requires the General Dental Council to ensure that dental schools meet the high standards of dental education at every stage. The aims of the dental curriculum are to produce a caring, knowledgeable, competent and skilful dentist. The current aim of the undergraduate dental education relates to the empathized importance of 'communication' and its effects in the best interest of patients at all times. Students must also be competent at managing fear and anxiety with behavioural techniques and empathise with patients in stressful situations (GDC 2002). Mataki (2000) established that there is less progress concerning the patient–dentist relationship, anxiety, communication and patients' satisfaction and suggests further studies in the future.

Framework proposals for primary dental services in England from 2005

When the item of service payment for dentists is removed and the primary care trust start to commission NHS dentistry, the new General Dental Service contract may improve the dentist–patient relationship; as it will allow the dental surgeon to spend more time with the patient. The care to be provided under the NHS contract aims to improve patient experience. This aim is to be achieved by permitting the patient to exercise informed consent and by providing patients with the necessary information to make informed choices about their health care (Health and Social Care Act, 2003). Under this proposed Act, the dentists are obliged to encourage patients to enter into a continuing relationship with them and to be flexible, if a patient does not wish to, by responding to their treatment needs as appropriate. This will address one aspect of the issue of utilization of dental health provision and may improve patient experience through supporting mutual participation in the dentist–patient relationship. However, important issues still need to be addressed. Although the Health and Social Care Act (2003) requires dentists to encourage patients into a continuing relationship, there is no information, training or suggestions as to how to achieve this. Therefore, it is suggested that the therapeutic relationship may do much for health provision, compliance, continuous care, changing patterns of disease, the social and psychological consequences of oral disease, behaviour, fear or anxiety, dental health education, reduction of occupational stress and improve the dentist–patient communication – just what the doctor ordered! Newsome and Wright (2000) find that a better understanding of patient satisfaction and the evaluation process that leads to satisfaction can only be achieved if patient perception, expectations and desires are considered.

Method of investigation

Aims and objectives

The study's application was to integrate the therapeutic intervention within complementary health care into a dental setting to ascertain the effect(s) of a therapeutic relationship on dental patients, the dental surgeon and the dental nurse. The study was also aimed at establishing the relevance of this intervention. The objective is to establish whether this intervention improved the participants' experience in the dental setting.

Design

A model of therapeutic intervention in a dental setting was devised by the principal researcher who correlate a current published working model of the therapeutic relationship in complementary medicine (Mitchell and Cormack 1998) and recommendations of 'patient management' in the dental surgery (Burke and Freeman 1994), which identified where opportunities arose for therapeutic alliance.

The principal researcher recommended that a psychiatric nurse coach the dental surgeon and dental nurse on achieving the features of therapeutic intervention. This was to ensure that the incorporated communication skills were conveyed appropriately and effectively to the dental patients. Current education guidelines recommend that dental students develop their skills through role play (GDC 2002). Therefore, the training programme for the therapeutic intervention consisted of a 'lecture' and role play so that the dental surgeons and the dental nurses were equipped with appropriate communication skills.

The principal researcher devised a letter, along with a 'suitable' information pack containing a literature review and a copy of the therapeutic intervention to be incorporated, and sent it to two dental practices. The letter was sent six months in advance and gave full details of the expectations of the dental surgeon and dental nurse. A time and date for professional training were provided, along with the study schedule. The dental surgeon and dental nurse were informed that five dental patients were required. The inclusion criteria consisted of a dental appointment for dental treatment of no less than twenty minutes. A prompt reply was requested.

A letter was also sent to a primary care psychiatric establishment six months in advance, inviting a psychiatric nurse to participate in this study. The letter attached a copy of the research proposal, providing full details on the nature of the study and requirements. Dates and times were provided as to when and where the psychiatric nurse would be required to attend. Again, a prompt reply was suggested. Within three weeks, a psychiatric nurse and the two dental practices had contacted the principal researcher and agreed to participate. The principal researcher arranged to meet the psychiatric nurse in Stamford, Lincolnshire and escorted the psychiatric nurse to the dental practices to conduct training.

One week after training, the study commenced. The principal researcher attended the dental practices at nine o'clock on different days, and was provided with a list of dental patients undertaking the study and their appointment duration. The dental patients were escorted to a private room where they were interviewed immediately after their dental treatment.

The context of this intervention was the dental practices, including surgeons and nurses. The conditions were the same for each patient, the only change being the application of the devised therapeutic model and the semi-structured interview process. The participants in the study had to have had previous experience of dental treatment. Their cultural background was also considered important in their treatment regime (Holloway and Wheeler 2002).

The dental surgeon and the dental nurse ascertained their application of the therapeutic intervention on the clients and were provided with a model of the therapeutic intervention for each dental patient to establish, indicate and validate the incorporated therapeutic processes. This was achieved by ticking the appropriate section. The dentist's objectives were to achieve all the phases of the therapeutic intervention during the clinical encounter. The dental surgeon and dental nurse were also able to refer to the tasks. The semi-structured questions were designed to extract the dental patient's interpretation of the clinical encounter. Therefore, detection of the application of the therapeutic intervention by the dental surgeons and dental nurses was reiterated, along with a recorded indication on the provided model. The initial question in the semi-structured interview ascertained a dental patient's general thoughts and feelings regarding dental visits.

The interviews took place at the dental practices for the safety of the dental patients, dental surgeons and the principal researchers, thereby reducing any potential hazards and risks.

The principal researcher introduced herself to the dental patients and described the nature of their participation, which was that they were to be interviewed regarding their experience of a dental setting. The principal researcher explained that all information was confidential and that personal details would be replaced by a code. The principal researcher also explained to each of the dental patients that they were one of ten dental patients being interviewed and that five patients were from a different dental practice. The principal researcher illustrated and reinforced the above to avoid any bias, which could prevail.

The dental surgeons and dental nurses had no foresight with regard to the semi-structured interview questions. The dental patients had no foresight with regard to the incorporation and application of the therapeutic intervention devised. The dental patients were aware they were being interviewed in relation to their experience in a dental setting and were encouraged to express ways of improving an experience. This was to avoid or decrease the Hawthorne reactive effect (Bowling 1997) and for reliability, concerning the effect(s) of the therapeutic intervention.

The research took place at a location in Lincolnshire in one of the four dental practices. The pilot study was undertaken at a location in Cambridgeshire in one of the two dental practices. The therapeutic intervention was applied to ten dental patients after the dental surgeon's and dental nurse's insight and training on the devised model. The dental patients were then interviewed immediately after their dental treatment, in order to evaluate the fundamental essence of their experience. The semi-structured interviews were conducted in a private area away from the dental surgery. The dental surgeon and the nurse were interviewed separately after all the subjects had participated. The dental patients, the dental surgeon and the dental nurse were required to produce a description of their experience for the semi-structured interview.

This study is attainable through a case study due to the indepth analysis of the organization involved. It is acknowledged that case studies may be challenged from rational and irrational perspectives and that perspectives and insights resulting from a case study may be under-appreciated. However, a case study is the preferred strategy when 'how' or 'why' questions are posed (Yin 2003).

A revelatory case study is functional in order to incorporate a detailed and intensive analysis of a case. The aim is to generate an intensive examination, whilst engaging in theoretical analysis. Therefore, an association is evident between theory, generation and theory-testing (Bryman 2001). In addition, a case study is potentially challenging, with a revelatory character that is often able to challenge the existing order of things. Moreover, a case study provides insight to people's lives; which is what is required for better understanding and an improved response or attitude. Therefore, the crucial role of pattern and context in achieving knowledge is within reach through a case study (Gillham 2000). Moreover, a case study has the potential to increase both prepositional and experimental knowledge (Denzin and Lincoln 2000).

A phenomenological approach was incorporated into this study. Phenomenology is primarily a philosophy; its applicability to this study is owed to its 'insightfulness' and its potential for illuminating the phenomenon under-study and to capture its essence (Holloway and Wheeler 2002). Using a phenomenological approach, the intention is to uncover and produce a description of the lived experience of dental patients, dental surgeons and dental nurses. This is to be achieved through semi-structured interviews, as semi-structured interviews have been established as being an important form of interviewing within a case study (Gillham 2000). Also, semi-structured interviews form an interrelationship between the method and sub-method incorporated. A semi-structured interview permits respondents to reply in their own words, allowing a range of reply, when an unaccounted response is expected (Bowling 1997) or invited.

Sample

A sampling strategy used by the qualitative researcher is the underlying principle of gaining rich, in-depth information (Holloway and Wheeler 2002). Purposeful sampling was applied as the objective was to sample a group of people within a setting (Bowling 2002) according to the criteria within this study. Individuals and groups within the dental setting were identifiable by the principal researcher. Informants who could provide information about the specific phenomenon were dental surgeons, dental nurses and hence dental patients.

A triangulated analysis is included in the study, which compared the views of patients, dental surgeons and dental nurses on the therapeutic intervention. The responses to the semi-structured questions are analysed additionally to identify any similarities in statements and impressions or in actions, language and views (Holloway and Wheeler 2002).

The pilot study identified that changes were required in the schedule of interview questions.

Ethical considerations

This study aimed to advance complementary medicine and orthodox medicine by ensuring patient satisfaction and supporting continuous care in a dental setting. It sought to improve the dynamics between the dental surgeon and patient through a therapeutic relationship. The study also aimed to benefit individuals by catering for their particular needs, and improving the clinical encounter would do much to support patients and their oral health. The subjects would be outpatients recruited from two dental practices. The selection criteria were dental patients who required dental treatment and who had an existing appointment. The procedures carried out on the subjects would be a form of dental treatment carried out by their dental surgeon and assisted by the dental nurse. There were no additional risks to the subjects as procedures remained as usual, the only changed factor was the additional therapeutic model incorporated by the dental surgeon, assisted by the dental nurse.

The subjects were approached by the dental practice with an interval between supplying the information and gaining consent (Thomas 2000). Willing subjects were sent a letter explaining what was being asked of them, along with a consent form and stamped addressed envelope. Their dentist had described the process of informed consent for their treatment previously. All subjects were informed of their right to withdraw at any time. There would be full compliance with the Data Protection Act (1989). The principal researcher would also be working within the research governance frame-work for health and social care (DoH 2001). The security precautions taken to safeguard the confidentiality of the subjects' data involved no identifiable information being passed to any other member of the dental team at the practice. Each participant was supplied with a code and referred to by a code rather than their name. The magnitude of risk for each subject remained consistent in a dental setting. However, the dental surgeons involved were extremely experienced in the field of dentistry and did much to reduce any risk to patients. Subjects benefited directly from this incorporation of a therapeutic relationship into the dental setting, especially whilst undergoing treatment. Future patients may also benefit from this therapeutic relationship model in a dental setting (Freeman and Tyler 1992). The therapeutic model was devised to ensure patient satisfaction and this devised intervention would be available to all existing dental surgeons who wish to develop interpersonal skills, improve communication, support their patients and develop their dental practice through the therapeutic relationship. The devised model would also be available for student dental surgeons as a researched teaching aid.

Plans for analysis

The collection of primary 'material' bearing on the question (and beyond) is analysed (Denzin and Lincoln 2000) in an idiographic manner (Bowling 2002). The seven-stage process is the approach for the 'data analysis' and occurs as follows (Colaizzi 1978). All the subject's protocols will be read in order to acquire a feeling for them and to make sense of them. Significant statements will be identified by studying every description and extracting phrases or sentences that directly pertain to the investigated phenomenon. Formulated meanings are produced by highlighting the importance and meaning of each significant statement, then repeating the above for each description and organizing the aggregate formulated meanings into clusters of themes. By referring to these clusters of themes and then back to the original protocols, the process of validation is established. This is so discrepancies among and/or between the various clusters can be noted. All the results, integrate into an exhaustive description of the investigated topic (Holloway and Wheeler 2002).

The themes that arose from the respondents are arranged methodically with subdivisions. The reported experiences are quoted to enable recurring analysis and validation of bases for interpretation. In addition, analysis is presented neutrally, with both supporting and challenging data (Yin 2003).

The reader can therefore reach an independent judgement regarding the merits of the analysis (Yin 2003). This also permits an increase in both prepositional and experimental knowledge (Denzin and Lincoln 2000).

Pilot study

The piloting of the semi-structured questions and 'the therapeutic intervention in a dental setting' was further under scrutiny by professionals in this field in order to establish any ambiguity relating to the content (Bowling 2002). A dental coordinator for an NHS primary care trust examined the research proposal and its contents fully understanding the aims of the study, the content and the importance, although it was suggested that the researcher revisit grammar errors. Two dental surgeons and two hygienists not involved with the study examined the research proposal and therapeutic intervention and found no ambiguity, suggesting that the study was interesting and appropriate. Although this procedure relies on solely subjective judgements, it will, along with other methods employed, increase the validity and reliability of the proposed questions, the therapeutic intervention and objectives of the study (Silverman 2000).

Although pilot studies are not always conducted in qualitative inquiry due to the research being developmental, as a 'novice' researcher the testing of semi-structured interviews and data was undertaken with colleagues and acquaintances in order for the researcher to become familiar, confident and developmental of necessary skills for data collection (Siliverman 2000).

The conduct of the pilot study in a different location, with different dental patients, a different dental surgeon and dental nurse, ensures the validity and reliability of the results presented. Their reliability can be equated with the stability, consistency or dependability of the measuring tool. The stability of measure will refer to the extent to which the same scores are obtained when the instrument is used with the same subjects (Silverman 2000).

The administration process of the pilot study also 'tests' the use of the incorporated therapeutic intervention and semi-structured interview questions. The pilot study was also conducted at a different dental practice to reduce the Hawthorne effect (Bowling 2002). The pilot study identified flaws in its design and improved the 'instrument' for replication (Reid 1993). Five dental patients, a dental surgeon and a dental nurse tested the use of the incorporated therapeutic intervention, the training applied and the semi-structured interview questions in context. The training also provided the dental surgeon and dental nurse with a place to ask questions relating to objectives and their role.

Training within the pilot study also permitted development and ensured satisfaction regarding the presentation of the devised therapeutic model. It became apparent that the model would best be reduced to only one or two pages to ensure efficiency with application and delivery during the research process. The therapeutic phases were narrowed down to one major application for each phase to ensure effectiveness. The pilot study also established that training consisted of information partaking, i.e., a 'lecture' on the psychological theories, by the psychiatric nurse, with a requirement for the principal researcher to describe and discuss the incorporation of therapeutic skills in the dental setting. This was a desired requirement by the dental surgeon and widened the principal researcher's role. In addition, the principal researcher and the dental surgeon collaborated on the devised therapeutic intervention with the psychiatric nurse's advice and expertise on the best way to achieve objectives through verbal communication. This pleased all participants involved.

The pilot study also addressed certain areas relating to the dental patient's interpretation of the semi-structured questions. Four out of the five patients interviewed in the pilot study did not identify with the terminology 'clinical encounter'. The term 'clinical encounter' was then changed to 'experience in the dentist surgery'. It also became evident through the pilot study that a conveyed therapeutic skill of mutuality by the dental nurse was misinterpreted. Although this did not provoke anxiety in the particular dental patient (in fact the opposite), a potential was identified. One stage of the therapeutic intervention asked the question: 'we need to provide you with a clothes protector. Would you like me to put it on or would you like to?' This was shortened to 'Would you like me to put it on or would you like to?' only. This is because during the semi-structured interview a dental patient pointed out that 'they [the dental team] even put a protector on you in case your clothes get messed up, but I told them these are my work clothes.'

The pilot study also enabled the principal researcher to identify and reflect upon interviewing techniques. Whilst transcribing the data from the pilot study, she recognized incongruity within the techniques and style of delivery. It became evident that the principal researcher completed the last word of a sentence, or displayed an understanding of interpretation, that inhibited and closed the respondents' response. In addition, data that may have presented were subsequently repressed. This occurred on several occasions, disappointing the principal researcher as what would have been effective data had to be disregarded, as it was a confounding factor (Bowling 2002) in the nature of the study.

Reflection of the process

The principal researcher participated in the training, firstly by introducing the team to each other as all parties involved initially appeared nervous. The principal researcher initiated the links between psychological theories and therapeutic skills in the study and encouraged the participation and collaboration of the dental team for two reasons: first, for the development of the devised therapeutic intervention and second for the additional benefits that involving professionals would bring to the nature of the research. The training demonstrated that the dental team involved had little knowledge of the suggested related psychology and therapeutic skills. The dental team were extremely interested and said that they were pleased to have found the training interesting. This provided modification and improvement as, although notes were taken, the dental surgeon was very interested in an information leaflet, and asked that the principal researcher and the psychiatric nurse send him one. Therefore, one was devised. The second time around, training had improved as a result of this process. However, there is always room for improvement: the layout could have been better organized to make the therapeutic tasks easier to follow.

The dental patients interviewed were very responsive and felt at ease with the interview process. These respondents appeared very willing to share their experiences and the interview process was developed and expanded by their description of their experiences. Little skill, if any, was required on behalf of the principal researcher in interviewing technique. The latter learnt to just ask the semi-structured questions and listen. However, she now acknowledges the importance of the interviewing skills required for such a study and that she failed to prompt patients for further description which would have enriched this study with a vast amount of information. The principal researcher felt comfortable about interviewing the dental patients, though once they had related their experiences after the interview process she felt a bit helpless, as it appeared to end the process which gave great insight into respondents' lives. The researcher wore casual clothes, a pair of jeans and a jumper and offered them a cup of tea – which they had to decline because of the local anaesthetic. The interview environment had comfortable sofas and was clear of clutter, tidy and private.

The principal researcher was under the impression that the dental patients interviewed seemed surprised at her age she felt that this assisted them in feeling comfortable, and with the descriptions they gave.

When the researcher interviewed health professionals, they all appeared nervous; one dental team remained so throughout the interview process in direct contrast to the dental patients. A dental nurse even tried to get out of it by explaining she had to pick her son up, and could she do this over the phone – though this was already arranged. The principal researcher had to assure the nurse that it would not take long and that she would be more than able to cope with the interview process and contents. The dental nurse then agreed but appeared nervous so that the principal researcher then also felt nervous. After the first question was asked, the dental nurse had to take deep breaths and both started to laugh nervously. The dentist also appeared nervous in interview. The interviewer also felt nervous, but had managed this nervousness previously and ensured that the dentist and dental nurse were as comfortable as possible. All then relaxed, though they were pleased when it ended. The other dental team interviewed were nervous initially, the dental nurse more so than the dental surgeon, but the researcher now felt fine about the interview process, as she had been exposed to this situation previously and so managed the situation.

Analysis

The names of the patients, the dental surgeons and the dental nurses were replaced with an identifiable code, to ensure confidentiality and anonymity within the dental practices.

Key
patients = PResponse
dental surgeons = DSResponse
dental nurse = NResponse

Whilst transcribing the data, the principal researcher obtained an idea of similarities and clusters. The data was read in the context of the particular dental surgeries and then as a whole. Responses were noted under related headings. These headings then either grew in content or did not. The plan for analysis followed, though it was adapted slightly; the researcher used coloured dots for identification and to ensure rigour. Data were then read in context and as a whole. This process was repeated, as each time the principal researcher began to recognize a deeper meaning and content. The data then became clearer and what was previously read and reread stood in a different light. Under scrutiny, existing data was shown to have more value than previously thought. The headings also grew, with relevant or what was assumed to be irrelevant data. This process was repeated. Different themes and clusters began to jump out from the data. Headings that did not appear to be related, often were but in a different way. Data from the dental team were subject to the same process; in addition, all this data was related and then interlinked and grew from previously scrutinising the dental patients' data. Therefore the initial clusters and themes developed in different directions. What the researcher started out with, was not what she finished up with. Data obtained became precious and dynamic and was then identified as research. Headings emerged and themes were developed from them.

Dental patients

A theme identified in dental patients consisted of apprehension.

Apprehension

Dental patients were asked what their general thoughts and feelings were about coming to a dentist.

Three of the dental patients interviewed readily expressed that they felt apprehensive.

> 'Well, I am always apprehensive when I come, but I'm not frightened or anything. I just made the appointment and I must go.' (*PResponse 1*)

These dental patients felt apprehension before a dental appointment, although apprehension existed at varying degrees.

> 'A necessary evil I think is perhaps the best way to describe it. Not something I particularly look forward to … Um, it is a necessary evil, you have got to do it – you have to look after your teeth, simple as that.' (*PResponse 4*)

Three patients who implied that they were fine about dental treatment revealed their concerns within the interview session.

> 'I take it as part of life and obviously as times progress people can have their teeth longer. It doesn't frighten me in the least – I've just had a wisdom tooth out. I was not bothered about having the tooth out. Yes, I was not bothered; they always call me by my first name anyway. It's more like a family relaxed atmosphere. I think that obviously relaxes patients.' (*PResponse 5*)

When this dental patient was asked what her expectations were when coming to the dentist, she replied:

> 'I think it went exactly as I expected … um. I was hoping that it – it would not be like it was years ago – I sat in the chair for an hour for that. I was hoping it was not going to be that bad and it was not so.' (*PResponse 5*)

The other dental patient stated similar views on coming to a dentist.

> 'I am open – I don't worry about it, the practice is brilliant here, you know the dentist and his assistant, the hygienist are all brilliant. I never felt a think in actual-fact. No-No, I can't fault them in anyway to be honest with you on that end. My – I don't worry about it, you know. I think they can't do enough for you here, and

you know as soon as you have an appointment you're in and that is it, sort of thing. I never felt a thing in actual fact.' (*PResponse 6*)

One of the ten patients interviewed, when asked what his general thoughts and feelings were regarding coming to a dentist, explained that he was pleased to get dental treatment.

'I am just pleased to get treatment. I'm not at all worried about coming to a dentist ur . . . you know if I need treatment I'm just glad to get it. So, I'm pleased to come to a dentist. I am pleased – I'm not unhappy about it . . . and – because I know I am going to get treatment and if I've got toothache I know it's going to be/do something about it, ur, so . . . what more do you want me to say [*laughs*].' (*PResponse 10*)

This particular patient felt pleased to attend a dental surgery and receive dental treatment, and felt no apprehension or fear nor expressed any information throughout the interview session that would correlate to emerging themes. The respondent had some difficulty with access to a dental surgeon.

'The treatment – it could have waited till July; um, I wasn't compelled to have it now, err, I decided it was worth paying the money now, rather than waiting till July/August whenever. Err, my previous dentist was the same situation, when I moved to this area he – he had not got a place on his national health list. So he took me as a private patient initially until there was room for me on his list. The treatment was just the same, whether it was national health or private and I'm sure the same applies to this practice too. I was prepared to pay quite a lot of money in order to get this done [dental treatment] as I felt I needed it, rather than wait eight months or whatever. Having had serious toothache – (when was it) about six weeks ago, um, I did not want a repetition of that.' (*PResponse 10*)

Fear

An emerging theme in the latter three patients was fear. These dental patients described their thoughts and feelings about coming to a dentist and the consequences.

'Scared stiff, really frightened, I mean not just frightened: absolutely, really terrified. I could not eat; well, you made my appointment [turns to husband]. I could not even make my appointment, I could not even ring up – I knew I had to come. I had pain on the left side of my tooth, and by the time my appointment came, of course the pain went. I was saying to my husband, I don't, I won't, need to go; I'll be alright – I'm not going to get really worked up. I couldn't eat and I couldn't sleep. I knew I had to come, so I thought don't be stupid, I will go; so I walked down from where I lived. I was petrified, really petrified. I had not been for a long time [47 years, says husband]. Yes, I had two teeth that had grown under the dentures and I thought what will the dentist think of me. I thought I might have this awful and what would this dentist think – he might be really awful to me and tell me I should have come sooner, what are you bothering me now for ... So there was a bit of that as well.' (*PResponse 7*)

The patients interviewed had varying degrees of apprehension or fear:

'Horror – because I haven't been for a long time. Um, yes, very nervous and apprehensive. Not nice.' (*Response 9*)

Some dental patients readily expressed their negative thoughts and feelings and others attempted to conceal them.

'Well, I'm always anxious when I come, but there is no need to be now. I don't lose sleep over it or anything; I sometimes think, oh gosh, I've got the dentist. I hope I don't have to have an extraction – that's what I really fear.' (*PResponse 2*)

All dental patients expressed the belief that there is a need to attend a dental surgery.

'Well, I am always apprehensive when I come, but I'm not frightened or any thing. I just made the appointment and I must go.' (*PResponse 1*)

The need to attend was seen as a health value:

'I can have anything done – I'd, I'll lie there for an hour if it [the tooth] can be repaired or built up – but otherwise not. But no, no, I am not too anxious. I'm a bit jittery when I get in the chair, but otherwise I'm ... I don't mind that much.' 'Cause it's for my good really.' (*PResponse 2*)

Or there was an acknowledged need for dental treatment, such as pain or cosmetic purposes.

'Err, he explained the problems, err, that, err, with regards to my mouth – various teeth – and I was well satisfied that he would be able to deal with it to my satisfaction ... err so that I wouldn't have any more toothaches, err, so that I would ... have a reasonable set of teeth with which to, err, eat.' (*PResponse 10*)

The patients' explanation for their 'apprehension/fear' was highly correlated to experiences as a child and school dentists. Eight of the ten patients interviewed described the effect of an experience with a school dentist:

'When I'd been before [to a dentist] it was really old fashioned and horrible-horrible, brown, brown things and instruments all over, really frightening and they are. But, when I came in it looked so different you see – it just looked so nice and different and he's [the current dentist] so nice to me. I still had this vision of this horrible old dentist, where I used to go that was horrible when we were kids. So, so you know I got a different one, when I came he was nice, really nice.' (*PResponse 7*)

The experience of school dentists by patients when they were children varied in consequence and effect.

'It's the normal psychological reaction to dentistry. I associate it for some reason or another ... go back to school when you had, um, quite considerable amount of pain when you went to a dentist [laughs] – cause we used to have school dentists in them days, but since then there's no real problem now.' (*PResponse 1*)

A 'better' dental experience provided a reduction in apprehension.

I've been coming here for years, it's nice, warm, relaxed, not like the dentists when I was a child – when you went in and it was all very severe. Waiting room with hard chairs, few magazines, and it always had a sort of disinfectant smell. It is far more relaxed these days. I think that is more important for today.' (*PResponse 5*)

Each dental patient's apprehension correlated to the prospect of replication of the past event. A patient who had booked an appointment for dental treatment, had a dental examination and returned later that afternoon to begin dental treatment described her expectations:

'Pain, I think, you know, um, because having um – when I was a child we had a school dentist who was horrendous. Er, and I think from that all dentists were, it – it all went with pain. As soon as you heard the word 'dentist' you associated it with pain.' (*PResponse 4*)

A subdivision within this theme correlated with a past experience, although not through an experience with a school dentist in two dental patients. One of the ten patients interviewed expressed his dissatisfaction with a previous dentist three years ago.

'Um, I actually left our previous dentist who was NHS, and the reason we did that – we were actually at that practice for three years and there was a continual change over amongst dental staff. And there were a couple of dentists I wasn't particularly happy with. I have experienced where you have not had it done quickly [dental treatment] and that is really distressing for me.' (*PResponse 4*)

Of most importance to this dental patient was:

'The very, most important, thing is the actual accessibility of the dentist, um, regularly. Check-ups are great 'cause they are always booked in the diary and there are occasions where you need tre-treatment quickly and I suppose to have that treatment done quickly is the single most important thing for me.' (*PResponse 4*)

One of the ten dental patients interviewed explained how his fear existed through recurring nightmares of a dentist when he was a child.

'I've had nightmares as a child that the dentist – the dentist screaming out to reception for somebody to come and stick something into my mouth to take out something.' (*PResponse 8*)

The same prospects of replication are evident in those two patients whose apprehension/fear does not correlate highly with a school dentist but with a past experience.

'I personally feel, their persona, their tones in their voices, the fact that there is constant communication of what is happening next helps to relax.' (*PResponse 8*)

'I think the beauty of it is – is I'm actually listening to what is actually happening now – you know I can sense if something is wrong or if there is something in his tone.' (*PResponse 8*)

'I've never experienced it here – but I would hate to come and something go drastically wrong or hear something in his tone which would make me think, oh, hold on something more going on here.' (*PResponse 8*)

Each patient's apprehension/fear or pleasure correlated to the prospect of replication of a past event.

Impression of the dental surgery and environment

An emergent theme related to impressions of the dental surgery and its environment. The dental patients were asked what their initial impression of the dentist were when they entered the dental surgery. All the dental patients interviewed described interpersonal skills in initial impressions that involved familiarization of the dental surgeon, politeness together with mutuality.

'Of the dentist himself, er, very polite, um, explained everything that wanted – what treatment wanted doing, um, very helpful and um, explained everything as he went along.' (*PResponse 9*)

Two dental patients interviewed also described the confidence the dental surgeon installed in them.

'Well, having met him before, ur, I, I, I am very content to getting him to deal with whatever-to trust him to do what is right as far as my mouth is concerned.

He seems to be most competent and, er, interested in what he is doing, err, conscientious, err, so, I am pleased that, that he is dealing with whatever the problem may be.' (*PResponse 10*)

The remaining subdivisions concerned the dental surgery and the dental environment.

'Initial impression is it is a professional set-up, efficient looking set-up, clean and tidy so.' (*PResponse 4*)

When the dental patients were asked what their initial impression was of the dental surgeon as they entered the dental surgery a subdivision of this theme emerged that illustrated that the initial impressions of the dental patients emerged with present impressions.

Well, the impression was that it was well laid out and it was quite a clean sort of premises. Well, I was interested in getting the dentistry finished – I must admit [laughs]. Yes, well apart from apprehension I think that was the main thing.' (*PResponse 1*)

Thus, eight dental patients (the latter two were PResponse 9 and 10) said that they were always seeking to revise their impressions of a dentist.

'The man – well, he is very nice; he, er, sort of very calming – when you look at him – when you see him. He – he seems to have this quite calm way when he speaks to you and everything; he puts me at ease. Well, I was thinking, I hope this is the last time and these teeth fit and that I will be OK really. I was just hoping they would fit alright cause we've had such a problem with them and for him as well you know. I thought, I hope they fit this time and they are alright – cause I've kept coming back and they were not – but everything was alright.' (*PResponse 7*)

'He explains exactly what he is doing. He reassures you, yes, he was fine. He's always welcoming. He smiles at you and talks to you but he doesn't try and hold a conversation that you can't answer, you know – he's got the touch really. Well I'd got a broken tooth at the back, I had a temporary filling that had come out and I just, just wanted it saved, that tooth. And I said I don't care what you have to do as long as I don't have to have it out and he said no, no, I can repair it, and he repaired it.' (*PResponse 2*)

'Um, very courteous, very helpful, um, I get a bit frustrated with delays as a private patient paying quite a bit of money – I would have expected to go in at the time I was supposed to be in where as I think too. I've waited an hour and a half today it was very, very frustrating. Apart from that a good dentist. Fine, just hoping he would be able to do what he said he'd do on the day.' (*PResponse 3*)

The initial and generally familiar environment of the dental surgery reassured patients. Familiarity on the background of optimistic impressions, such as politeness, appeared to be an important aspect of reassuring patients and reinforcing initial good impressions. All patients could describe their initial impressions of the dentist, no matter how long ago.

A subdivision within the dental surgery environment category established the role of members of the dental team. This was positive in only one dental practice. One dental patient from the other dental practice, when asked if there was anything he felt might improve experience in the dental setting, said:

> 'I think that, you know, looking over the treatment, the only thing which wasn't so bad this time but the previous time the amount … the assistant who assists. Who puts the suction thing in your mouth – she seemed to nearly choke me [laughs]. So I found that most uncomfortable initially. That was the only thing. I suppose that just was one of those things, that's happened to me I – I don't know.'   (*PResponse 1*)

The corresponding dental patients from the former dental practice pointed to the role of the receptionist and dental staff as influential to their experience of a dental setting. One dental patient described members of the dental team in the context of their general thoughts and feelings on coming to a dentist.

> 'You know (the dentist) and his assistant (hygienist) are all brilliant.'   (*PResponse 6*)

The same patient describes initial impressions of the dental team:

> 'Like I'm talking to you – that's how the practice is like what's her name downstairs … [receptionist] is always very pleasant, very good.'   (*PResponse 6*)

The patient also describes the dental team in the context of his experience of dental treatment.

> 'Very well 'cause they make you feel at home, your part and parcel of their life – as you are to a point, in a roundabout way.'   (*PResponse 6*)

A dental patient at the same practice describes how he was supported emotionally and physically.

> 'Between the dentist, the dental nurse and the receptionist, they make me feel very relaxed.'   (*PResponse 8*)

Another dental patient from the dental practice described the dentist and dental nurse being emotionally and physically supportive:

> 'Very helpful, both the dentist and the nurse. They both have a nice calm approach which is reassuring.'   (*PResponse 4*)

Another dental patient describes the role of the dental team in their dental treatment.

'I do like the friendly ... we have a joke and the nursing staff and the reception staff ... personally I think it relaxes me. I come in quite relaxed, the treatment goes better 'cause you are not all tensed up.' (*PResponse 5*)

The patient describes the role of the dental team as of key importance to her during a visit to the dentist.

'Whenever I walk in to the surgery, it's that friendly. You go in, it's relaxed – they are friendly, first-name terms. It is socially that, really ... When you are first greeted, that is what relaxes you. It does make a difference.' (*PResponse 5*)

When asked whether this experience would affect her perception, thoughts or behaviour in any way, and why, in future appointments, the patient said:

'It has a positive effect on me, 'cause if it did not I would not return. I think it does ... .' (*PResponse 5*)

Reaction to dentist/treatment

Expectations of the clinical encounter were derived from past and current experiences of dentistry, either positive or negative.
    Dental patient expectations were derived largely from the dental surgeon.

'I have a full understanding of what is going to be done. So I'm not sitting in the chair not knowing what to expect. The general persona, I think they make you feel relaxed; when you are getting an injection, they are telling you it's going to be a small little scratch. Just the tone in their voices helps you to relax. Because, I think, all of a sudden, um, I was taken sort of back – I used to sit in the chair completely clenched and so tight and not really taking in what was happening around me. My eyes were very closed and, um, ears and thinking about birds twittering in the distance. Whereas now ... it's difficult to explain. I can sit in that chair and have a conservation with them – obviously I have got my mouth full of something. So, although I still probably clutch the arms – I can sit there and basically not feel how I used to.' (*PResponse 8*)

This dental patient described what his previous expectations had been.

'I walk in; I could actually talk you through the whole process. I walk in, I go in, I get an injection, I come back out in the reception. I read a magazine for a few minutes and I go back in and it's done.' (*PResponse 8*)

Being aware what to expect made patients less apprehensive or fearful.

'You come to a dentist and you are never quite sure what's going to happen. And there is always an element of ... your not quite sure ... .' (*PResponse 1*)

The dental patients were asked how they feel they were supported emotionally and physically throughout the dental treatment. Apprehensive patients described, interpreted and reacted to the dentist's application of the therapeutic intervention in dental treatment.

'Alright because he kept saying 'you're doing well' – 'cause he knows that I had four teeth taken out here once, and I think it's on my notes. And, um, er, but I've had really good treatment, 'cause I was very, very anxious. I didn't know that I was going to have these four teeth out until I got there. It was a tremendous shock, that was a long time ago, probably ten, twelve years ago. But then he, no, was fine. He said he knew I was nervous, and, um, he said I was doing really well. He said ... oh and I had lots of little rests in between which was good. 'Cause sometimes you want to swallow or spit out and you can't. But, he just said 'Raise your left hand if you want me to stop or if you want a breather' – that was good. Well it – I was just calm in there, I didn't feel nervous at all. I just felt calm.' *(PResponse 2)*

Interpretation and reaction to the dentist's application was obtained from fearful dental patients.

'Very ... well he explained everything to me, if I had any discomfort or anything to raise my left hand and he would stop and he kept saying ... he was ... um, how can I explain it, he helped me through it by, by saying what he was doing and how well I was doing 'cause he knew I was nervous. And, he gave me the confidence to [*laughs*]. It made me feel a lot easier, not so nervous, a lot better.' *(PResponse 9)* '

Patients who claimed that they were fine about going to the dentist reacted to the dental surgeon's applications and treatment.

'Um, I suppose there were regular questions to as to whether I was alright, to raise an arm if there was any pain, so you know it wasn't as if he wasn't caring about ... you know, me as a patient. So that was good. It made me feel very relaxed while the treatment was being done – that's good.' *(PResponse 3)*

The patient who was pleased to come to a dentist, and did not feel the need for emotional support, responded to the dental surgeon's applications and treatment.

'I didn't need to be supported emotionally as far as I'm aware. However, I was told if I was in any pain to raise my left hand (I didn't need to). And, um – ur – every so often the dentist would stop and say 'Is this alright? How are you doing?', and, er, he'd say 'I think you are doing very well.' Um he said this several times – at different times, because I was in there seventy minutes. Err I've had longer times than this in the distance past err, but today everything was done to make me as comfortable err as I could be in the circumstances. Err – whenever my mouth was filled, they kept using the – what's it called? *The Suction (principle researcher).* Yes, that's it. Emotionally there was no problem at all, it was physical discomfort that's all I can say but they did the best they could in the circumstances, it wasn't painful. It gave me confidence, that's I think that would be the best thing to say. I felt confident that er, what was happening was happening under control, and I was well satisfied.' *(PResponse10)*

The dental patients interviewed placed emphasis upon being supported emotionally, synchronizing emotional support with physical support.

The therapeutic intervention incorporated by the dental surgeon had positive affects on nine dental patients.

The tenth dental patient expressed ambiguity with regards to reaction to the dentist, though the response is contradictory. When this patient was asked whether they (the dentist and himself) reached a shared agreement, the response established an aspect of uncertainty.

'In terms of today, I fully understood what was going to happen today: always feel that they are very informative here. So they are actually telling you what they are going to do. Sometimes that does not help. I'd rather not know and get my head down and just get it over and done with ... I think the experiences I've had with previous dentists it was very much not really knowing what they were doing in there. There was very little communication ... Or if I turned up for treatment it was not knowing you know ... so here you currently get a full understanding of what treatment is about to take place. It makes me understand that I'm not going for something totally unexpected. So I suppose it helps all the nervousness ... concerns I have on the build up.' *(PResponse 8)*

The dental team also acknowledged this (see below).

Dental patients were asked to describe their experience of the dental treatment and seven dental patients expressed similar views:

'Today, top class. It was really good. You couldn't have got any better if you had paid, if you had paid a lot of money. You know you're treated like an individual, you know. Time did not seem to matter to him. He was not hurrying to say, thinking, I am sure he wasn't thinking about the next person. He was only thinking that you were in there.' *(PResponse 1)*

A dental patient described his experience of dental treatment as

'As usual very good, no pain, in and out very quick.' *(Response 8)*

Another dental patient described either uncomfortable or horrible elements of dental treatment:

Er, painless – I must admit it was painless, um ... I don't really know what happened, it was just ... just said what he was doing as he went through it. I mean I had the injections and that, and everything just went perfect, not a, nothing at all. The only horrible thing was having an impression taken. But apart from that it was very painless and ... very well.' (*PResponse 9*)

Dental patients were asked if their experience today would affect them in any way when returning for future appointments and why. Eight of the patients said that the experience today would not have any effect on them.

'No, I was more than satisfied with today, with his performance today and I would come back in six or eight months or whatever it is.' (*PResponse 1*)

When asked this question, one patient said:

'Oh no, I am not bothered about coming back, no, no, not at all. Because of the way you are treated you're an individual and, um, treatment's good, it's painless and those things matter a lot.' (*PResponse 2*)

One patient said that he is comfortable to attend a dentist anyway:

'Um, no I feel comfortable; I come to the dentist anyway so, no, fine, fine. Um, I mean I've always felt comfortable, nothing was, er, carried out today by the dentist to make me feel otherwise bothered by that. The only thing that would bother me again was coming in thinking am I going to be seen or am I going to wait for an hour and a half to see a dentist and as a private patient that is quite a concern for me.' (*PResponse 3*)

The dental patient who was pleased to come for dental treatment also describes how the experience would not affect him and why:

'Um, not really, because I shall be glad to come anyhow. So, so if I'd had a bad experience today I would not want to come. I've had a good experience. Not a comfortable experience and err a long time, but I feel this was the right thing to do, rather than having to come several times for perhaps twenty minutes. It was all done in one go. And that's good as far as I'm concerned. So I'm very happy with the experience today ... it makes me feel in a fortnights time I shall look forward to coming to get the crown fitted and all will be done.' (*PResponse 10*)

One dental patients describes the positive effect the experience has on her:

'It has a positive effect on me, cause if it did not I would not return. I think it does.' (*Response 5*)

A fearful dental patient who booked an appointment in the morning and returned in the afternoon describes

'Um ... [Laughs] You're asking me to come back to the dentist [laughs]. Um, er, I'm coming back for fillings and new dentures to give me a better appearance. Um, especially with the new dentures and tidying all the fillings up. That I've got a better appearance than what it is now.' (*PResponse 9*)

Dental patients were asked what was of most importance to them during a visit to the dentist.

'Everything he does is valuable to me. His attitude, his work, his patience um personality.' (*PResponse 7*)

'The way he makes me feel relaxed and comfortable and am not being a nuisance to him. 'Cause sometimes you go to the doctors and that you feel like you, feel like you're being a bit of a pain don't you sometimes, and we've had this problem but he is just so nice about everything.' (*PResponse 7*)

'Well the most important thing I I suppose is the confidence in your surroundings – providing that you are comfortable – you can relax then. And there was no problem at all. It was three quarters of an hour late but – that was one of those things. You know somebody before me obviously needed more treatment then first in visited.' (*Response 1*)

'That's quite difficult ... [laughs] 'cause you can't have one without the other really can you. Um, good treatment – I want good successful treatment. Um well to be just treated well and today you are treated well in all things, doctors–dentists; it's much better than when I was a child.' (*PResponse 1*)

'To be told that there is no further treatment required [Laughs] ... That the treatment goes well, I think that's the most important thing. I think for my point of view it's to turn up and know that everything is going well.' (*PResponse 8*)

'Just that relaxed atmosphere, I think that's what is important. Perhaps it is the familiarity of me being a patient here for several years. Um I don't quite know what they are like with new patients but for me they are friendly – that obviously goes on through out the years. It built up over a period of time.' (*PResponse 5*)

'That it's efficient and the work that I expect will be done on the day.' (*PResponse 3*)

'H ... h ... h ... interesting question, er ... the most important thing I think is to have confidence in your dentist. Er, to feel secure that er, you're in the safe hands of someone who knows what he or she is doing (as the case may be) and that the outcome will be satisfactory to the both of us.' (*PResponse 10*)

'Um, I think having confidence in the dentist if he is talking to you all the time and saying how you are progressing and your progressing with it, with the pain or what ever he is doing. I think it is the confidence he gives you is the most ... .' (*PResponse 9*)

Dental surgeons and dental nurses

Reaction to therapeutic intervention

The dental surgeons and dental nurses were asked to describe their initial feelings on taking part in the therapeutic relationship in a dental setting. Similar views were expressed by dental surgeons and dental nurses. A dental surgeon describes how he felt apprehensive initially:

> 'Apprehensive, well I was not sure what was going to be involved in it or how difficult it was going to be – as it turns out it was quite straightforward.' (*DResponse 1*)

The dental nurse who was employed by the dental surgeon above expressed similar feelings regarding taking part.

> 'It has been very interesting, I've learnt that we do do a lot of these things any-way – I've just been aware what we're doing really [laughs nervously]. [*Principal researcher rephrased the question: How did you feel?*] I initially felt slightly nervous. Wasn't quite sure what it entailed – um, that's it really. [*Principal researcher: You felt nervous?*] Because of the way the questions were set, the way we had to ask questions to the patients – especially patients that have been coming here twenty years or whatever and they know us and we know them. It was quite hard to say different things to them ... It's nice to be involved to see what comes out of it, really.' (*NResponse 2*)

The dental nurse had mixed feelings concerning taking part in the study. The dental nurse's response was very similar to the dental surgeon's response, though the dental nurse had some concern regarding practising styles and refers to the relationships built with the dental patient: 'they know us and we know them.' However, in the same instance, the dental nurse felt it was nice to be involved and appeared keen to observe the outcome.

The dental surgeon was asked how he found the integration of the therapeutic intervention into his job role.

> 'Oh, you will have to run that one by me again ... [*Principal researcher repeats question: How did you find the integration of the therapeutic intervention within your job role?*] How did it all fit together – Oh, I thought it all went really well – yer. Yes, I'm sure we did a lot of that anyway. It was nice to have it compartmentalized and realize what you're doing, the stages ... yes. Well, it tends to be a bit stinted to start off with but I think by the time we got to the fifth one we were doing quite well actually.' (*DResponse 1*)

The dental nurse was asked how she found the integration of the therapeutic intervention into her job role. The dental nurse had a question to ask in stage one, about mutuality: 'Would you like me to put it on for you or would you like to?' The dental nurse describes how she found the question hard and appeared concerned with this particular question.

> 'Certain questions I found quite hard. Because you do ask them – but you ask them in a different sort of way – so the way you're asked to say them I found quite difficult – but, er, once you've done it a couple of times you sort of get used to it, get in the swing of it – it sort of comes more naturally. You're all the time thinking, like, what am I going to say here, I've got to say this and that. It is no different from normal really – you are just aware you are thinking of it all the time, have we said this – have we said that – but we have said them.' (*NResponse 2*)

The dental surgeon at the other dental practice described his initial feelings:

> 'Er, my initial feelings were good, OK, you know, er, obviously we like to try something that can help our patients. So it was quite positive.' (*DResponse 2*)

The dental nurse employed by the dental surgeon above describes how she found the integration if the therapeutic intervention into her job role:

> 'Er, I thought that it worked, and the patients were happy afterwards ... [*Principal researcher: How did you feel initially when you were asked to take part*]? I didn't mind – I felt OK about it.' (*NResponse 1*)

The dental surgeon from the other dental practice describes how he found the integration of the therapeutic relationship into his job role:

> 'I think, um, you know, most of the things we obviously went through in this study we were doing already. But I think since we obviously went through this study we are doing it in a more constructive, more ordered manner. Before that we were doing things, we were not doing all of them. OK maybe we were doing a few things, but we will now try and do all the things. So we have actually implemented these things. Quite positive. We were able to order it and integrate it within our normal practice. Most of the things we were doing already but we were not doing them in a constructive manner; it was not ordered, we were doing it sometimes, or we were probably doing a few bits. But now we are doing it to all our patients. But sometimes you're a bit busy then we might miss a step, but generally we will do it to all our patients now. The patients appreciate – the patients like being in control.' (*DResponse 2*)

His dental nurse describes how she found it:

> 'It was easy, it fitted in quite well. 'Cause it made the patients' more comfortable and they knew what you were doing and he explained it better. They were more comfortable 'cause normally he doesn't explain, he just gets on with it. It's easy, it

only takes about five seconds to explain what you're doing, put a bib on and make a patient feel more comfortable with you.' (*NResponse 1*)

The dental surgeon described his experience of the training received:

'I think, I think obviously initially – initially the training – um the first time we had training we didn't obviously get to know exactly what we needed to do, but we had all the information on paper as well, so when we went through that then it became quite clear. So the training was good. Cause, it was one off training we had to reinforce it, the way we reinforced it was that we had handouts didn't we. I think the only way to do it better is if um we did it again, closer to the time we were seeing the patients.' (*DResponse 2*)

The dental nurse employed by the dental surgeon above describes how she found the experience of the training received:

'Er ... I didn't feel that much different.' (*NResponse 1*)

Insight

The dental surgeons and dental nurses were asked what insight they felt they had gained through incorporating the therapeutic relationship. Both dental teams felt they had gained insight. As the dental surgeon put it:

'Well, I guess it's quite interesting to realize the patients know what you are actually doing – they actually appreciate that you are actually doing these things. Not actually saying them but they are actually – actually – getting something out of it. It seemed to be the result of what we were doing today. People seemed to recognize that we were trying to calm them down and, er, give them a chance to respond. So yes – it's – it's quite interesting actually. 'Cause you often think it goes over their head. Obviously, it does soak in.' (*DResponse 1*)

Asked the same question, his dental nurse says that she has learnt how important it is to take patients into consideration.

'I have learnt that you have got to take the patients into consideration which you do to a certain extent, but obviously you have never thought what they are thinking. You think they are thinking something, but you have to be more aware of what they are actually thinking.' (*NResponse 2*)

The other dental surgeon describes the insight he gained:

'Hum, I think, again, because obviously I have been in dentistry for quite a while now. I think the major aspect is we've given more control to our patient. Yes and obviously we've realized if the patient is in control they feel more comfortable. And, um, I think we didn't realize how important that was. 'Cause normally when patients come in you just get on with it, don't you. Time constraints [laughs uncomfortably], financial constraints but that way we have learnt quite a few things.' *(DResponse 2)*

His dental nurse describes what she has learnt:

'I learnt that the patients were more comfortable if they got told what they were doing, [the dentist] explained what he was doing, they liked it better. And, er, what else did we do – oh – put the bib on and things, instead of just wacking a tissue over them. They said, oh, you don't normally do this, putting the bib on and things [explanation] one patient said that.' *(NResponse 1)*

However, only one dental practice acknowledged any significant aspects of behaviour they felt they altered through the therapeutic intervention:

'A lot more positive. The patients were – like, this last patient you've interviewed, she was very nervous. Because we went through the steps she felt, like, she was in control. And she actually enjoyed the experience. I think she was very happy. When she came in the morning, I saw her in the morning 'cause I had a gap today. When she came in she was very nervous – apprehensive, very negative, she did not really want to be here. She had not been to a dentist for seven years. I'm not sure how long, did say how long? So – so by the time she left today she was quite happy. Very positive. Again, it is to do with patient control. Yer, we've given the patients more control and, er, you know and also we explain things to them exactly what's going on. Very good.' *(DResponse 2)*

His dental nurse adds:

Yes, they spoke to [the dentist] a bit more because they knew what he was doing, and they, er, I think they were more comfortable, 'cause they knew what you were doing. They started talking a bit more. They came across less nervous; they felt more comfortable.' *(NResponse 1)*

The other dentist when asked this question said:

'Um – not particularly, I think we tend to do those things anyway – people are quite used to us chatting anyway. So I did not particularly notice they were reacting differently. Except one chap – [PResponse 8] who found me sitting in front of the chair and obviously looked at me and thought – seemed to think – what was I doing there. I thought he thought I was going to give him some bad news or something. Oh well, that is the only thing I noticed different. Everyone else seemed to react quite normally to me sitting in front of them and not behind.' *(DResponse 1)*

His dental nurse replied:

'No, not really.' (*NResponse 2*)

When this dental surgeon was asked what he thought patients' overall opinion is of the incorporation of the therapeutic relationship, he answered:

'That's a difficult one, because you don't know what they thought before they did it, do you really? I would hope it was positive. They noticed we were doing a few things differently. As I say, they may as well have been happy with what we were doing before … it's a bit difficult really – you will have to tell me that.' (*DResponse 1*)

His dental nurse also describes similar views:

'I do not know really – um – it's hard to say, 'cause all these patients are old patients. I don't know really. I think it is a positive sign. Because … er I don't know, because we just talked to them and [the dentist] talked to me more, really.' (*NResponse 2*)

Both the dental surgeons were keen to know the outcome and asked the principal researcher for information concerning their dental patients.

This dental surgeon describes what has been of most value from participation in the study:

'I think, er, the biggest values have been, you know, that we have participated in something, it's been ordered, we've tried it, we like it and implemented it. I think the biggest aspect we like about it is spending time with our patients, going through the therapeutic steps from the study. Like I said before, most of the things we were doing before but we weren't doing them on a regular basis, with everybody. We weren't doing it in an ordered manner. We were probably saying to a patient like, um, if you feel anything raise your left hand, that's what we were doing. But now we are being more positive, we are saying to them what we are going to do before we start. You know we obviously tell them to raise their left hand, but we also ask them how the treatments progressing, how they are, if everything's OK. So, so all these things I think are quite a few-a lot of things that have been positive in our practice for our practice for our patients. I mean, I mean for example, in the study, what did the patients say to you about the most important thing to them?' (*DResponse 2*)

His dental nurse describes:

'Making, er, the patients a bit more comfortable, they feel a little at – er, more at ease with [the dentist] and me.' (*NResponse 1*)

The dental surgeons were asked whether they would recommend acupuncture to reduce dental anxiety for their very nervous patients:

'Um, I don't know that much about it. To be honest, if I found out it was good for people, I probably would.' (*DResponse 1*)

The dental surgeon then explains:

'I tend to, my practice tends to be, I assume people don't need to have that intervention. I will always give them a chance to come in and try and have things done as we normally do them without sedation, without accessory methods. But if we find that they cannot cope with it, then, yes. I would certainly look into referring them to people elsewhere. But that does not happen very often. We just tend to give those people more time, um, usually get round the situation or they don't come back. I attract the same, similar patients to the practice. So, I don't get a huge number of patients petrified. We have a narrow intake here.' (*DResponse 1*)

When asked if he would consider referring very anxious patients for acupuncture, the other dental surgeon replied:

'Er, I would say definitely, I would say, you know acupuncture, hypnosis, whatever can help patients. Um, er, you know, different things work for different people. Some people would prefer hypnosis, some people would prefer acupuncture. Other people would prefer either sedation: very few people would have nothing done without general anaesthetic.' (*DResponse 2*)

The dentists and dental nurses were asked what they think is most important in a clinical encounter, and what they thought their patients felt was most important. One dental surgeon said that he thought most important to dental patients was:

'Probably they want to be listened to, I imagine.' (*DResponse 2*)

His dental nurse answers:

'A happy environment where they can feel at ease, and not this dentist they're scared of.' (*NResponse 1*)

The other dental surgeon describes what he feels is of most importance to dental patients:

'They want a good smile; they want the treatment done, minimum sort of discomfort, that they know the costs, the dentist explains the options to them, and the treatment works.' (*DResponse 2*)

His nurse adds:

> 'To be able to talk to the dentist, at ease, have their treatment done, and they feeling comfortable with the dentist and not nervous.' (*NResponse 2*)

The dental surgeons and nurses were asked if participating in this study had altered their views of complementary medecine in any way. A dental surgeon says:

> 'To be honest, I did not even realize that was complementary medicine – it's just common sense really. What we have done today? If that is what complementary medicine is, I am all for it. Is that it? Oh, thank you very much.' (*DResponse 2*)

The related dental nurse adds:

> 'Oh yes, because it is not all these herbal things; it's really – there's psychological ... yes.' (*NResponse 1*)

The other dental surgeon says:

> 'I think really I have known obviously that complementary medicine is very important. At college we are taught about hypnosis; we are not taught about acupuncture but you can go on acupuncture courses. That's something that I have thought about but I definitely was aware that they are very important, probably not as aware as I know now but obviously aware of their importance.' (*DResponse 1*)

His dental nurse adds:

> 'Yes, 'cause it did work, and it's quite simple. It's not hard to do, is it?' (*NResponse 1*)

The dental team and their patients

The dental surgeon and dental nurse did not acknowledge any particular behaviour they felt they had altered through the therapeutic intervention. The dental surgeon describes how his dental patients may well have been happy with what they had before. However, the therapeutic relationship improved their dental patients' experience, by providing additional support. Both the dental surgeon and dental nurse felt that there were positive effects, but ascertaining them proved difficult.

The dental nurse points out that the dentist

> '... chatted to the patients and spoke more to me, really.' (*NResponse 1*)

Their dental patient explains:

> 'I think, how he communicates with the dental nurse, I think that helps as well because I mean both are working in tandem. I think the actual sort of relationship that the two of them have is very much ... You can vision it as a doctor working in theatre putting his hand out and being given the right bit of equipment. I had this vision of him just putting out his hand and all the right equipment just landing in the palm of his hand. So, you know, again it's just although you can sense that things going – it seems to be seamless. The two of them just seem to be working together.' (*PResponse 8*)

The dental surgeon admits that he gained insight:

> 'People seemed to recognize that we were actually trying to calm them down and, er, give them a chance to respond.' (*DResponse 1*)

His dental patient said:

> The dental surgeon – well he is very nice he, er, is sort of very calming when you look at him – he – he seems to have this very calm way when he speaks to you and everything. He is really nice.' (*PResponse 7*)

Another dental patient says:

> 'His confidence – he is defiantly reassuring, so, I always get the impression and I suppose it helps with the layout that this is a professional at work. Again it's all in their personal tone. Very calming, and it is also – I know completely what I am doing here, you are in safe hands, you have got no need to worry sort of thing.' (*PResponse 8*)

A dental patient describes his experience of the dental treatment as

> 'Very helpful, both the dentist and the dental nurse. They both have a nice calm approach, which is reassuring.' (*PResponse 4*)

The dental surgeon in this dental practice describes what he feels is professionally most important to a dental patient:

> 'I think it is explaining what you are doing really and doing it in a friendly manner really.' (*DResponse 1*)

Four of his dental patients refer to what their dental surgeon feels is most important to a dental patient, and describe 'explanation' in the interview process. A dental patient describes mutual participation:

'He has explained everything as we have gone along and shown me things. He has been good like that.' (*PResponse 7*)

A dental patient also describes this within his experience of the dental treatment received:

'When he injects me, he tells you, it will be a tiny little prick he said, just a little bit sore – that's it. You know it's coming then, don't you? They don't just jab it in; you know everything that's going on.' (*PResponse 6*)

A dental patient describes 'explanation' within mutual participation and also how he felt he was supported emotionally and physically:

'The fact that when you get an injection they are telling you it's going to be a small little scratch, just generally the tone in their voices helps you to relax.' (*PResponse 8*)

Another dental patient says:

'What happens here which is really good is that you are told what is happening as it does happen, rather than lying back and you have all these things in your mouth and you're not quite sure what's going on. So a little commentary is very useful. Makes you feel more relaxed and confident with the situation.' (*PResponse 4*)

Interestingly, the dental surgeon describes how he found his experience of training:

'Um, oh yer – I thought it was well explained to us.' (*DResponse 1*)

In contrast to the dental surgeon, there was a similarity of impressions and statements between the dental nurse and the dental patients. The dental nurse refers to the environment within the dental practice:

'A happy friendly environment.' (*NResponse 1*)

All the dental patients at this practice describe a friendly environment and include the role of the dental team significantly in their experience of the dental setting.

'Everybody has been really, yes, the receptionist has been really nice, um, the dentist and and the nurse today. Yes, they have been really nice.' (*PResponse 7*)

The dental surgeon from the other dental practice describes that he has given his patients more control and explains that they (the dental surgeon and nurse) have realized that the patients feel more comfortable if they are in control. The dentist explains that before they were probably saying 'If you feel something, raise your left hand'. The dental surgeon also says that now they (the dentist and nurse) are additionally asking their patients

> 'How is the treatment's progressing? How are they? If everything's OK?' (*DResponse 2*)

Four of these dental patients describe an instance where the dental surgeon asked them to raise their hand if they had any pain or wanted a break. For example:

> 'If there was any pain, I was to raise my left hand, which fortunately there was no real problems. So I didn't have to. I had to raise my hand once and that was it. There were no real problems. Well, that just put my mind at ease really. I suppose that just eased the whole position 'cause you know after being apprehensive and then he told me to raise my left hand, which meant that I had some form of signal to him without shouting. So I would have done if it hurt.' (*PResponse 1*)

One dental patient says that she had rests:

> 'He said he knew I was nervous, and, um, he said "You're doing really well." He said, oh, and I had lots of little rests which was good. 'Cause sometimes you want to swallow or spit out and you can't.' (*PResponse 2*)

The dental surgeon describes why he would implement the model in his practising style and refers initially to explaining things to dental patients.

> 'Again for the reasons already explained [*laughs*] all the reasons we've explained, so like, explaining things to patients, patient control, er, patient reassurance, yes, awareness, um, er, and the overall experience for the patient. All very positive.' (*DResponse 2*)

The patient who was pleased to attend the dentist refers positively to an 'explanation' involving the treatment process, and used the words 'explained' and 'explain' six times while describing his experience. The dental patient describes his expectations:

> 'Um, well, I knew because they told me beforehand that, er, he would be removing this crown. And he, er, had to remove it because behind it and under it there was decay. So I was aware – they made me aware – of what was going to happen and I think that is very important. Having spent many years [laughs] in dentists' chairs (not many years but many hours) at different times in dentists' chairs. Er, my previous dentist who had the same qualification as this one – very good, he always explained as well what he was doing – he is now retired. And he always explained what he was going to do. But in the ... past when I was a teenager for example,

they didn't explain. They just did it. When I was in the forces it was explained what they were going to do – er but not a great deal … of er …help was given as far as … um … pain was concerned. Er, when I was a teenager for example, er, I had to go I was in the Lake District, um, there was no electricity, it was just a foot drill. And, er, it wasn't a pleasant experience having a filling in those circumstances. When I was in the forces, again they had electricity and, er, so on but er … they removed a nerve with no anaesthetic of any kind. Which took a long time and wasn't very comfortable, er, it was quite painful. They weren't unpleasant, er, they weren't in anyway, they – it was just what happened. I remember those occasions um and I am pleased that nowadays … the modern techniques are much better.' (*PResponse 10*)

All of these dental surgeon's patients said how they valued the explanations the dental surgeon provided. In initial impressions this dental patient describes:

'Of the dentist himself, er, very polite, um, explained everything that wanted what treatment wanted doing, um, very helpful and, um, explained everything as he went on.' (*PResponse 9*)

This patient also positively describes the dentist's explanations throughout the semi-structured interview. The dental surgeon and the nurse had acknowledged that all his dental patients benefited from his explaining things to them.

The dental surgeon describes what he thinks is most important to a dental patient as a professional.

'What is the most important thing to me? [*Principal researcher repeats question – what do you feel is important as a professional?*] Um, I can't really say one thing is more important than the other. I think you know the overall thing is more important, yer, from diagnosing to treatment planning, to explaining to patients, that's important. So I can't really say one thing is more important than the other. Um, obviously most things are measured by outcome, OK the outcome only derives from what we have done before. So I would say everything is important. To get a good clinical outcome you had to have a good examination, diagnosis, treatment plan, consulting the patient, explaining what needs to be done, so the whole cycle from beginning to end is important. Each step is important. So times as clinicians we only feel that the clinical aspect is important, treatment, diagnosis element is probably just as important as if not more so.' (*DResponse 1*)

Interestingly, his dental patients had similar views and impressions:

'And that the outcome will be satisfactory to both of us.' (*PResponse 10*)

'That it's efficient and the work I expect will be done is actually done on the day.' (*PResponse 3*)

'No, I was more, more than satisfied with today, with his performance today.'
(*PResponse 1*)

'That's quite difficult ... [laughs] 'cause you can't have one without the other really, can you. I want good treatment, I good I want good successful treatment.'
(*PResponse 2*)

'I'm coming back for fillings and new dentures – so to give me a better appearance.'
(*PResponse 9*)

What the dental surgeons believe is of most importance to their patients appears to be subconsciously anticipated by the dental patient.

Discussion

Locker (1989) describes how patients judge dentists on their personal qualities rather than their technical competence and are more satisfied with those dentists who are successful at relieving anxiety. This relates partly to the study, though the dental patients were appreciative of the dental surgeons' application in reducing their presenting apprehension/fear as well as of their technical competence and this correlated with overall patient satisfaction.

Gale et al. (1984) establish that limited verbal interaction between dentist and patient leads to less anxiety reduction, less positive attitudes and lower levels of satisfaction and it has been found that positive and negative communication influenced patient's anxiety (Rouse 1990). It has been suggested that a willingness to listen, to explain and to deal with patient's concerns are taken as an indication of a general interest in patients and their welfare; and that these qualities are most appreciated by patients (Locker 1989). Though the study verifies that the therapeutic relationship within a dental setting is not confined to a general interest in a patient's welfare, and although these qualities are 'most' appreciated by patients, the therapeutic intervention significantly reduces apprehension or fear in within patients undergoing dental treatment. These qualities are most appreciated and responded to optimistically.

Freidson (1988) believes that the patient is personally involved with illness and assesses its significance in terms of its social and psychological impact, and its implications or the patient's life as a whole, which relates to similar experiences of the dental patients within the study. However, it was also suggested that a doctor views the patient's condition in a scientific manner and evaluates its severity and significance according to clinical criteria, which is not so precise. Both the dental surgeons viewed the application and capability of the therapeutic intervention in a personal manner, challenging both their previous practice and existing practice. A dental surgeon was either apprehensive regarding ability or an inclination for further training was required, to feel confident to apply therapeutic skills. Freidson suggests that a physician should at least act like a member of the therapeutic team, and his suggestion is borne out by the outcome of this study as a physician who is therapeutic and influential in oral health care, and able to achieve positive outcomes.

Chapple et al. (2003) find a high preference for mutual participation, placing emphasis on patient and dentist sharing equal responsibility for decision-making, and that patients have distinct preferences in relation to this. The study illustrated patients' preferences for an explanation rather than for a share in decision-making. The dental patients in the study placed emphasis on and benefited from mutual participation throughout their diagnosis and dental treatment, rather than on decision-making.

Locker (1989) explains that encounters between dentist and patient are constrained by the patient's condition and the nature of the treatment offered, and that the relationship between them is highly variable. The study acknowledged this to an extent; although it illustrates that this is manageable when responded to appropriately. It is, however, readily observable how variable the dentist–patient relationship is.

Corah (1988) establishes that dentists' views are influenced primarily by those patients' characteristics that are manifested during treatment, It is suggested that patient characteristics observable during treatment are limited, not independent of nor personal towards the dentist and are definitely not a true representation of the particular patient. Therefore, this implies that these dentists may be stripped of psychological, interpersonal and therapeutic skills, and these findings reinforce a personal involvement concerning attitudes towards patients. The study demonstrates that patient characteristics manifesting themselves during treatment result primarily from the physical and interpersonal application of the dental surgeon.

Locker (1989) describes how it is not unreasonable to suppose that health professionals offer less information to those whom they assume do not share their values with respect to oral health. This study suggests that dentists offer less means of support because they may be unaware of the potential consequences their behaviour permits.

It is held that cognitive processes have their origins in experiences of failure, comprehension, interpretation and memory and, even when professionals make 'special' efforts to communicate more effectively, many patients remain dissatisfied. Certain features, such as the delivery of technical language incorporated in dentistry and anxiety (anxiety has a negative effect on memory), may contribute to dental patients remaining dissatisfied (Locker 1989).

While it is acknowledged that dissatisfaction may present, the study demonstrates that comprehension, interpretation, memory and satisfaction present even when a dental patient is apprehensive or fearful. However, this is when such manifestations have been attended to and reduced. Moreover, fearful dental patients can still remember an unhappy encounter with a dental surgeon, even the colour and layout in a surgery forty-seven years ago.

Gale et al. (1984) found that it takes no more time for dentists to interact with patients than for them not to; 'busyness' does not hinder information-sharing, and the dentist's practising style does play a role. The study also suggests that a dental surgeon's attitude, and familiarity, together with the necessary skills, are contributing factors in the practising style and its consequences.

Lahti et al. (1995) asserts that patients want more interaction and encouragement during the dental treatment. Corah (1988) establishes that empathy, friendliness and support are closely linked to patient satisfaction. Kankin and Harris (1985) found that patients are sensitive to dentist behaviour, and findings in the study support this. The therapeutic intervention in a dental setting obtains those components, with substantial positive effects.

Locker (1989) identifies communication as being important to the patient, as it allows the patient to understand, manage and feel at ease with their health problems. In addition, communication throughout dental treatment reduces apprehension and fear, supports and encourages dental patients, increases satisfaction potentials and facilitates continuous care which is not only of assistance and valuable to dental patients, but also to the dental surgeon and the dental practice.

It is evident that those dental patients who have had an opportunity to experience contemporary dentistry obtain an advantage in their oral health care. Although it has been acknowledged that dental anxiety prevents regular oral health care, the anxiety may arise from expectations associated with a past experience. Addressing this aspect through advertisement or other media may reassure potential patients who avoid the dental setting. The dental environment is significant and along with the members of staff the practice layout contributes to overall patient experience. This may not help, however, as a coping strategy if accessory methods are not employed by the dental surgeon.

The study emphasizes that the role of a dental nurse is also influential. It is suggested that a dental nurse has contributing qualities that could be exercised further in the dental setting. In this study, a majority of dental patients discussed associated fear. In addition, all the patients responded to the semi-structured interview in this manner. This suggests the importance of efforts to improve an experience within the dental setting and letting society know about it.

The new framework for the NHS intends to improve patient experience by providing more time for the dental surgeon to spend with them. However, lack of time was not criticized by the dental patients in this study; rather, it is what a dental surgeon does within the time.

The devised model of the therapeutic intervention has assisted in the development of the relationship between the dental surgeon, dental nurse and the dental patients and met the need of the dental patients. This has occurred because the dental surgeons have applied features within the model. The first stage permits the dentist to discuss the patient's views and provides an opportunity for the patient to consider. This replicates past research on mutual participation, and contains the therapeutic skill mutuality. A dental patient is then treated as an adult and is participating in the treatment planning with the dental surgeon. In the first stage, the dental surgeon describes the treatment process and provides an explanation of it (before treatment). The dental patient then has an opportunity to acknowledge the reasoning behind what is about to take place. The dental surgeon can therefore ascertain the patient's thoughts regarding the process. The patient is able to illustrate what those thoughts might be. They may include fear, apprehension, cost and worry. This is also an opportunity for the dental patient to raise any issue that may contribute to a negative experience of treatment. The dental patient has the chance to acknowledge that the dental surgeon is interested in their welfare and can manage and tolerate their concerns and also appears conscientious. The model further provides for this, as in stage two the dental surgeon is able to respond accordingly, and support and encourage dental patients appropriately. The dental surgeon increases verbal interaction so the dental patient is aware of what is happening, and the dental surgeon provides a means whereby the dental patients feel they can trust the dentist. For example, the dental surgeon explains that if they raise their hand, he will stop, at any time; this is conveyed in a supportive manner. The dental surgeon also encourages and supports the client by saying they are doing well. This encourages a two-way process during treatment. The dental surgeon is to remain aware of the patient throughout this process and his or her attention and interpersonal skills are focused upon the patient: this is stage three, that is, care. Stage four's challenge is to respect and behave courteously to all members of staff at all times since patients may form an impression of the dental surgeon from interaction with the dental team members. The dentist is encouraged to be positive with his dental nurse, due to the nature of dental treatment. This reinforces a positive and safe environment when patients cannot speak or interact with the dental team. It provides an insight for the dental patients and conveys that everything is running smoothly and is managed accordingly. Stage five of the model is performance, and the end and a return to mutuality. Here the dentist gives the patient credit for any positive outcomes. This reinforces what the dental team and the dental patient have accomplished; it provides for mutuality and further encourages collaboration between the dental surgeon and the dental patient. At this point, any aftercare advice that is usually given is emphasized. The dental patient is then positively aware and has the means and encouragement to manage their oral health. This encourages compliance with the dental practice.

Summary

(1) The model provided for all these patients' individual needs:

> The way he makes me feel relaxed and comfortable and am not being a nuisance to him. The dentist just wanted everything to be right. He just said and wanted the

teeth to be right and he said I had been very patient but I said so had he. That's all really. The man – well, he is very nice, he is, er, sort of very calming when you look at him – when you see him – he seems to have this quite calm way. He speaks to you and everything. He is really nice. He puts me at ease. Well, I was thinking, um, I hope this is the last time and the teeth fit and that will be OK for the – well, just that really. I was just hoping they fit alright, cause we've had such a problem with them and for him as well you know. I thought I hope they fit this time and they are alright 'cause I've kept coming back and they were not but everything was alright. I thought I should have, it's awful and what will the dentist think; he might be really awful to me and say you should have come before. What are you bothering me now for; so there was a little bit of that as well.

(2)

They gave me these extraction instructions. Oh yes. Well, you do not just go away and think I can have a cup of tea or anything. You know to take your time and just relax. If it starts bleeding again he tells you what to do in there, get a hankerchief, roll it into a square. He talks to you, the assistant put the apron on – I cannot fault him. When he injected me he says, "It will be a tiny little prick", he said, just a little bit sore, that's it. You know it's coming then, don't you – they don't just jab it in; you know everything that's going on my love. It felt, um, I think er, having trust in the bloke doing the job, isn't it, and no fear you know him. He is very good at his job and the assistant as well. They are all there they make you feel at home. This is it. It's not in the chair, bang. They sat me down, had a word with me. They talked to me like I'm talking to you in a roundabout way ... He injected it; he tells you everything that is going to happen, he said back and forwards and he is talking to you all the while. It's strange really a few years back I had to take my brother to Peterborough to a dental surgeon. The dentist there had been on the beer; he was screaming blue murder, my brother was – he pulled – I thought he was going to pull his head off when he pulled it out, strapped him in virtually. But Stephen in actual fact he just wiggled it, he said it's on its way. He said, it's coming and it was out, as simple as that. I never felt nothing, I heard it just crack a little bit and that was it. You set yourself to a point, no matter who you are. I could have sat in the armchair, 'cause he said I'm a star patient that's it. So I, as I say, I got on the settee and he had a look, checked it all out, and then we had a few words about it; we had a chat as he looked at the tooth. He always asked, 'Do you want it out or to keep it?' Fair enough. I let him decide. I never felt a thing in actual fact.

Limitations of study

The limitations of this study include the sample size, which comprised five dental patients, their dental surgeons and their dental nurses (in total four-teen participants). The incorporation of further dental patients might have provided for further similarity or deviant data. The study ascertained the short-term effects of the therapeutic relationship and did not look at the long-term improvements or development; and it addressed treatment process only.

The dental patients interviewed were existing dental patients at those dental practices; potential dental patients i.e., those who do not access a dental setting were not included.

The principal researcher did not incorporate observational methods within the study and there proved to be many observations which would have been beneficial.

The training proved sufficient regarding the nature of the study the second time around and this therefore affected the comprehension and application of the therapeutic relationship in a dental setting. One dental practice gained further insight and were better equipped with training reflecting the therapeutic skills.

Conclusion

- The therapeutic relationship in a dental setting affects dental patients, the dental surgeon and the dental nurse.

- The extent is positively and substantial.

- The dental patients experience is improved.

- Apprehension and fear is significantly reduced. Dental patients feel relaxed and calm during dental treatment.

- Dental patients feel safe as they can exercise their right with means of stopping the dentist if required. Dental patients are able to trust the dental surgeon.

- Dental patients are involved throughout the dental treatment.

- The dental patient is encouraged to return for further dental treatment.

- The dental surgeon and dental nurse are able to gain insight to their practising styles, and are given the means to manage their patients effectively. —

- The therapeutic relationship in a dental setting is not a model in its own right. It is a tool, which facilitates positive improvement for all within a dental setting.

- The therapeutic relationship in a dental setting can be used during dental treatment by an appropriately trained dental surgeon and dental nurse to reduce varying degrees of fear and apprehension and to improve the experience for dental patients.

References

Bailey, J. and Baillie, L. (1996) Transactional analysis: how to improve communication skills. *Nursing Standard*, **10** (35): 39–42.

Barnard, P. (1997) *Effective Communication for Health Professionals*, 2nd edn (London: Chapman and Hall).

Bellet, P. and Maloney, M. (1991) The importance of empathy as an interviewing skill in medicine. *Journal of the American Medical Association*, **266**: 1831–32.

Berne, E. (1964) *The Games People Play: The Psychology of Human Relationships* (London: Penguin).

Bowling, A. (1997) *Research Methods in Health: Investigating Health and Health Services* (Milton Keynes: Open University Press).

Bowling, A. (2002) *Research Methods in Health Services: Investigating Health and Health Services*, 2nd edn (Buckingham: Open University Press).

Burke, F. J. T. and Freeman, R. (1994) Psychological aspects of patient management: behavioural science in dentistry. *Dental Update*, **21** (4): 148–53

Bryman, A. (2001) *Social Research Methods* (Oxford: Oxford University Press).

Cartwright, A. and Anderson, R. (1981) *General Practice Revisited: A Second Study of Patients and their Doctors* (London: University Press, Tavistock Publications).

Chapman, H. R. and Kirby-Turner, N. (2002) Visual/verbal analogue scales: Examples of brief assessment methods to aid management of adult patients in clinical practice. *British Dental Journal* **193** (8): 447–50.

Chapple, H., Shah, S. and Caress, A. L. (2003) Exploring dental patients' preferred roles in treatment decision making. *British Dental Journal* **194** (6): 289.

Cohen, S. M., Fiske, J. and Newton, T. (2000) The impact of dental anxiety on daily living. *British Dental Journal* **189** (7): 1–12.

Colaizzi, P. (1978) Psychological research as a phenomenologist views it. In R. Valle and M. King (eds), *Existential Phenomenological Alternatives for Psychology* (New York: Oxford University Press).

Cole, A. and Bird, J. (2000) *The Medical Interview*, 2nd edn (New York: Mosby).

Corah, N. L. (1985) The dentist–patient relationship: mutual perceptions and behaviours. *Journal of the American Dental Association* **113** (2): 253–5.

Corah, N. L. (1988) Dental anxiety: assessment, reduction and increasing patient satisfaction. *Dental Clinicians in North America* **32** (4): 779–90.

Corah, N. L., Oshea, R. M., Bissel, G. D., Thines, T. J. and Mendola, P. (1988) The dentist–patient relationship: perceived dentist behaviours that reduce patient anxiety and improve satisfaction. *Journal of the American Dental Association* **116** (1): 73–6.

Dailey, G. M., Humphris, G. and Lennon, M. A. (2001) The use of dental anxiety questionnaires. *British Dental Journal* **190** (8): 1–7.

Data Protection Act (1984) Acts of Parliament, in *General Principles of Record Keeping and Access to Health Records* (2000) Part 3, Appendix 15.

Davis, M. (1997) *Scientific Papers and Presentations* (New York: Academic Press).

Department of Health (2001) *Reseach Governance Framework for Health and Social Care* (London: HMSO).

Denzin, K. and Lincoln, L. (2000) *Handbook of Qualitative Research*, 2nd edn (New York: Sage Publications).

Elstein, J. (1995) Psychological research on diagnostic reasoning. In M. Lipkin, S. Putnam and A. Lazare (eds) *The Medical Interview: Clinical Care, Education and Research* (New York: Springer).

Freeman, R. (2002) Communicating effectively: some practical suggestions. *British Dental Journal* **187** (5): 1–7.

Freeman, C. and Tyrer, P. (1992) *Research Methods in Psychiatry: A Beginner's Guide*, 2nd edn (London: Royal College of Psychiatrists).

Freidson, E. (1988) *Profession of Medicine: A Study of the Sociology of Applied Knowledge* (London: University of Chicago Press).

Gale, E. N., Carlson, S. G., Erikson, A. and Jontell, M. (1984) Effects of dentists' behaviour on patients' attitudes. *Journal of the American Dental Association* **109** (3): 444–6.

General Dental Council (2002) *The First Five Years: A Framework for Undergraduate Dental Education*, Part 1, 2nd edn (London: General Dental Council).

Gillham, B. (2000) *Case Study Research Methods* (London: Continuum).

Gross, R. D. (1992) *Psychology: The Science of Mind and Behaviour*, 2nd edn (London: Hodder & Stoughton).

Johns, C. (1993) Professional supervision. *Journal of Nursing Management* **1**: 9–18.

Holloway, I. and Wheeler, S. (2002) *Qualitative Research in Nursing*, 2nd edn (Oxford: Blackwell Publishing).

Humphris, G. (1999) Dealing with highly anxious dental patients. *British Dental Journal*, **186**: 1.

Kankin, J. A. and Harris, P. (1985) Patient preferences for dentists' behaviours. *Journal of America Dental Association*, **110** (3): 323–7.

Lahti, S., Tuutti, H., Hausen, H. and Kaariainen, R. (1995a) Opinions of different subgroups of dentists and patients about the ideal dentist and the ideal patient. *Community Dentistry and Oral Epidemiology* **23** (2): 89–94.

Lahti, S., Tuutti, H., Hausen, H. and Kaarianien, R. (1995b) Comparison of ideal and actual behaviour of patients and dentist during dental treatment. *Community Dentistry and Oral Epidemiology*, **23** (6): 347–8.

Lahti, S., Tuutti, H. and Kaarianen, K. (1996a) Patients' expectations of an ideal dentist and their views. *Community Dentistry and Oral Epidemiology*, **24** (4): 240–4.

Lahti, S., Verkasalo, M., Hausen, H. and Tuutti, H. (1996b) Ideal role behaviours as seen by dentists and patients them selves and do they differ? *Community Dentistry and Oral Epidemiology*, **24** (4): 245–8.

Lazare, A. (1987) Shame and humiliation in the medical encounter. *Archives of Internal Medicine*, **147**: 1653–8.

Ley, P. and Spelman, A. (1988) *Communicating with Patients: Improving Communication, Satisfaction and Compliance*, the Psychology and Medicine Series (Cambridge: Cambridge, University Press).

Locke, F., Spirduso, W. W. and Silverman, S. J. (1993) *Proposals that Work: A Guide for Planning, Dissertation and Grant Proposals*, 3rd edn (San Francisco, CA: Sage Publications).

Locker, J. (1989) *Behavioural Science and Dentistry* (London: Routledge).

Maciocia, G. (1997) *The Foundations of Chinese Medicine* (Edinburgh: Churchill Livingstone).

Mataki, S. (2000) Dentist–patient relationship. *Journal of Medical Dentistry and Science*, **47** (4): 209–14.

Miller, G. and Dingwall, R. (1997) *Context and Method in Qualitative Research* (London: Sage).

Mitchell, A. and Cormack, M. (1998) *The Therapeutic Relationship in Complementary Health Care* (Edinburgh: Churchill Livingstone).

Newsome, P. R. and Wright, G. H. (2000) Qualitative techniques to investigate how patients evaluate dentists: a pilot study. *Community Dentistry and Oral Epidemiology,* **28** (4): 257–66.

Newton, J. T. (1995) Dentist/patient communication: a review, *patient management: Dental Update,* **22** (5): 118–21.

Nuttall, N. M., Bradnock, G., White, D., Morris, J. and Nunn, J. (2001) Dental attendance in 1998 and implications for the future. *British Dental Journal,* **190** (4): 177–82.

Parsons, T. (1951) *The Social System* (London: Routledge & Kegan Paul).

Polit, D. F. and Hungler, B. P. (1993) *Essentials of Nursing Research: Methods, Appraisals and Utilization,* 3rd edn (Philadelphia: J. B Lippincott).

Reed, J. and Procter, S. (1995) *Practitioner Research in Health Care: The Inside Story,* Part One: *Basic Issues in Practitioner Research* (London: Chapman & Hall).

Reid, N. (1993) *Health Care Research by Degrees* (Oxford: Blackwell Scientific Publications).

Rouse, R. A. (1990) Dentists' technical competence, communication, and personality predictors of dental anxiety. *Journal of Behavioural Medicine,* **13** (3): 307–19.

Schouten, B. C. and Vinkesteijn, F. J. (2002) Complaints of patients concerning obligation to inform and consent requirements. *Ned Tijdschr Tandheelkd,* **109** (12): 481–4.

Schouten, B. C. Eijkaman, M. A. and Hoogstraten, J. (2003) Dentists' and patients' communicative behaviour and their satisfaction with the dental encounter. *Community Dental Health,* **20** (1): 11–15.

Seoane, J., Varela-Centelles, J., Guimaraes, M. J., Garcia-Pola, N. Gonzalez-Reforma and T. F. Walsh (2002) Concordance between undergraduate dental students and their lecturers in their attitude towards difficult patients. *European Journal of Dental Education,* 6 (4): 14.

Silverman, D. (2000) *Doing Qualitative Research: A Practical Handbook* (London: Sage Publications).

Sondell, K. and Soderfeldt, B. (1997) Dentist–patient communication: a review of relevant models. *Acta Ondontal Scandinavia,* **55** (2): 116–26.

Thomas, S. A. (2000) *How to Write Health Science Papers, Dissertations and Theses* (Churchill Livingstone).

Tuckett, D., Boulton, M., Olsen, C. and Williams, A. (1986) *Meeting Between Experts* (London: Tavistock).

Veldhuis, B. and Schouten, B. C. (2003) The relationship between communication styles of dentists and the satisfaction of their patients, *Ned Tijdschr Tandheelkd,* **110** (10): 387–90.

Willis, T. (1982) Non-specific factors in helping relationships. In *Basic Processes in Helping Relation* (New York: Academic Press).

Yin, K. (2003) *Case Study Research, Design and Methods,* 3rd edn, vol. 5 (London: Sage Publications).

CHAPTER 11

Mentorship in Practice: Student Nurse Perspectives

KATIE COOK

The history of mentorship has its origins in Greek mythology: in Homer's Odyssey 'mentor is seen as an advisor to the young Telemachus' (Earnshaw 1995). The role of the mentor at this time was that of 'a wise, trustworthy counsellor or teacher' (Ryan and Brewer 1997).

Mentorship was introduced into nursing in Great Britain in the 1980s, having originated in America where it was said to be a product of the feminist movement (Morle 1990; Armitage and Burnard 1991). There is still much controversy over the definition of mentorship to the extent that a 'definition quagmire' is described by Hagerty (1986; cited by Andrews and Wallis 1999). Furthermore, nursing has been criticized in the literature for readily pursuing mentorship with little idea of what the process is about (Armitage and Burnard 1991). However, in exploring this phenomenon, clarifying existing mentorship roles and considering the classical mentor is advocated by Morton-Cooper and Palmer. They suggest that this in turn will lead to 'the discovery of the richness of the relationship and facilitate an explanation of the various mentoring approaches that exist' (Morton-Cooper and Palmer 2000, p. 40)

The classical mentor is therefore defined as someone who 'facilitates personal growth and development and assists with career progression, while guiding the mentee through the clinical, educational, social and political networks of the working culture' (Morton-Cooper and Palmer 2000, p. 40). Morton-Cooper and Palmer go on to describe three main elements of classical mentoring. These are:

- repertoire of helper functions;
- mutuality and reciprocal sharing;
- duration, identified stages and transitional nature of the relationship.

These three elements link specifically with findings from a study by Darling (1984) describing specific qualities of the mentorship relationship, and these will be discussed in greater detail later in this chapter. Where exactly, then, does mentorship in nursing fit in with the concept of the classical mentor? The mentor in nursing is currently defined by the English National Board and Department of Health as 'the role of the nurse, midwife or health visitor who facilitates learning and supervises and assesses the students in the practice setting' (ENB and DoH 2001a).

It can clearly be seen from this that one of the main roles of the mentor in nursing is to assess student practice. Assessment is not one of the roles considered applicable to 'classical mentoring' as Morton-Cooper and Palmer (2000) state: 'It is our considered opinion that formal assessment and documentation procedures have no place in this type of mentoring.' Mentorship in nursing is therefore classed as a form of pseudo-mentorship, (Morton-Cooper and Palmer 2000, p. 46) and 'has probably arisen due to the initial lack of understanding of the roles, purposes, processes and formal application of mentoring' (Morton-Cooper and Palmer 2000, p. 47).

Pseudo-mentoring relationships:

- focus on specific tasks or organizational issues of short-lived duration;
- include guidance from several mentors for short periods;
- do not demonstrate the comprehensive enabling elements of the true classical model;
- specify clinical placement;
- have a probable duration of six weeks to one year.

(Morton-Cooper and Palmer 2000, p. 46)

In 1986 a document entitled 'Project 2000: A New Preparation for Practice' (UKCC 1986) was published, describing a way forward for nurse education based on the principle of training a 'knowledgeable doer'. Due to the lack of formal clinical skills training given during the academic part of the course, mentorship for the student nurse in practice was of much greater importance, however little thought was given to the preparation of mentors (While 1996). For a number of reasons, Project 2000 did not deliver (Lord 2002) and was criticized for 'failing to produce practitioners who are fit for practice at the point of qualification' (Bradshaw 2000).

With New Labour coming into power in the late 1990s, major reform of the National Health Service (NHS) and Higher Education provision was undertaken. Of particular relevance was the paper 'Making a Difference: Strengthening the Nursing, Midwifery and Health Visiting Contribution to Health and Healthcare' (DoH 1999). This paper called for a review of nurse training to ensure that it was 'more responsive to the needs of the NHS' (DoH 1999). The paper also highlighted the report commissioned by the United Kingdom Central Council (UKCC) that would 'propose a way forward for pre-registration education that enabled fitness for practice based on health care need' (UKCC 1999). The 'Making a Difference' (MaD) curriculum emerged as a result of the report and heralded significant changes to nurse education. A competency-based curriculum was the main change to be wrought and, though criticisms of this type of curriculum have been made (Webb 2002), it was felt to be a better option than the previous apprentice style of training.

Of particular importance to this study were the implications this new curriculum would have for mentors and for student experience in practice. 'Fitness for Practice' (UKCC 1999) stated that: 'Students, assessors and mentors should know what is expected of them through specified outcomes and competencies which form part of a formal learning contract, give direction to clinical placements and are jointly negotiated between the health care providers and Higher Education Institutions.'

In support of this, two documents were produced by the ENB and DoH. In the first document, 'Preparation of Mentors and Teachers' (ENB and DoH 2001a), there is a clear description of the mentor's role. This is to:

- facilitate student learning across pre- and post-registration programmes;
- supervise, support and guide students in practice in institutional and non-institutional settings; and
- implement approved assessment procedures.

The document also provides clear guidelines on the preparation of the mentor to undertake their role.

In the second document, entitled 'Placements in Focus' (ENB and DoH 2001b), a practical guide is offered to all those involved in placement learning with the purpose of 'enhancing the quality and innovative development of practice placements.' 'Placements in Focus' (ENB and DoH 2001b) also suggests that the appointment of placement coordinators can help to improve the quality of mentorship available to the student by ensuring mentorship support and training is available.

Finally, in respect of changes to mentorship, the Nursing and Midwifery Council (NMC) updated the requirements for mentors and mentorship in July 2003. In this update, the NMC stressed that standards are no longer advisory but are now 'required'.

How then does this all fit in with the study undertaken? The local university commenced the MaD curriculum three years ago, and at that point also assigned a number of staff to joint appointments as Practice Placement Facilitators (PPF) with the local NHS trusts. Initially these posts were second-ment opportunities only and were in essence the Placement Coordinators advocated by the 'Placements in Focus' document. Over the last three years, mentorship training and support has been available to all mentors within the Trust and a large number of staff have attended for mentorship skills updates. Due to this and other aspects of the PPF role, the profile of the PPF and mentorship in general has risen over the last three years to the point where there are now two full time substantive posts as PPFs within the Trust. During this time there has been no formal investigation into any aspects of the mentorship received by the student in practice and the researcher felt that this was an ideal opportunity to undertake such an investigation into this fascinating phenomenom.

Literature review

A comprehensive review of the literature was undertaken and the following databases were searched:

- Cumulative Index to Nursing and Allied Health Literature (CINAHL);
- Royal College of Nursing (RCN);
- OVID;
- Medline.

Literature was first sought dating back over the last 20 years and from studies specifically related to mentor–student relationships. From this initial search, the researcher found that the quality of mentorship was predominantly based around the qualities of an effective mentor and a number of studies have focused on this particular area. A subsequent search identified other aspects that might affect the quality of mentorship experience for the student nurse in practice. Overall, though it would appear that the mentor's role is influential in a number of areas (Earnshaw 1995; Watson 1999). However, as Merriam (1983; cited by Gray and Smith 2000) found, 'there was little evidence of quality research' and 'there was a bias towards reporting positive aspects of mentorship.' Cameron-Jones and O'Hara (1996) subsequently found a similar problem when researching into mentorship and raised concerns about how little reliable research was available.

The researcher's own review of the literature found that more recent studies around mentorship reported both positive and negative aspects of mentorship and it is the author's intention to reflect this in the following text and to assess the quality of that research. Furthermore, in order to ensure that all aspects relating to the quality of mentorship received by student nurses in practice were addressed, the author decided to focus specifically on two areas.

Firstly, the student nurses' views on the qualities of an effective mentor will be reviewed along with the effects these qualities have on the mentor–student relationship. Following this, a review of any other factors that may affect the quality of mentorship for the student nurse in practice would also be carried out. Original research reports were obtained for the literature review and a critical evaluation of each made.

In what would appear to be one of the most significant research studies in relation to qualities of an effective mentor, Darling (1984) describes how a series of 150 interviews was undertaken with a range of health professionals including 50 nurses. From the results, Darling identifies that nurses' views on the qualities of an effective mentor are the same as other health professionals views in the study. Darling (1984) states that: 'The absolute requirements for a significant mentoring relationship are attraction, action and affect.' Darling continues by describing a total of 14 characteristics of the effective mentor, three of which are essential to the basic mentor role. These are 'inspirer', 'investor' and 'supporter'. Using this, the 'Darling MMP: Measuring Mentoring Potential' (MMP) tool was devised. This MMP tool, Darling suggests, can be used to assess one's own mentoring ability and the ability of mentors that student nurses may have worked with in practice.

It would seem from this study that a number of researchers have taken a similar view after investigating this subject and the author therefore felt that she needed to compare Darling's findings with other researchers' more recent work. In particular, the author was interested in whether student nurses in the 21st century had the same needs in a mentor as the student nurses of 20 years ago. With the ever-changing face of the National Health Service (NHS), was it possible that the personal attributes of an effective mentor had remained the same?

Cameron-Jones and O'Hara (1996) undertook an interesting study, investigating specifically the questions that the author was asking. In this study, an adapted version of Darling's (1984) analysis is used, with a further four aspects of the role of the mentor being added to the original MMP. These were 'friend', 'assessor', 'intermediary' and 'tutor'. These four roles were identified by a total of 30 nurses, rather a small number of participants compared to Darling's initial 150. From the point of view of the student nurses' experience, they agreed with mentors that the three core essential requirements of the mentor were 'supporter, feedback-giver and model.' This compared very closely to three essential sub-roles identified in Darling's study, qualities such as 'model', 'feedback-giver' and 'supporter'.

When questioned about what might in future be considered essential qualities for a mentor, student nurses also felt that the roles of 'problem-solver, assessor and energizer' should be developed. The 'challenger' role of mentors was not highly important on their list; however, they did feel that 'a more challenging role' for mentors will be expected in the future due to the 'demanding organisational cultures increasingly encountered by health professionals in modern times' (Cameron-Jones and O'Hara 1996), showing a shift in student perspective from Darling's analysis.

Although there is some criticism of the research study undertaken in so far as it had a sample size of only 39 student nurses and no evidence of limitations, it is still interesting to note how student nurses' views might be beginning to change over time to reflect current trends, but that they still saw the fundamental role of the mentor as 'supporter, feedback-giver and model'.

A further study along similar lines was undertaken by Andrews and Chilton (2000). They compared differing views about the mentor role from both mentor and student perspectives and again used Darling's Measuring Mentoring Potential (MMP) scale as an investigative tool. The researcher felt that again too small a sample was taken; however, a pilot study was undertaken with minimal changes needed to the final questionnaire. From the student nurses' perspective, they rated the quality of mentorship higher than the mentors did and felt that the mentorship they had received had been effective. The three essential qualities of the mentor identified by Darling all received high scores from a large majority (82 per cent) of the students. This, the author feels, showed that not only had an effective experience been received but that the students agreed that these roles were high on their list of how they perceived the mentor's role. Similarly, other roles such as 'eye opener' and 'standard prodder' were all rated highly. Andrews and Chilton suggest this could indicate that 'mentoring is a personal process and that formal teaching aspects are less important.' Certainly, at a time when nurse education was based on fostering the so-called 'knowledgeable doer' of Project 2000, the author agrees with Neary et al. (1996) and Phillips et al. (1996) that the 'teacher' role would in fact be quite a significant part of the mentor's role. On the other hand, the roles of 'challenger' and 'counsellor' scored low. It is interesting to note the lack of importance that student nurses place on the need for counselling support. This may be due to the short-term nature of the mentor–student relationship; however, further evidence of this has been found in other studies (Atkins and Williams 1995).

From the point of view of the 'challenger' role, Darling (1984) advocates this as essential for developing critical thinking in the student nurse. Without this, Andrews and Chilton warn that the learning environment can lack stimulation. It is unfortunate, as Andrews and Chilton (2000) go on to say, that nurses do not recognize the need to be challenging as, 'they are socialised to be compliant'. Evidence in a study by Earnshaw (1995) supports this. He suggests that: 'Many of the students seemed to view the mentor as a matriarchal figure whose purpose was to smooth their passage through training rather than provoke, challenge and present them with the unfamiliar.'

Myrick and Yonge (2001), however, highlighted the importance of the challenging aspect of the mentor/student relationship, in particular to encourage critical thinking. In their study, they state that: 'In the process of enabling students to think critically, it is as important for the preceptors to know when to provide them with unconditional support as it is to know when to challenge them.' The author therefore suggests that the 'challenging' role of the mentor is an important quality and may become more so in the future.

Further evidence of this is found in a commentary by Northcott (2000), who describes 'specific actions that the mentor can provide to fulfil this role'. These actions are identified in the work of Daloz (1987) cited by Northcott, (2000). 'Challenging, supporting and vision' are seen as the three components central to the role of the mentor, clearly supporting the argument that a challenging mentor can provide an effective experience for the student nurse in practice.

Certainly, in relation to the qualities of an effective mentor identified by Darling, it is difficult to determine whether student nurses views have changed over time. With the recent changes to the current curriculum, evidence from the author's study may be gained to support or refute this but there is still clearly a need for further investigations of this subject.

Further literature on the subject of developing the mentor–student relationship was also found, again partly focusing on the qualities of the effective mentor, but clearly emphasizing that: 'Compatibility of the mentor and mentee is central to effective mentorship' (Woodrow 1999).

Spouse, who undertook a longitudinal naturalistic study of eight student nurses during a four-year degree programme, states: 'During the data collection and analysis it became evident that the influence of the clinical mentor and the nature of the relationship were central to the students' knowledge and growth' (Spouse 1996). In particular, five roles were identified by the student nurses as being significant in the mentor–student relationship. These were, 'befriending', 'planning', 'collaborating', 'coaching' and 'sense-making' (Spouse 1996).

'Befriending' by the mentor was highlighted strongly as helping the student cope with the adjustment to the busy clinical environment and students soon came to realize that the mentor was the 'gatekeeper' to their learning experience and acceptance in the placement community. The importance of 'befriending' is highlighted by Suen and Chow (2001) during a multiphase study of students' perceptions of the effectiveness of mentors, again in an undergraduate programme. Their study also shows the detrimental effect the mentor can have on student learning when 'befriending' is ineffective. In this study, the English National Board's definition of mentorship states that 'Mentors are there to assist, befriend, guide, advise and counsel students' (ENB 1988, p. 17; cited in Suen and Chow 2001). This was used to explore the students' perceptions. Results showed that mentors did not always achieve the befriending role adequately and this left the students feeling more like guests on the wards rather than team members.

Spouse (1996) also cites 'planning' and 'collaborating' as essential elements for the mentor–student relationship. This helps to ensure that the student is part of the team and is particularly important when the student is new to the area. A 'thoughtful, democratic approach' by the mentor helps the student to develop both interpersonal and professional skills. Watson (1999) supports the view that student nurses value the 'planning' aspect of the mentor role. Ensuring a learning menu is available could help to support and focus the students' learning, especially when the mentor is absent. Effective 'planning' and 'collaboration' with the student is cited in other studies as essential requirements in the building of an effective mentor–student relationship (Cahill 1996; Coates and Gormley 1997).

Evidence from these studies showed that a lack of these elements could go as far as creating an environment of social control for the student, to a point where students had to judge when it was safe to ask questions 'depending on the "looks" given by members of staff' (Cahill 1996). This type of behaviour by staff is particularly distressing for students and has been highlighted as one of 'the hardest acts of aggression to deal with' (Freshwater 2000). This is a major concern, especially when the student feels that if they do not comply, negative responses will be given and, at worst, an unsatisfactory report could result. This supports the evidence that the major stress on the placement is not the work but the people that the student has to work with (Baillie 1993; Cahill 1996).

Evidence contrary to this is found in a work by Earnshaw (1995) who undertook a study of 19 third-year student nurses, by way of a questionnaire. Limitations to this study are well documented and Earnshaw does tend to draw some conclusions beyond the limits of the study. A number of themes drawn from the research should however be noted. In this study in particular, the mentor was seen as 'reducing stress, helping with orientation and settling in'.

Yet more interesting data around the subject of mentor–student relationships can be found in a study by Gray and Smith (2000) where the mentor is described by students again as 'the gatekeeper of learning'. Here, the qualities of an effective mentor from the student nurses' perspective are investigated using a longitudinal qualitative study. Although again only a small sample of 10 student nurses was used, they were interviewed five times throughout their three years. This offers a good insight into how their views on mentorship changed over time. Ethical considerations are noted and the need to gain consent from the student nurses prior to each interview. In this study, again, similar qualities to Spouse's (1996) study were highlighted that would constitute an effective mentor. These were that the mentor 'should be nice, approachable, be a good communicator, be understanding, allow them to try things, and be respected by other members of the ward team' (Gray and Smith 2000).

The reality in practice for the students, however, proved to be somewhat different. Firstly, the researchers found that the student nurses had unrealistic expectations of their mentors prior to their first placement and soon found that 'their mentor had competing priorities'. What they also, rather unfortunately, found was that 'having a good mentor and a good placement (was) associated with luck'. The student nurses were quick to identify traits of a poor mentor, and dealt with this by 'more commonly engineering their off duty to reduce the times they work with their mentor' (Gray and Smith 2000).

Clearly, student nurses are fully aware of which attributes they do appreciate in a mentor. However, it is an unfortunate fact that student nurses are at times disappointed by the support received in practice and somewhat worrying that 'luck' plays such a significant part in the quality of the mentor–student relationship developed during practice experience. Student nurse practice experience will vary in length and it certainly cannot be easy to build an effective relationship with a mentor in a short space of time. However, as Spouse (1996) states, 'only through a sharing of self and the development of mutual positive regard' can an effective relationship be established.

At this point, it is appropriate to move on to the second part of this literature review, looking at other factors that may affect the quality of mentorship received by the student nurse in practice. As previously stated, the development of the mentor–student relationship is vital in supporting student learning in practice and, as Spouse (1998) states: 'students' learning was severely affected in the absence of effective mentorship'. One of the main issues linked to this is the amount of contact the student actually has with the mentor during their allocation period. It is suggested that 'students and mentors work together for at least three out of five shifts', each week (Royal College of Nursing 2002). A local policy further recommends that 'students work a minimum of 40% of their placement experience hours in direct contact with their nominated mentor' (University of Hull 2002).

Of particular interest in relation to this issue is a study by Lloyd Jones et al. (2001). Here a quantitative study was undertaken with a qualitative element, using an activity diary for both mentors and student nurses to complete. A good sample size was used – 125 students and 117 mentors – and there was a 40 per cent response rate. Relevant statistical testing was used to analyse results that highlighted a number of issues. Firstly, even when the student nurse and mentor were on the same shift they were not always directly in contact with each other. This was partly due to 'pressure of work or because an alternative arrangement had been made to broaden the student's educational experience'. Secondly, 'the diary data demonstrated that students spent a substantial amount of time in the placement area without their mentor' and that mentors felt that available time to mentor effectively was a major problem.

Although this study had its limitations and possible bias (some mentors and students chose to complete the diary during a week when they were working together), there clearly is an issue around students gaining sufficient contact with their mentor. Further evidence of this is found in a number of other studies (Barlow 1991; Gordon and Grundy 1997; Watson 1999). However, something that is most interesting is the precise reason for lack of contact between mentor and student. Darling (1985) describes one of the characteristics of the so-called 'toxic mentor'. This is the mentor known as an 'avoider', which in reality means the mentor is either unavailable or inaccessible. In this case it is the mentor that is purposefully causing difficulties with contact with the student. Wilson-Barnett et al. (1995) found a similar problem in their study as did Cahill (1996). Interestingly, in this study, the students felt that the reason for lack of contact with the mentor was 'attributed to lack of interest on the part of the mentor, poor organisation of shift patterns, or a combination of the two' (Cahill 1996).

Another viewpoint has found that the problem is the student nurse who has difficulty coming to terms with working shift patterns (Morgan 2002). As the mentors' duty rota is written before the student arrives on the ward, it is to some extent the student's responsibility to work around this to ensure effective contact is made, (Gordon and Grundy 1997; Watson 1999). As Gordon and Grundy (1997) state, 'Attempting to achieve a compromise between the off-duty the student wants and the supervision that can be offered can cause many difficulties, especially if changes in the off-duty result in supervisor and student having different days off.'

In terms of off-duty arrangements within this researcher's areas of practice, a system called the 'helix' system is in place. Here, each student works a total of 37.5 hours per fortnight. During this time, there are set days in university on a strict patterned basis of Monday and Tuesday one week and Wednesday, Thursday and Friday the next week. Any other days can be spent in practice but the university days are fixed. Compromising this issue further is the fact that the majority of mentors in the Acute setting work a 12-hour shift system and so will only work three days per week. This can potentially lead to difficulties, matching mentor and student off-duty.

Moving on from this to another very pertinent subject, the researcher found that a large number of studies investigating effective mentorship highlighted the issue around time and resources as a major concern. These studies will now be discussed.

Phillips et al. (1996) describe this situation clearly when stating that 'A conflict of interests was prevalent when mentors were faced with dual tasks of teaching and supporting students in addition to providing quality care for patients.' From the student nurses' point of view, their expectations of mentorship are vital in analysing this issue. Gray and Smith (2000) describe how student nurses prior to their first placement experience viewed mentorship 'positively' and believed that the mentor would play a crucial role in their learning in practice. Unfortunately, as Gray and Smith (2000) go on to say: 'Once experiencing a practice placement they (the students) very quickly realised that their mentor had competing priorities.' This inevitably leads to a reduced quality of mentorship (Wilson-Barnett et al. 1995; Lofmark and Wikbald 2001) and has been found to lead to students being 'condemned to repeating mundane, routine tasks of which they are more than capable whilst missing out on more complex care activities' (Spouse 2001).

Although some studies have found that regular interaction between the student and mentor is not always necessary for effective mentorship to take place (Lloyd Jones et al. 2001), the most effective way of developing a student's learning has been found to be through effective support mechanisms and 'adequate resources especially in the form of manpower' (Marrow 1997; Neary 2000). In general, it has been found that students are aware of the workload pressures that mentors are under and often feel a burden to staff because of this (Dolan 2003). This can only have a detrimental effect on the student's learning and service providers need to recognize this to ensure adequate support is available. Sadly, this does not happen and very little thought is given to how to support a student when a mentor is absent or how to support resource problems in ward areas (Marrow and Tatum 1994; Watson 1999; ENB Research Highlights no. 43 2000). Similarly, evidence was found to indicate that Project 2000 courses did not provide the clinical skills training required for student nurses to have the confidence in the practice setting. Bradshaw (2000) points out that: 'This in turn is interpreted by permanent staff as a lack of motivation who then fail to offer students the support needed for them to practice competently.' Furthermore, as service providers do not employ the students during training, the amount of interest taken in the student was variable (Bradshaw 2000). Student nurses need support in the practice environment and can only be assured of this when mentors have the time to do the 'job'. As Spouse (1996) states: 'To help clinical staff to fulfil the mentor role effectively it is important to ensure that the clinical workload is adjusted to recognise the time and energy required.'

As a final issue, the author felt that the effects of the gender of both the mentor and student should be considered in relation to the quality of experience for the student. Although a number of studies were found to investigate issues relevant to gender, there was little in the way of evidence in relation to mentorship.

As approximately only 10 per cent of nurses are male (Waddell 1995), it is often suggested that nursing is 'traditionally viewed as an occupation for women' (Muldoon and Reilly 2003). Irrespective of this, men do enter the profession for a variety of reasons, yet have had little influence in redefining the stereotypical view of nursing as being 'an extension of the female domestic role' (Muldoon and Reilly 2003). As a result, male student nurses can at times find discrimination against them during placement experience (Waddell 1995). However, there was no evidence in any other study as to whether students were male or female. Certainly, the attitude of staff was at times negative towards the students, seemingly irrespective of their gender (Freshwater 2000).

Arguments for and against having a male nurse as a mentor are cited. Donovan (1990) suggests that having a male mentor could alienate a female nurse from the usual belief systems and from other women. Similarly, he suggests that as it is the male view that they should support themselves rather than others, this could affect the support offered to the student.

Evidence contrary to this is found in a study by Gilloran (1995) who suggested that: 'males were seen to be more rational and academic in their approach in comparison to females who were perceived as more often acting upon feelings'. One could argue from this that the academic approach of the male nurse would be of greater benefit to the student for their learning in practice, although this would need to be balanced by providing appropriate support. Certainly, as Fields (1994) suggests, it is vital that, should there be a gender difference between mentor and student, each recognizes that the way in which men and women learn from experience can differ.

However, having a mentor and student of different genders is not necessarily a detrimental experience, as Fields goes on the say: 'indeed it can be enriched, particularly where acknowledged diversity is combined with sensitivity'. Surely, it should be our aim as nurses to reduce internal issues of identity and exploitation, especially as it is bad enough that nurses are seen as an 'oppressed group' (Freshwater 2000). As Mackenzie (1997) states, 'without some concerted effort to move towards solidarity and the sharing of ideas, nursing as a profession dilutes its own potential to optimise patient care.'

In conclusion, this literature review has addressed a number of issues that have been found to affect the quality of mentorship received by student nurses in the practice environment. Firstly, the qualities of an effective mentor were identified and focused on a number of key roles or attributes that the mentor has. Secondly, evidence focused on factors other than the mentor that may affect a quality experience for the student. Building a relationship is seen as a crucial component; however, the difficulties in student contact with the mentor can seriously affect this. Having time to mentor effectively and to fit mentorship in alongside numerous other important roles is highlighted as a major problem. The lack of protected time to support students has been found to cause severe pressures on mentors and subsequently to have a detrimental effect on student support. Finally, the issue of gender again has been found to influence the quality of mentorship received by a student.

The research study undertaken provided further insight into the subject of mentorship and helped to support or refute the evidence already in the literature. The study also aimed to uncover new data and so it should be noted that this literature review is by no means exhaustive.

Methods

Introduction

The aim of this study was to explore student nurses' views on the quality of mentorship they was received in practice during their Diploma in Nursing course. It is the intention that, with the information gathered, recommendations could be made, if need be, to pursue the improvement of this support system.

Study design

For the purposes of this study, a form of qualitative research was used called 'phenomenology'. The use of qualitative methods is often found within the nursing literature and has become increasingly popular since the 1970s (Burnard 1991; Holloway and Wheeler 1998, p. 1; Van der Zalm and Bergum 2000). Qualitative research is in its broadest sense a 'method which focuses on human beings within their social and cultural context, not just on specific conditions. It is in tune with the nature of the phenomena examined: emotions, perceptions and actions are qualitative experiences' (Holloway and Wheeler 1998, p. 3). Qualitative research has been criticized for its flexibility and lack of structure (Silverman 2000, p. 2). However, in reality, the choice of method should be based on the type of research to be undertaken, not on which method appears to be more reliable (Silverman 2000, p. 2). This can be more clearly understood when comparing qualitative and quantitative research techniques.

Quantitative research is described as 'a formal, objective, systematic process in which numerical data are used to obtain information about the world' (Burns and Grove 2001, p. 18). Objectivity is essential for this type of research and, as Burns and Grove (2001, p. 19) go on to say, 'values, feelings and personal perceptions cannot enter into the measurement of reality.' Silverman (2000, p. 2) agrees with this by stating that 'quantitative research simply objectively reports reality'. Quantitative research can, however, 'conceal as well as reveal basic social processes' (Silverman 2000, p. 8). Comparing this to qualitative research, here a methodology that is based around the 'meaning of social interactions by those involved' (Burns and Grove 2001, p. 19) is used.

Qualitative research provides a setting where 'truth is both complex and dynamic and can be found only by studying individuals as they interact with and in their socio-historical settings' (Munhall 2001; cited by Burns and Grove 2001, p. 19). As this research study was based on student nurses' interactions with their mentors, it was felt that qualitative research would be most appropriate for the intended study with, in particular, a phenomenological approach.

Phenomenology is described as having its disciplinary roots in both philosophy and psychology and focuses on the lived experiences of human beings (Hallett 1995; Baillie 1996; Polit and Hungler 1997, p. 200; Burns and Grove 1997, p. 70). The history of phenomenology is certainly complex and, although a number of philosophers have described their views on this research method, it remains at times somewhat difficult to understand (Burns and Grove 1997, p. 71; Crotty 1996, p. 1). The work of two philosophers is cited in many texts as being fundamental to understanding phenomenology (Holloway and Wheeler 1998, p. 118; Polit and Hungler 1999, p. 246). These are Edmund Husserl and Martin Heidegger who, during the 19th and 20th centuries, described their at times differing views on the essentials when using phenomenology to guide research. Broadly speaking, however, their views focus on one specific goal – 'that is to gain knowledge about phenomena' (Holloway and Wheeler 1998, p. 121).

When comparing the beliefs of the two philosophers, the researcher felt that a Heideggerian approach was the most appropriate for her study. This was specifically for the following reason. Firstly, the Husserlian viewpoint 'has as its focus a description of the lived world that conceptualizes people as detached subjects existing in a world of objects' (Dreyfuss 1987; cited by Walters 1995). This compares with the Heideggerian view that phenomenology 'is interested in the origin of knowledge embedded in our everyday activities' (Walters 1995). More specifically, Heidegger believed that humans are people who 'are in and of the world, rather than subjects in a world of objects' (Reed 1994). This, the researcher believed, fitted most comfortably with her own views on where humans fit into the world. As Walters (1995) goes on to say, 'Heideggerian hermeneutics is interested in the origin of knowledge that is grounded in our everyday ready-to-hand practical experiences.' As the researcher's study was based around the 'everyday' experiences of student nurses in the practice setting, this again suggests that this was the most appropriate approach for the study.

Subjects

A purposive sample of third-year student nurses was interviewed, using a semi-structured interview schedule. Purposive sampling is described by Silverman (2000, p. 104) as allowing us to 'think critically about the parameters of the population we are interested in and choose our sample case carefully on this basis'. The aim was to 'deliberately reduce variation and allow a more focused inquiry' (Polit and Hungler 1997, p. 237). Purposive sampling is the type of sample most often used in phenomenological research (Clark 1998) and it is essential for the sample to include participants who have experienced the phenomena under investigation (Corben 1999).

For these reasons, the following specific eligibility criteria for inclusion in the sampling frame were devised.

- The student nurses identified to take part in this study must be from the February 2002 cohort of student nurses within the adult branch of nursing.
- They must have had a minimum of four placement experiences within the researcher's Hospital Trust.
- They must have been in training consistently since February 2002 and must not be a student nurse that has re-entered following a period of intercalation.

As there were more than 15 student nurses who fitted this category, the actual sample was picked randomly from the number of students available. The services of the Programmes Office at the Students' University assisted in the selection of students by identifying those that fitted the above criteria and from this 15 participants were randomly chosen by placing all the names in an envelope and 15 names were chosen blindly by a member of the Programmes Office staff. As soon as student names were available, the researcher contacted each student individually to see if they were willing to participate in the study.

Sample selection

It was intended for the purposes of this research to interview 15 student nurses. However, as 'there is no firmly established criteria or rules for sample size in qualitative research' (Polit and Hungler 1997, p. 237), the researcher determined sample size on the guiding principle of 'data saturation' (Polit and Hungler 1997, p. 238). As stated again by Polit and Hungler (1997, p. 238) and by Clark (1998), a small sample of possibly less than 10 may well be enough. The final sample size was therefore determined at the time of the study.

Measurements

The way in which data was collected subsequently reflected the quality of the phenomenological work that was undertaken (Hallett 1995). For this reason, interviewing was decided upon as the main investigation technique. As Miller and Glassner, cited in Silverman (1998, p. 104), states, 'a strength of qualitative interviewing is precisely its capacity to access self-reflexivity among interview subjects, leading to the greater likelihood of the telling of collective stories.' The taped interviews would then be transcribed verbatim and the material analysed using a phenomenological technique.

The main weakness of using this technique was the fact that the researcher was a novice within this field, and as stated by Guba and Lincoln (1989; cited by Whitehead 2004), 'Hermeneutic phenomenology recognises the influence of the researcher on the conduct and presentation of a study.' However, the researcher does have a nursing background and, having worked with student nurses in practice for a number of years, felt that she understood some of the issues students may have. The researcher is also a student herself and working full time, which again adds credibility to her understanding of the interviewees' situation. Hopefully this helped to refute one of the problems highlighted by Miller and Glassner, cited by Silverman (1998, p. 101) when they state that: 'Particularly as a result of social distances, interviewees may not trust us, they may not understand our questions, or they may purposely mislead us in their responses.'

In preparing for the interviews, questions were prepared in advance and designed to 'be sufficiently open that the subsequent questions of the interviewer cannot be planned in advance but must be improvised in a careful and theorized way' (Wengraf 2001, p. 5). The author hoped that these questions would elicit the information she would need to gain good insight into students' views on the phenomenon of mentorship.

Having a high level of interviewing skill is advocated for producing a true phenomenological investigation (Corben 1999). However, interviewing the participants proved difficult at first and the researcher was glad of the opportunity to pilot the interviews in order for her to practise the questioning technique. It was intended that the interviews would last no longer than one hour. Interviews took place in a room adjacent to the researcher's office, where complete quiet could be guaranteed and away from the practice setting and its many distraction. This is advocated by Wengraf (2001,

p. 200) who highlights the importance of a quiet area to conduct interviews along with sufficient time to complete the interview and debrief without being hurried.

The interviews were taped for transcribing and analysis later. However field notes were taken during the interviews and each tape was listened to immediately after completion and time allocated for the debriefing of the session as suggested above. The aim of this was to prevent data being lost Wengraf 2001, p. 222) and a process that the researcher found of particular value. Following the interview with each participant, the tapes were handed to an audio-typist for transcription which was carried out verbatim and as soon as possible after each interview so that the researcher could receive the data back quickly.

Validity and reliability

Validity of the research process was secured by careful analysis of the data that was obtained. Silverman (2000, p. 177) suggests that 'thinking critically about qualitative data analysis' can lead to more valid findings.

Enhancing validity through analysis was the researcher's aim. In particular, confirming the researcher's interpretation of transcriptions with the participants would be a vital component in ensuring validity of the study.

Reliability of the study really was dependent on the transcriptions of the tapes, ensuring that 'apparently trivial, but often crucial, pauses and overlaps' (Silverman 2000, p. 187) were included.

It could be argued that the researcher should have transcribed the tapes herself and, time allowing, she would have preferred to do this. However, a professional audio-typist was employed to undertake this task. The researcher did need to carefully read and re-listen to the tapes a number of times, again however increasing the reliability of the analysis.

A further issue that the researcher did have concerns about in relation to validity and reliability of the study related to her position as a Practice Placement Facilitator within the trust where the students were working. Although her primary responsibility is with providing support to mentors, the researcher had at times over the duration of her employment been involved in cases where students failed their practice. The researcher was therefore concerned about how she would be perceived by the students participating in the research and that the inequality in power might affect responses from the students. As described by Stew (1996), 'Researchers do have a responsibility to describe where they stand in relation to the issues covered, in terms of their own position, interests and hunches.' The researcher needed to ensure that this power struggle would not affect the data collected and aimed to prevent this by careful explanations of the research and intended use of results, along with making the participants feel at ease by introducing general discussion around day-to-day events.

Pilot study

By ensuring that the pilot study was carried out on the interview schedule, the researcher would 'determine insofar as is possible whether the instrument is clearly worded and free from major biases and whether it solicits the type of information envisioned' (Polit and Hungler 1997, p. 257). The intention within the pilot study was to undertake five interviews with student nurses from the same cohort but studying the child branch of nursing. The researcher hoped that this pilot study would provide her with an opportunity to practise her questioning technique. She was also keen to use students for this purpose in the hope of creating a setting as close to the real study as possible. Again this would help the researcher to build confidence when faced with new situations.

The pilot study proved to be invaluable for the study for two reasons. Firstly, it allowed the author to test out environmental factors. Tarling and Crofts (1998) advocate the consideration of these factors prior to the main undertaking of the study. This included the temperature of the room. As this was the summertime, it was necessary to have the windows open; however, there was a significant amount of outside noise which could be heard on the tape recordings and which distorted the students' responses. The author therefore obtained a fan so windows could be left closed. Interviews were also scheduled, where possible, for the cooler parts of the day, either early morning or late afternoon.

It was also noted that noise from nearby offices could be heard so signs saying that interviews were in progress were posted and colleagues were asked to reduce the volume of telephone ringtones. The positioning of the tape recorder was also adjusted to ensure it was facing the respondent. This ensured that where possible the respondents' responses could be heard clearly on the tape.

Secondly, the pilot study allowed the author to test out the interview schedule as described above and to practise her interview technique.

The first interview only lasted approximately 20 minutes and after the tape had been transcribed and analysed, the author felt that she was asking too many closed questions without delving further into a student's thoughts. The author believed that she needed more interviewing practice at this stage and she should consider further her interview technique. Robson (1995, p. 232) suggests when interviewing to take particular note of the following: 'Listen more than you speak ... put questions in a straightforward, clear and non-threatening way and eliminate cues which lead interviewees to respond in a particular way.' After analysis, the author felt that certain topics, such as the definition of mentorship and factors affecting the quality of mentorship, had produced limited data and that vital details could be missing.

For the second pilot interview, the author prepared a developed interview schedule and included considerations as an *aide memoire*. This was particularly useful and allowed the author to consider issues as the interview was progressing.

A third interview was undertaken for the pilot and at this point no further alterations were made to the interview schedule. Undertaking this third interview gave the author a further opportunity to practise her interview technique and ensured that her questioning elicited rich data. After undertaking this third interview, the author felt that she was ready to commence the main study.

Data analysis

Following interviewing of the participants, the tapes were transcribed verbatim as soon as possible. Qualitative data analysis has been described as controversial, which is in the main due to the researcher's 'conceptual capabilities, coupled with ambiguity about the process of analysis' (Whitehead 2004). Both structured and unstructured frameworks of data analysis are cited; however, there are criticisms of each type of framework. For example, unstructured analysis has been criticized for its lack of rigour (Whitehead 2001), whereas structured analysis is criticized for leading phenomenology to a methodical rather than a philosophical approach, (Hallett 1995).

Having reviewed the evidence for the different types of analysis, the researcher decided that, as she was a novice in the field, a structured approach would be the most appropriate. She therefore used a system of data analysis based on Colaizzi (1978; cited by Holloway and Wheeler 1998). This involved a seven-stage process of analysis, which in brief is as follows:

1. The participants' narratives are read to attempt to understand their ideas.
2. Extracting significant statements relating to the phenomena under study is then undertaken.
3. The researcher then formulates meaning for each significant statement.
4. Clusters of themes are then sought.
5. An exhaustive description of the phenomenon is then developed.
6. The next stage is described by Colaizzi as 'an unequivocal statement of identification of the fundamental structure of the phenomenon'.
7. Participants are then asked for a further interview to elicit their views on the findings and to validate them. (Colaizzi 1978; cited by Holloway and Wheeler 1998)

The researcher's overall aim was to remain true to the data (Whiting 2001), and returning to the participants for confirmation that the researcher's interpretations were correct was vital to validate the study (Whitehead 2002).

In reality, this type of analysis did not prove to be ideal. As the research was being undertaken during the summer break, it was difficult to contact student nurses for a second interview. The author therefore had to limit the number of students contacted and use the telephone as a means of discussing the analysis. This clearly became a limitation of the study.

Ethical issues

In order to gain access to the university setting and student details, ethical approval was sought from the university ethics committee. Ethical approval is required before conducting any research study to ensure that institutional approval of the research has been obtained as well as ensuring other considerations have been made such as protecting the subjects' rights, balancing benefits and risks and obtaining informed consent (Burns and Grove 2003, p. 161).

The student nurses have the right to refuse inclusion within the study simply by non-attendance at interview. However, each student nurse was contacted individually by phone to discuss their inclusion in the study, giving informed consent at this time. A formal consent form was also signed by each participant at the time of interview. The student nurses were advised on specific information as to how much of their time the interview would take and their commitment to the research process in general. This is essential to ensure that participants will agree to take part (Holloway and Wheeler 1998, p. 44). As stated above, an information sheet and consent form were provided for the student nurses to read and sign if they chose to take part in the study. Confidentiality was guaranteed as there were no student details on any of the transcriptions or names used in writing up the study. To help achieve anonymity, each student was identified by a number only and this number was used throughout the research process.

Students were also asked to ensure that they did not disclose personal information of any particular mentor or placement area during the interview. Although this was at times difficult it was essential in maintaining confidentiality within the research study (Polit and Hungler 1997, p. 138).

Time was allowed after each interview to debrief students. This was particularly useful as some of the content of the interviews elicited data on difficult situations that had involved the student.

Following completion of the study, students were asked if they would like their tape to be returned to them, and if they did not want it, the researcher informed them that she intended to destroy the tapes herself.

Results and analysis

Defining mentorship and first experiences

Results from the first question,

'How would you define mentorship?'

are as follows.

Of the 12 students interviewed, a total of 39 different responses were elicited in their attempts to define mentorship. From the responses gained, the author felt that four themes in particular emerged. Interestingly, in their attempts to define mentorship, the students described the roles of the mentor in their answers but did not include any qualities that they felt a mentor should have.

Firstly, the students described statements in regard to the 'relationship-building' (Theme 1) part of the mentorship process. The supportive nature of the relationship was highlighted by seven students with such responses as:

'I'd say mainly to support ... talk about any worries or anything on the ward or wherever you were on placement ...' (*Student No. 4, Response 2*)

and:

'Mentorship is a qualified nurse supporting a student ... supporting emotionally ...' (*Student No. 5, Response 1*)

Belonging within the relationship was also described as an essential aspect of mentorship, with five students stating that the mentor would be 'assigned to them'. Furthermore, the students felt that the mentor would work with them on a 'one-to-one basis' (*Student No. 7, Response 2*) and would:

'Follow you through, through your whole placement ...' (*Student No. 2, Response 3*)

Ten of the 12 students interviewed described aspects of the second theme, that being 'quality of teaching and assessing'. Four students in particular highlighted that mentorship involved the mentor teaching them to impart their knowledge and:

'help you understand things and go through things with you.' (*Student No. 2, Response 4*)

Aspects of assessment were identified by three students with statements such as:

'Fills in the CAP (Continuous Assessment of Practice) document ... supervises what we're doing ...' (*Student No. 11, Response 1*)

and:

'Go through things with you like learning objectives ...' (*Student No. 3, Response 2*)

Student No. 6 described what a mentor would need in order to undertake this role, that being:

'.. quite a wide range of knowledge, relevant to where you're working, and a fair bit of experience ...' (*Response 2*)

'Professionalism' was the third theme to emerge. Here, five students identified that the mentor would be a 'qualified nurse', and in particular Student No. 3 commented on how the mentor would be a:

'support for me maintaining my professional conduct.' (*Response 3*)

Finally, the theme around 'clinical skills training' emerged with six students stating that mentorship meant to them that they would be:

'... learning new skills' (*Student No. 10, Response 1*)

and:

'basic day-to-day activities ...' (*Student No. 2, Response 6*)

Clearly, the students interviewed had a good understanding of the process of mentorship and the author felt they were well equipped to discuss issues of quality around this subject.

In response to the second question:

'What were your expectations of mentorship at the start of your training?'

An overarching theme soon emerged and that was that the students all had 'unrealistic expectations' of mentorship at the start of their training. To further describe this, the author felt that two sub-themes were linked to the overarching theme of 'unrealistic expectations'.

Initially, unrealistic expectations of the amount of time spent with the mentor was highlighted by eight students in the theme 'time spent with the mentor', with such statements as:

'I think I was expecting to be with them all the time ... expecting them to work with me most of the time and to introduce me to everything.' (*Student No. 4, Response 1*)

and:

'I expected to spend practically all my time with someone, for them to show me you know, everything really ...' (*Student No. 6, Response 1*)

Secondly, the 'quality of teaching and assessing' theme recurred throughout eight of the interviews, again demonstrating an unrealistic perspective as acknowledged in these extracts from Student No. 8:

'Somebody ... who would teach me how to be a nurse, who would teach me the practical skills needed to be a nurse, somebody that I could look upon as a role model and be supportive and patient with me, you sort of picture your mentor as being the perfect nurse.' (*Response 1*)

Shortly after making this statement, the student goes on to say that:

'As you go along you realize that's not always the case.' (*Response 3*)

Further evidence of how unrealistic these expectations were was shown in the responses to how the students found the mentorship they actually received during that first experience. In relation to 'contact with the mentor', five students emphasized that their experience did not meet their expectations. This appeared to be mainly due to the off-duty rota and the days that students were expected to be at university. For one student, mentor contact was particularly poor as she comments:

'To be honest, my very first mentor, I saw her twice.' (*Student No. 2, Response 4*)

Support for this student was provided by unqualified staff, which was also the case for Student No. 5. She states that:

'it was the auxiliaries who took you under their wings, and said, "Here I'll show you how this ward works".' (*Response 7*)

The experience of working with auxiliaries was not viewed positively, mainly due to the lack of theory behind the practice of undertaking clinical skills. This student in particular felt that a clinical support worker would have been more appropriate in supporting the student at this time, as they have knowledge of the theory behind practice. This produced a second theme for this question, 'taught by others'.

The theme 'quality of teaching and assessing' revealed a different view of why students' expectations of mentorship were not realized in their first placement. Here five of the students interviewed realized very quickly that they were actually responsible for their own learning on the placement and that the role of the mentor was to support the student in this. The mentor also ensured that the student was learning at the right level for their stage of training. Although at the time this seemed to create feelings of frustration for students, they could now reflect and see the value of the experience. As Student No. 3 says:

'Sometimes I felt like I was being held back. I often wanted to learn more from the clinical environment ... but thinking back now, I can understand how in that first experience the mentor did guide me through, and she said, she guided me through the clinical skills that she thought were more appropriate for my level of training.' (*Response 1*)

A final theme to emerge from this part of the interview was the 'attitude of the staff'. Of the 12 students interviewed, five did not comment on the attitude of the staff and one student commented positively, stating that:

'I didn't feel in the way or anything ... I didn't feel like a cold reception or frosty or anything ... with being a new person.' (*Student No. 9, Response 2*)

Five students, however, commented negatively on the attitude of the staff, although they justified the staff's attitudes by recognizing the workload on the wards. For one student in particular, this had been a very distressing experience. She describes how a comment by a nurse made her feel unwilling to return to the placement.

'I do remember somebody saying to me on my first placement "well, fancy sending a first-year student here, you're not much use to us" and I sort of went to the toilet and cried.' (*Student No. 11, Response 8*)

'I was so frightened it really knocked me' (*Student No. 11, Response 14*)

'I went home and said I'm not going back ... it's terrifying when somebody says something like that to you ...' (*Student No. 11, Response 15*)

Student No. 2 describes equally well how she found the staff in her first placement, and why the staff did not help with her lack of confidence at this stage of training.

'Intimidation' (*Student No. 2, Response 22*)

She describes this further:

'... they don't intentionally intimidate you but ...' (*Student No. 2, Response 23*)

'It's just that they are because they're ... they've been there for years, they know what they're doing, and it's very busy and you just, you daren't speak up, 'cos you're just going to give them extra work really.' (*Student No. 2, Response 24*)

Mentor as assessor

Considering the issues raised by the previous question, the author then asked if the students felt that the mentor was the best person to assess them. Eleven students agreed that the mentor was the best person to assess them, and five students unequivocally thought this, one student in particular stating that:

'I see them as a peer and I value their opinions and their assessments' (*Student No. 3, Response 4*)

Six students again highlighted issues that might affect the quality of this part of the mentorship process and one student was unsure if the mentor was the best person to assess them.

The themes of 'contact with the mentor' and 'time spent with the mentor' were described by two students. They felt that the mentor was the best person to assess them as long as there were enough opportunities to work with them, but that sometimes the mentor was too busy. Interestingly, Student No. 8 highlighted another issue of concern, stating that:

'It depends on whether they're a good mentor, because who assesses the mentors? In an ideal world, yeah, that would be a good system but it's not an ideal world and there's not all ideal nurses and mentors out there so possibly not in some cases but I don't know how you would differentiate.'   (*Response 1*)

This response clearly defines the whole issue of the study and will be explored later in the discussion.

Qualities of an effective mentor

The author then asked the students what their experience so far had taught them about the qualities of an effective mentor. In response to this, there were 36 different statements. These responses were categorised into three themes. It should be noted that the students didn't always describe the mentors' qualities when answering this question but described what the mentor should do to be effective.

Firstly, the 'relationship' between student and mentor was described; in particular, seven students stated that the most important factor is that the mentor has time for them. As Student No. 10 says:

'Be able to give you the time, even if it is on a busy unit.'   (*Response 2*)

The other main qualities highlighted by students around the relationship theme were that the mentor should be 'friendly', 'approachable' and 'supportive', each of which was cited by five students. Seven students cited being taught by their mentor as a key part of the effective mentor role, again linking the 'teaching and assessing' theme. Alongside this, the students felt that the mentor should be able to give 'praise', 'encouragement' and 'feedback' to students. Also seen as important by five students was that the mentor understood the assessment documentation and learning outcomes that the student had to achieve.

The final theme to emerge from this category was around the 'attitude' of the mentor. As Student No. 9 puts it:

'the attitude, where they include you in everything, helpfulness, willing ...'
(*Response 7*)

Another important quality described within this theme was that the mentor was empathetic towards the student in training. This was described by four students, and was particularly important to Student No. 7. She states that the mentor should be:

> 'Somebody who's got empathy, knows what it's like, remembers what it's like to be a student ...' (*Response 2*)

Whilst responding to this question, it was noted that three of the students felt that the mentor should 'ask you everything'. With this in mind, the author pursued this area of questioning by asking whether students thought the mentor should challenge their practice.

Challenging practice

All 12 students felt that their mentor should challenge their practice and although they had all experienced this throughout their training, the extent of challenge at times was limited and often perceived as a questioning of practice rather than challenge. The whole concept of challenging practice, however, was seen as a positive aspect of mentorship by eight students.

Being 'safe to practice' was the first theme to emerge from this question, as challenging practice was identified as a good way for the mentor to test out the students' ability and be sure they were safe to practice with different levels of supervision.

As Student No. 9 found:

> 'obviously they've got to know that I'm capable of doing my own things ... and I think, yeah, they have to push so far to make sure we are capable of you know doing something, carrying a practice out.' (*Response 2*)

Similarly, Student No. 8 described her reasons for feeling the mentor should challenge her practice:

> 'You're more aware of what you're doing and you tend to look at the whole picture, and be more questioning in what you're doing rather than just getting on and doing the job.' (*Response 2*)

This was definitely seen as a good thing as the student goes on to say:

> 'In this day and age because, you know, there's so many issues in nursing now, nursing is not just the solely caring profession that it was, there's a push to, to make it a profession you know, and plus nurses are more accountable nowadays so you need to question what you're doing.' (*Response 3*)

Other positive statements around this were such things as:

'It makes you learn as well that way.' (*Student No. 2, Response 5*)

and:

'I think it gives you confidence in a way.' (*Student No.11, Response 5*)

Four students did, however, have reservations about the mentor challenging their practice, but this was around the way the challenging was done and also the stage of training they were at. As Student No. 6 describes:

'I think that the way they challenge your practice should be the correct way and not like screaming at you in front of all the patients or putting you down in front of the patients; I think there's a way to do it but yeah, I definitely expect people to challenge my practice.' (*Response 1*)

Student No. 4 describes how she could at times find challenge intimidating:

'I sometimes find that a bit intimidating ... I'd be more comfortable with it now, than what I would be in the first year, I used to panic when my mentors did that to me, or even doctors as well.' (*Response 3*)

The interview progressed by asking students if they would challenge their mentor's practice. Varying responses were given to this question but clear themes emerged around the following issues.

Firstly, the theme of 'confidence to challenge' was identified. All the students felt that they should challenge the mentor's practice but their lack of confidence in their own knowledge, especially in the early part of training, hindered them from doing this.

The following extract from Student No. 11 illustrates this clearly:

'And you think, oh well, they're the qualified ones, I don't know, and even though I probably, in my first year, came across things where I'd been shown in clinical skills how to do it and they would do it probably different, I wouldn't have said anything.' (*Response 12*)

Following on from this, again student reluctance to challenge practice was seen in the second theme, 'attitude of the staff'. Four students in particular felt that their mentors' attitude was such that it would have been very difficult to challenge their practice, and the one student who had done this felt they were criticized for doing so.

He mentor's attitude so affected one student that she felt it would be very difficult to challenge any aspect of their practice. She said that it:

'Depends who's the mentor that you've got, some mentors are lovely and some of them you think, oh God ... you just sort of do as you're told and get your head down.' (*Student No. 5, Response 6*)

Finally, the theme of 'how to challenge' was highlighted by four students, all of whom had had experiences where they had felt it necessary to challenge the mentors' practice. Each felt that using a questioning approach was received positively by mentors and one student even found that the practice on the ward had changed due to her challenging what she had witnessed.

Student No. 11 provided a good example of this when describing an incident with her mentor who was not using a sterile technique for a dressing. The student had been taught that a sterile technique was needed so she questioned the mentor. When asked how the mentor had responded to this, the student said:

'Fine because she didn't know any different, and she said "Well, let's look it up".' (*Response 6*)

and:

'Yeah, she accepted it, that's fine ... I think if I'd said "Oh you're doing this wrong, that's not the way you do it" she probably would have took the hump, wouldn't she? Which is fair enough.' (*Response 7*)

Mentor preparation

Considering some of the responses to the previous question, the author wanted the students to consider whether they found that mentors were prepared for their role. This question again received a mixed response. However, a main theme around the mentor's lack of understanding of the assessment documentation was highlighted in the theme 'unprepared' by nine of the students interviewed. The majority of students were keen to point out that in most cases, it was not that the mentors were not bothered about the documentation; it was just that they had not had any training in this aspect of mentorship, especially as the documentation changed with each new course. As one student put it:

'... it wasn't that she wasn't bothered'. (*Student No. 9, Response 4*)

One thing, however, that the students did find frustrating was when they had to go through documentation with the mentors. Often the students found that the mentor was unsure what to write for their interviews, which made the students feel like the whole process was a waste of time. Student No. 11 describes her experience of this:

'The interviews always sort of throw them, they never know what to say at the interviews; they should have some sort of I don't know, thing to follow or something.' (*Response 5*)

She goes on to say:

'It's only when you get a very experienced nurse who says I expect you to do this, this and this and to learn about this that you get a particularly good interview I think … you talk to student nurses and lots of them say the mentor asked them what they should put, and it's a waste of time when you've got to tell them what to put, isn't it.' (*Response 7*)

Another pertinent theme to emerge from this question was again the 'attitude of the staff'. Some students had found that their mentors made it quite clear that they felt the paperwork was a waste of time. Some mentors even signed off the paperwork without reading it which was particularly upsetting for the student, considering the amount of work they had put into completing the document. Student No. 12 had problems with this issue:

'But I had one mentor who, I felt quite insulted really 'cos I'd spent all my time filling it in and they didn't even bother to read it … I asked him about it and he said "Oh, I just come to work to do my job. I don't come to, you know …".' (*Response 5*)

As a new Mentor Preparation Programme had been running at the local university, some students had come across mentors who had attended this course and found that they were up to date with the paperwork. Similarly, another student found that their mentors had a good understanding of the CAP document.

'Whenever they've gone through the CAP document with me, they've always had a good understanding of what learning outcomes … I've needed to meet and if I've ever been in trouble, they've always come up with some examples that I could have maybe used.' (*Student 3, Response 7*)

Organization of mentorship support

'Gaining perspectives on and support in practice' was the main theme to emerge from analysing the students' views on the organization of mentorship support. Nine students described how beneficial it was having two mentors assigned to them. The main reason for this was that it solved the problem of having mentor contact. Often they found that of the two mentors, one would take the main responsibility for their CAP document and the other would be there to work with and support them when the main mentor was off duty.

Other benefits were described, particularly in respect of 'gaining perspectives on practice'. Student No. 8 describes how having two mentors made her consider different ways of adapting her practical skills:

'... gives you an opportunity to see you know how more than one nurse works in the same practical setting.' (*Response 5*)

Similarly from the mentors' point of view Student No. 7 felt that it would also be beneficial for them.

'I think for the mentor it must be beneficial because they're seeing you sort ofbetween two people ... they could share what's going on ...' (*Response 4*)

Only one student found a problem with this system, pointing out how having two mentors means that no one takes responsibility.

'It can seem like "oh well, so-and-so is your mentor as well, why don't you ask her about it?" and it might sometimes seem like, well, yeah, but you're my mentor as well.' (*Student No. 6, Response 2*)

Overall quality of mentorship

When asked about this, three students described a high quality of mentorship support throughout their training. The other nine students described varying levels of quality although overall they had found more good than bad experiences during their training. Comments such as:

'They've been more good than bad definitely. And they do get better as you go along.' (*Student No. 11, Response 3*)

and:

'If I had to say on the scale of one to ten, I'd say eight.' (*Student No. 3, Response 1*)

were made, clearly identifying student views around the quality of mentorship.

An interesting theme to emerge throughout six of the interviews was 'ways of coping with bad experiences'. All these students recognized the need to be realistic about mentorship support and, if a bad experience occurs, to be pro-active in resolving problems. This extract from Student No. 6 illustrates this clearly:

'I think that no matter what you do, you're going to get good and bad at everything, I mean I've had some absolutely brilliant mentors, and I've had some not so good ones but I think it's also down to the students to seek out knowledge and if there is a problem then you know help to sort it out yourself ... and I think as long as you're fairly flexible ...' (*Response 3*)

Alongside this, it was recognized that the student needs to make the effort to work with the mentor and where possible work the same shifts as them. However, in some cases, even when the student had arranged their shifts to coincide with the mentor, there was still little contact during the shift because the ward was busy. Student No. 4 describes this:

'A lot of the time, though, they just don't have the time to spend with you on the ward as well.' (*Response 4*)

'Because in my last ward, I barely went on shift with her, but I tended to work with auxiliaries because she just didn't have time.' (*Response 5*)

'It's not, I don't mind doing, working with auxiliaries, its part of my job but when you want to like learn how to do things like that, some just don't have the time, and sometimes I get the appearance that they don't want to, 'cos they're just so stressed.' (*Response 9*)

Similarly, some students recognized how other staff on the placement could support them even if their mentor was not wholly supportive.

'Even when I had the bad mentor – well they weren't bad but, the bad experiences – the other nurses would help explain things and let you take on a couple of patients, and let you do drug rounds and care plans and things like that.' (*Student No. 2, Response 1*)

Factors affecting the quality of mentorship

The main factor affecting the quality of mentorship in practice was 'time'. This was identified by nine students and has emerged as a theme at some point in all the interviews with the students. As Student No. 1 describes:

'You don't have time to sit down and have your interviews sometimes when you're supposed to have them and you know you want to ask things and be shown things and just, there just physically isn't the time ... to do that.' (*Response 3*)

Linked to this, students highlighted the difficulties of finding time during a shift to work together with their mentor:

'The busyness of the ward ... I mean on a normal general ward your mentors responsible for ten patients, and if it's a busy day ... or it's a busy ward ... I'd say it affects it sometimes because they can't always let you do the medication round ...

I found that on one placement I was kind of counted in the numbers and they were short of auxiliaries and you were doing the auxiliary's job really.' (*Student No. 12, Response 1*)

The second theme to emerge from this question was again the 'attitude of the staff'. Six students felt that their mentors or the ward staff's attitudes had negatively affected the quality of mentorship, along with in some cases an obvious lack of willingness to support student learning. As this student found:

'I think willingness just to be a mentor, if they're in a frame of mind where they think right I've got a student, I'm going to help them to do this, this and this, it just makes such a huge difference from someone saying "I've been put down as your mentor so it looks like you're going to be working with me" sort of thing 'cos, and then not providing you often with the opportunities that another mentor might have provided, I think that really just willingness to be a mentor and obviously act in that role.' (*Student No. 6, Response 1*)

Another issue highlighted was the 'organization of mentor support and the off-duty rota'. At times, it was found that a mentor had not been allocated to a student at the start of the allocation period or sometimes a student would find that the mentor had changed their shifts, was on holiday or off sick. This meant that the student struggled to find someone to work with and this affected their confidence in asking questions and their learning in the placement. Student No. 2 describes the effects of this:

'If your mentor's not there, then you don't know who you're with, you're just willy nilly anywhere, so you daren't ask much.' (*Response 6*)

Finally, the theme of 'numbers of students' was highlighted by three students who identified that there are large numbers of students allocated to each ward and if students are not willing to work shifts, then it can lead to large numbers on a particular shift at any one time. This can be particularly stressful for the mentors. For example, there may be an imbalance in staff ratios for late shifts compared to early shifts as early shifts were more popular because of the less unsocial hours. Student No. 4 describes her experience of this:

'The amount of students that we have on as well, so many students just aren't willing to do any weekends and come in on a week day when I, when my mentor was on, and I'd have to … on a week day or something, there was that many students on she'd had to share between us and things like that.' (*Response 2*)

Student No. 11 describes a similar experience:

'I think if you get a very busy mentor … sometimes it can be, you get a lot of students on a ward as well, the mentors tend to tear their hair out a bit don't they?

Because you know if they've got six or eight students, it's a bit of a nightmare for them isn't it really?' (*Response 1*)

Age, grade and gender of the mentor

In order to further investigate factors that might affect the quality of mentorship received in practice, the author asked the students to describe their views on three factors: age, grade and gender of the mentor.

In relation to age, the main theme, 'it's willingness to mentor and experience that counts' was identified from the respondents. The experience in question related either to the mentor's experience as a nurse or their experience in life.

Four students felt that the age of the mentor made no difference to the quality of the mentorship they had received. Four students felt that younger staff were better mentors as they had empathy with the students, were more enthusiastic and used evidence-based practice. One student in particular describes her feelings about the age of the mentor:

'I think when you've got a nurse, an older nurse that's worked for a long time in say the NHS, it's very difficult to shrug off what they've done for a long time and although the NHS has changed, you've got a nurse that's perhaps worked on a ward for twenty years and its difficult not to become tunnel visioned and not know what's going on outside that ward' (*Student No. 8, Response 2*)

When asked how she viewed the younger staff, she called them:

'A new breed of nursing.' (*Response 1*)

Two students preferred an older mentor to support them, but state this is because of their own age and the fact that they are mature students. Student No. 12 describes her views here:

'Because otherwise if you have like a mentor who's like 22, 23, that's like the same age as my children and I find that quite, not intimidating but, you know, I just think, well for me personally I think that the older mentors, I like my mentors to be either my age or older, I find that a lot better than having someone who's too young.' (*Response 2*)

Finally, three students claimed that it was not the age that affected the quality of the mentorship but the mentor's experience and how long they had been qualified. Student No. 6 explains this further:

'I mean, you get some mentors that are older and qualified only two years ago or whatever but then you get people that have qualified 20 years ago and often, well may not have moved on with the times ... I think that there isn't a problem with the age but if they see students as someone to help skivvy and do ... the jobs they don't want to do then I think, yeah there often is a problem.'   (*Response 3*)

In relation to the grade of the mentor, again the theme, 'it's willingness to mentor and experience that counts' could be identified in the students' views.

Five students felt that the grade of the mentor made no difference. They had all experienced mentorship from different grades of nurse and focused on the individual and their willingness to mentor as being the important factor not the grade. Newly qualified staff were seen as less effective as mentors mainly because both student and mentor were still learning at this stage. 'D' and 'E' grade mentors were seen as equally effective and in some cases more so than 'F' grade mentors. This was underlined by five students who recognized that although the role of 'F' grade was usually taken by an experienced nurse, they had even more conflicting responsibilities which left even less time for formal mentorship. Student No. 5 explains this further:

'The higher the grade, they seem to be more experienced but more like over the top, they seem to have too much information for you and then they're too busy flying off answering the phone, speaking to relatives and they don't really have time to like speak basic nursing cares to you and they don't, they're too busy, they've got too many stresses and pressure like bed management and things.'   (*Response 1*)

Student No. 11 describes a similar experience:

'The further up the ladder, the better the mentors, but they maybe don't want to do it when they get to that point because they've got so much stuff on.'   (*Response 6*)

The gender of the mentor was the last factor to be discussed with the students. Eight students had had experience of a male mentor and of these, six felt that they had been equally well supported as by a female mentor. Of the two students who felt that the gender of the mentor had made a difference, this was really about 'other factors' affecting the mentor or student and not specifically about the mentor being a male nurse. For example, Student No. 12 described her only experience of being mentored by a male nurse and the problems this presented:

'I think it could have been the fact that he had a lot of problems at home and he never stopped going on about them.'   (*Response 1*)

'Every day all I used to get was about his problems at home, and I never used to kind of elaborate on it, I just, I used to just, wished that he'd stop talking about it really and pay more attention to what he was supposed to be teaching me.' (*Response 2*)

The four remaining students never had a male mentor throughout their training so were unable to comment.

Discussion

First, it can be said that the student nurses interviewed had a reasonable understanding of what mentorship was; the key words they used to describe this process were 'supporter' and 'teacher', as found in previous studies (Darling 1984. Cameron–Jones and O'Hara 1996; Philips et al. 1996a). Two aspects of this part of the interview in particular need further discussion. Firstly, five students indicated that the mentor helped the students develop their clinical skills. Clinical skills training by a mentor is not specifically identified as one of the mentor roles in Darling's (1984) study. Similarly, more recent studies (Cameron-Jones and O'Hara 1996. Andrews and Chilton 2000) make no specific mention of clinical skills training, only of the role of 'teacher'.

Secondly, challenging practice was seen as a vital element of the mentorship process due to the changing roles of nurses within the profession. This particular part of the role is identified in the literature, particularly in later studies (Daloz 1987, cited by Northcott 2000; Myrick and Yonge 2001). The importance of enabling the student to think critically is vital to ensure that the learning environment is stimulating and interesting. On further questioning, it became clear that, for the students in this study, there are implications challenging practice that will be discussed later.

Mentors were also seen as the most appropriate people to assess the student in practice, even though this is not defined as part of the classic mentor role (Morton–Cooper and Palmer 2000, p. 40). It should be noted, however, that none of the students interviewed experienced any other form of mentorship or assessment from anyone else so were unable to compare systems in any way and could only comment on their particular experience.

Finally, students evaluated the effectiveness of the mentorship they had received in practice quite positively, acknowledging that there were a number of specific issues that were clearly influential in affecting the quality of mentorship they had received throughout their three years in training. Such positive comments surprised the author as, in her role as PPF, she is only witness to difficult mentorship situatons involving either a failing student or a complaint from a student about a mentor. This helped the author to question student responses and support an objective view throughout the interviews and analysis.

The issues arising from mentorship will now be discussed. The NHS Plan (DoH 2000) had pointed out that one of the main problems within the NHS was the lack of available nursing staff. To this end, the document highlighted the need to invest in more nurse training places. An increase in the number of student nurses is now being realized and it has affected the quality of mentorship as remarked by some of the students interviewed in this study. Student No. 10 describes what she felt affected the quality of mentorship she had received:

'It could depend on how many students the mentor's got ... like on some places they've got maybe ten students on one ward ...' (*Response 2*)

Providing adequate support for the numbers of students in practice is an ever-increasing problem (While 1996; Lord 2002) and to some extent 'full capacity is now being reached,' in practice placements (Lord 2002). Dealing with the issues around the recruitment and retention of existing staff is advocated by Macleod Clark (1998) as being one crucial way of providing a solution to this problem and she suggests that so called 'bottom loading is short-sighted and doomed to failure.'

A further salient point is that some of the students within the study maintained that they preferred younger mentors to work with and that older mentors were less effective. Student No. 5 describes her experience:

'The older mentors ... some of them are bored and they're bored with their jobs ... "Oh I've been working here years, oh I just do it like this, 'cos I've always done it like that ...".' (*Response 3*)

Evidence of this was also found in a study by Dunn and Hansford (1997) where student nurses stated that: 'There are older [RNs] that haven't gone through university and they just hate students.' Older nurses surely have a wealth of experience to offer to the student nurse; valuing these staff and supporting them to maintain their interest must surely be vital in maintaining the workforce. As Buchan (1999) states, 'Against a backdrop of increasing likelihood of skills shortages, there will be a need to maximise the actual contribution that these older nurses can make.'

Connected with this, an overarching theme throughout the study was the attitude of the staff or mentor towards the student. Negative attitudes were an issue in two specific areas. These were, firstly, when a student attempted to challenge practice and secondly, the mentor's or ward staff's apparent lack of desire to support students in the practice environment. Some students experienced this negativity from their first placement onwards and felt they were seen as:

'... foreign bodies coming in' (*Student No. 4, Response 9*)

On some occasions, negative comments were made directly to the student. One student in particular had challenged their mentor's decision over patient care and the mentor subsequently intimated that a poor reference would be given if such behaviour continued. Student No. 3 describes their experience:

'I got quite concerned in the end, because things were mentioned about references and I didn't think it was fair really. She said, "Don't forget, if you ever need a reference, I would give a reference ...".' (*Response 18*)

Similarly, other students found that both the general attitude of the staff in placements and sometimes even that of their mentor was negative towards them. As Student No. 4 states:

> 'I think it's the attitude of the staff ... some of them are just not interested, just don't seem to be willing to assist us in learning.' (*Response 10*)

Supporting evidence for this is found in a number of studies (Spouse 1998; Lofmark and Wikbald 2001; Jackson and Mannix 2001), where students were not wholly welcomed by the mentor. This led to poor relationship-building between student and mentor and caused the student to spend more time trying to 'fit in' with the team than learning in the clinical environment.

Farrell (1997) describes the 'hostile undercurrents' as 'horizontal violence' and states that 'intra-staff aggression was more upsetting for them [staff] to deal with than patient assault or the aggression they sometimes experienced from other disciplines.' Of greater concern is that, rather than focusing on patient care, the student may learn negative behaviours themselves from this so-called 'hidden curriculum' (Welsh and Swann 2002, p. 46).

This need to 'fit in', known as professional socialisation, is described as 'teaching workers at both a subliminal and conscious level which values are likely to bring them acceptance and reward within their chosen profession'(Ewan and White 1996, cited by Morton–Cooper and Palmer, 2000, p. 15).

Gray and Smith (1999) and Stuart (2003) suggest that it is both the mentor and the learning environment that best facilitates the professional socialization of the student nurse. It is vital that staff in the clinical environments are aware of this and see the value in supporting student nurses. Mentors should also be aware of their part in relationship-building with the student, ensuring that the student is welcomed to the placement and quickly made to feel part of the team. Supporting evidence for this was found in studies by Dunn and Hansford (1997) and Nolan (1998). They found that making the student feel part of the team ensured that the student nurse felt safe to develop their skills, knowledge and attitude about registration and that they were able to challenge practice whenever they felt it appropriate. This must surely lead to improved standards of practice.

Closely linked to the theme of staff–mentor attitudes is the preparation of the mentors. The study shows that some students felt that their mentor was unprepared for the role, specifically in relation to knowledge of the students' curriculum, paperwork completion and accountability within the role of the mentor. This was noted by the students in particular in such practices as mentors not reading students evidence in CAP documents and subsequently signing CAP documents without taking due care to follow the mentorship process to the letter. The following extracts from two students' interviews describe these issues well.

'They don't know what they're doing and I'm having to tell them what they're doing ... what to look at, they don't understand the criteria for assessment.' (*Student No. 4, Response 3*)

'She (the mentor) just signed it and I thought I aren't, I can't be bothered to tell you 'cos it's just more work. So she just signed it.' (*Student No. 2, Response 4*)

Such practices described here could lead the mentor to sign off a student who would not necessarily be competent to pass their placement. Further evidence of this has been found in a recently published study by Duffy (2004).

Major issues indicated in the study were, first, that mentors struggled with paperwork due to the use of academic jargon and, second, that it went against the mentors' caring nature to fail a student in practice. Even when the mentor felt a student should fail, they would often give them the benefit of the doubt in the hope that the student would improve over time. There also appeared to be little support for the mentor who had to fail a student. Similar problems were found in earlier studies, again highlighting mentor difficulties in completing paperwork and general lack of preparation for the role (Neary 1999; Calman et al. 2002).

From a professional perspective, advisory standards for mentorship were, until recently, available in the document 'Preparation of Mentors and Teachers' (ENB and DoH 2001a). These standards have since become mandatory and there is currently ongoing consultation aimed at developing a standard to support learning and assessment in practice (NMC 2004), which will in turn replace the recommendations made in 'Preparation of Mentors and Teachers' (ENB and DoH 2001a). The NMC (2004) recognized that mentor standards in particular should be agreed, become mandatory and be in place by September 2005. It states that: 'The argument for this short time scale is the considerable evidence base the NMC has accumulated of concern that the mentor standard is weak and needs urgent review.' The consultation document (NMC 2004) suggests that there should be a four-level 'framework of progressive skill development' for the preparation of mentors and teachers, including an 'associate mentor' level as a starting point prior to formal mentorship preparation and undertaking of the role. The author hopes that the new standard will support the development of strategies to address some of the issues highlighted from her study and give greater credence to mentorship support than ever before.

From the point of view of student assessment paperwork, there is currently a revalidation of the pre-registration course being undertaken locally. Issues around difficulties in completing paperwork have already been highlighted and future documents aim to be more 'user-friendly'. To support the process of development in assessment documentation, consultation with practice staff is being included in the revalidation process. A number of studies (Neary 2000b; Watkins 2000; Calman et al. 2002; Dolan 2003) have pointed to difficulties with assessment documentation. These have shown that designing and understanding assessment documentation is often complicated and problematic. Although the NMC is currently consulting on mentor and teacher roles, there is no national standard on assessment and one wonders if this is something that will need addressing in the future in order to ensure quality assurance in the assessment process.

A final point to discuss here in relation to mentor preparation is one particular finding from the study. When asked if a mentor should also be the assessor for the student, as stated above, one student voiced her concern by stating:

'It depends on whether they're a good mentor, because who assesses the mentors? In an ideal world yeah, that would be a good system but it's not an ideal world and they're not all ideal nurses and mentors out there so possibly not in some cases but I don't know how you would differentiate.' *(Student No. 8, Response 1)*

Discussion earlier focused on the preparation of mentors and the NMC has identified that mentors will need regular updating of both skills and curriculum development (NMC 2003). Darling (1984) developed the 'Measuring Mentorship Potential' scale, which assesses the mentoring potential of the mentor. However, there is no proposal at this stage by the NMC for any formal assessment of mentor skills.

From the author's perspective, there is currently a system in place whereby a percentage of students' CAP documents are reviewed by a 'scrutiny panel'. The panel consists of Adult Branch of Practice Placement Facilitators (PPFs), and its aim is to assess the effectiveness of the implementation of the mentorship process in relation to completion of the documentation. Feedback from this panel is given to mentors in general via mentorship workshop study days run by the PPFs. This system can be said to address some issues in relation to assessment of mentor ability. However, there are shortfalls. In particular, the documentation does not always reflect the discussion that has taken place between mentor and student. The written content will not always provide a clear picture of how the material has been interpreted by the mentor and on what they have subsequently based their assessment. Also in some ways the mentor is asked to assess academic rather than practical work which is not the aim of placement experience.

The emphasis on practice assessment is growing. This needs to account for 50 per cent of a student's marks for the course (Bradshaw 2000) and therefore needs to be both reliable and valid. Having a clear strategy for assessing mentor ability must surely be a way of promoting further quality assurance in practice assessment.

Moving on from this point to what is probably the main issue highlighted by the students in this study, that of time/contact with the mentor. As stated earlier, nine of the twelve students interviewed cited time as the main factor affecting the quality of mentorship they had received. Two of the students that didn't specify time as an issue identified the off-duty rota and contact with the mentor as a problem. Examples of the students' experience are:

'I think time plays a big part as well ... and I can realize that [the mentors] it isn't always possible to dedicate time to your students, and you've got to be more autonomous in your own role as a student and think, well, I can get on with this and that within your own limitations.'   (*Student No. 3, Response 2*)

'Time. They're just ... too busy to have a student under their wing. Shift patterns as well.'   (*Student No. 5, Response 2*)

'I'd say the rota and who they put you on with.'   (*Student No. 2, Response 1*)

'It's like for example the last mentor, they didn't give us mentors until I was like Week Three and then they gave me someone who was off on holiday for two weeks.'   (*Student No. 2, Response 2*)

Issues of time and contact with the mentor have been investigated in a number of studies (see Marrow and Tatum 1994; Wilson–Barnett et al. 1995. Spouse 1996; Coates and Gormley 1997; Gordon and Grundy 1997) and it is the conflicting roles and responsibilities that are identified as the cause of this by both the mentor and student. Time required to mentor a student has been found to be extensive, especially when the student is not achieving (Duffy 2004), therefore strategies to support time for mentoring need to be available.

Protected time for mentoring is not something that has been built into the mentor role. However, structuring the allocation of students to mentors may help to solve this issue. Students interviewed for the study asserted that having two mentors was particularly useful in redressing contact and time problems for the mentor. Here they give examples of their experiences:

'I had my mentor, who was fantastic and I had an associate mentor who was even more brilliant so I always worked with my mentor or associate mentor, and if they weren't on ... they arranged for me to go off somewhere to observe, say, the alcohol advisor.'   (*Student No. 5, Response 3*)

'Definitely the two mentors ... sometimes it's difficult, especially with a lot of nurses working the long days now, they might be at work (at the) beginning of the week and you're in at the end of the week, so it makes it easier actually to work with a mentor, and it gives you a bit more ... a couple of different perspectives to nursing.'   (*Student No. 8, Response 4*)

'Because you're only on the placement like two days one week, three days the other week, if they're part-time or they're working a weekend, you can't always work their shifts with them so I think when you've got two, you can play around with their shifts a bit more and then you've nearly always got a mentor ...'
(*Student No. 10, Response 2*)

The literature also presents arguments for and against the organization of mentorship on a two-mentor basis. Woodrow (1994) advocates the use of 'diffuse mentoring' whereby a system of mentor and associate mentor is used for each student. However, this system is described as less effective by Andrews and Chilton (2000), as neither mentor takes complete responsibility for the mentoring process.

Lloyd-Jones et al. (2001) found that, from a contact point of view, if a mentor was on duty with a student, the latter spent significantly more time in education-related activities. Currently, the 'helix' system is in use in the researcher's local area and until this is changed with the revalidation of the course, a two-mentor system would appear to be the most appropriate in ensuring more effective mentoring of the student. Once the 'helix' system is replaced and the students undertake a block system of allocations, the students should then find it easier to work the same shift pattern as the mentor. Using the two-mentor system at this time would still be useful from the point of view of providing the student with extra support and the mentor with feedback on the student's performance. This would also help mentors manage mentorship alongside all their other roles and responsibilities. Taking responsibility for the student must however be seen as a priority for mentors.

Specifying which mentor is assigned to which student may also help. Students in the study identified that the more senior staff, such as 'F'-grade mentors, had even greater responsibilities within the placement setting. Students felt that 'D'- and 'E'-grade mentors were more effective because of this. One student describes her experience of being mentored by an 'F'-grade nurse:

> 'I think that it means that the student can actually miss out on some … aspects of medicine rounds and things like that 'cos coordinating the ward, there's no way they can also go do like ward rounds … or medicine rounds … or do dressing changes … 'cos obviously they're busy coordinating the ward, so I think that makes a difference between like D grades or E grades …' (*Student No. 6, Response 2*)

Supporting evidence for this is again found in the literature (Earnshaw 1995; Andrews and Wallis 1999).

The study showed that there was no specific system for allocating students to mentors in specific grades and it appeared rather that whoever might be available to mentor at that time was allocated to the student. As all the students interviewed were only halfway through their third year, they seem to have preferred more junior grades of staff to mentor them so far. Certainly, there is clear evidence from this study that certain issues are affecting the quality of mentorship in practice. To some extent, these could be easily resolved if a more structured approach to the mentorship system was put in place.

Limitations of the study

The main limitation of this study was the sample size used. Burns and Grove (1997) suggest that 'a small sample size may better serve the researcher who is interested in examining the situation in depth from various perspectives.' This author, however, would have preferred to have increased the number of student nurses interviewed to ensure that data saturation had been reached. Unfortunately, due to time constraints in completing the study, this was not possible. A further 13 students will be interviewed over the next two months in order to further this research.

The author also recognized that the 'Hawthorne' effect may compromise the study. Polit and Hungler (1999) describe how 'the knowledge of being included in a study may be sufficient to cause people to change their behaviour, thereby obscuring the effect of the variable of interest.'

Also, the fact that the students were from the same cohort meant that a number of them were on the same placement at the time of interviewing. This meant that they had every opportunity to discuss the interviews and possibly influence each other's responses. On reflection, the author did not believe that this had occurred as very open discussions took place during the interviews and each individual student had clearly had very different placements and very different experiences.

Another limitation to the design of the study was in the chosen analysis. In the analysis by Colaizzi (1978; cited by Holloway and Wheeler 1998), it is suggested that participants are asked for a second interview in order to validate the findings of the original interview. The author found this particularly difficult as some students were unavailable when a second interview was requested, due to summer annual leave. Telephone discussions were therefore used to discuss findings with a limited number of students only.

The author being a novice researcher also limited the study. In particular, she felt that her interviewing technique might not have been wholly effective at eliciting the required data and she was conscious of over-clarifying what students were saying. It would have been useful to observe another experienced researcher prior to undertaking this study or to have read interview transcripts to see another researcher's technique.

Recommendations for practice

The Department of Health document, *Making a Difference* (DoH 1999), underlined the need to enhance student nurse competence in order to ensure 'fitness for practice at the point of registration'. An essential component in achieving this was identified as the supervision and support that was available to the student in the practice environment. Since the publication of this document, a number of strategies have been put in place aimed at enhancing the delivery of effective mentorship support for student nurses. This research project aimed to evaluate the effectiveness of the situation to date and its results clearly highlighted a number of conclusions that can be drawn, along with some key recommendations for practice.

Overall, the quality of mentorship that students received in practice was in essence more positive than negative. From the author's perspective, the study proved to be a valuable exercise in clarifying that there is some excellent support in placements for students.

Students were aware of what the mentorship role involved, although they seemed to have gained this knowledge through being involved in the system rather than through formal instruction. The mentorship role has remained fairly unchanged over the last twenty years although, with the new curriculum based on the 'Fitness for Practice' (1999) recommendations, there was a clear requirement to be competent in clinical skills and to develop critical thinking in order to question practice.

Most student nurses felt that the mentor was the best person to assess them although they highlighted a number of difficulties associated with this. Firstly, the large number of students now in training and subsequently allocated to each placement meant that there were not always enough mentors to support them. Sometimes students did not have the required level of supervision from a qualified mentor. Working alongside unqualified staff was often the solution to this. Although the students recognized that there was value in working with unqualified staff, they felt they were missing out on the theoretical component of practice experience.

Of great concern is that staff and sometimes mentor attitudes towards student nurses were not always positive and some students found that such negativity affected their confidence to perform and challenge practice. As students are the workforce of the future, it is difficult to understand this. Challenging practice is clearly a vital element for both student and mentor to undertake and needs to be a positive and welcome experience for both. Being unable to challenge practice can lead to a frustrating and dangerous situation and will inevitably compromise standards of practice.

Mentor preparation programmes have not always provided a national quality of mentorship training (Chambers 1998); however, the NMC (2003) has made recent recommendations as to the level of these courses. Although the majority of mentors will have attended such courses, the study shows that this does not always equip them to mentor the student effectively. Changes to curriculum and confusing documentation continue to make assessment in practice difficult. The study showed that at times the mentor had become blasé about the assessment process and this was often due to the numerous other roles and responsibilities that the mentor had.

Assessing the mentors' ability to mentor was considered in the study and, although local systems such as the scrutiny panel are in place, there are potential pitfalls as described earlier. The supervision and assessment of practice is crucial in ensuring fitness for practice and it will be interesting to see if the NMC feels that assessing mentors is necessary.

Time and contact with the mentor was probably the most common problem identified within the study as affecting the quality of mentorship. Recognizing early on in training that mentors had conflicting responsibilities, students realized that they had unrealistic expectations of the process. Student nurses subsequently learned strategies to accommodate this, some of which did not always enhance their experience.

With these issues in mind the author felt that the following recommendations would be useful in supporting the mentorship process in the future. Most student nurses at the start of their nursing career currently have limited education and training on the role of the mentor and what to expect in practice. This is currently delivered mainly by PPFs. A more informative and realistic information session needs to be included prior to students' first placement experience with a troubleshooting section to help with known problems that may arise.

As part of the author's role, campaigning to encourage staff onto mentorship training is an ongoing process. The aim of this is to increase mentor numbers in the future. However, only a limited number of places are currently available at the local university for this training and an increase in place numbers is recommended to enable as many staff as possible to enter formal mentor preparation. Recruitment and retention of all staff is vital to maintaining the workforce and in particular the older workforce needs to be valued and recognized for its wealth of experience. Strategies to support this should be put in place through appraisal systems and a focus on retention of staff. The implementation of *Agenda for Change* (DoH 2003) is imminent and may support the recommendation here. In reality, there may always be times when unqualified staff need to support student nurses in practice. It is therefore recommended that training should be available at this staff level. This may also eliminate some of the attitude problems and help unqualified staff recognize the importance of the student nurse training.

Streamlining the allocation process of mentor to student may have a more immediate effect on solving some of the issues related to time and contact with the mentor. Making better use of available mentors with consideration given to the grade of the mentor could help to make more effective use of all staff. Student coordinators are in place in all placement areas locally, and recommendations for this process can be made at time-out days in the future.

Again as part of the PPF role, the author reviews the availability of new placements for students. Also, in partnership with the university, the ability of placements to increase the numbers of students is dependent on numbers of mentors. Using placements in innovative ways needs to be pursued, again with staff education and training, to see how, for example, rotating students to other areas can help both to support the student experience but also to increase available places.

Ensuring that all changes to student practice documentation are made in partnership with practice staff is highly recommended and limiting the academic jargon of these documents is vital for the mentorship process. Using different strategies to assess practice, such as the OSCEs (Objective Structured Clinical Examinations), is also recommended so that practice assessment is not always undertaken by a mentor. This is currently under discussion with the local university as part of the revalidation of the course.

Finally, the NMC's (2004) current 'Consultation on a Standard to Support Learning and Assessment in Practice' can only help to give greater credence to mentorship roles. With support from the professional body, this author feels that in time mentors will value their role more and understand how implementing the mentorship process can lead to a higher standard in practice throughout the profession.

Recommendations for further research

The author found the undertaking of this research to be a fascinating process and has identified a number of research questions that could be investigated in the future:

- further exploration of students' first experience in practice would be useful to investigate, including identifying the numbers of students that leave training at this time due to placement experience;
- investigating the mentors' views on the quality of mentorship they are able to provide would be interesting as a comparison with the students' evaluation;
- investigating the effectiveness of the Practice Placement Facilitator role and asking mentors to identify what they want from this role;
- investigating whether older nurses feel valued in the workplace;
- investigating whether recommendations from this study, once implemented, are effective in raising the quality of mentorship in practice.

References

Andrews, M. and Chilton, F. (2000) Student and mentor perceptions of mentoring effectiveness. *Nurse Education Today*, **20**: 555–62.

Andrews, M. and Wallis, M. (1999) Mentorship in nursing: a literature review. *Journal of Advanced Nursing*, **29** (1): 201–7.

Armitage, P. and Burnard, P. (1991) Mentors or preceptors? Narrowing the theory-practice gap. *Nurse Education Today*, **11**: 225–9.

Atkins, S. and Williams, A. (1995) Registered nurses' experiences of mentoring undergraduate nursing students. *Journal of Advanced Nursing*, **21**: 1006–15.

Baillie, L. (1993) Factors affecting student nurses' learning in community placements: a phenomenological study. *Journal of Advanced Nursing*, **18**: 1043–53.

Baillie, L. (1996) A phenomenological study of the nature of empathy. *Journal of Advanced Nursing*, **24** (6): 1300–8.

Barlow, S. (1991) Impossible dream. *Nursing Times*, **87** (1): 53–4.

Bradshaw, P. L. (2000) Fitness for practice. *Journal of Nursing Management*, **8** (1): 1–2.

Buchan, J. (1999) The 'greying' of the United Kingdom nursing workforce: implications for employment policy and practice. *Journal of Advanced Nursing*, **30** (4): 818–26.

Burnard, P. (1991) The student experience: adult learning and mentorship revisited. *Nurse Education Today*, **10**: 349–54.

Burns, N. and Grove, S. (1997) *The Practice of Nursing Research: Conduct, Critique and Utilization* (London: Sage).

Burns, N. and Grove, S. K. (2001) *The Practice of Nursing Research: Conduct, Critique and Utilization*, 4th edn (New York: W. B. Saunders).

Cahill, H. A. (1996) A qualitative analysis of student nurses' experiences of mentorship. *Journal of Advanced Nursing*, **24**: 791–9.

Calman, L., Watson, R., Norman, I., Redfern, S. and Murrells, T. (2002) Assessing practice of student nurses: methods, preparation of assessors and student view. *Journal of Advanced Nursing*, **38** (5): 516–23.

Cameron-Jones, M. and O'Hara, P. (1996) Three decisions about nurse mentoring. *Journal of Nursing Management*, **4** (4): 225–30.

Chambers, M. (1998) Some issues in the assessment of clinical practice: a review of the literature. *Journal of Clinical Nursing*, **3**: 201–8.

Clark, A. M. (1998) The qualitative–quantitative debate: moving from positivism and confrontation to post-positivism and reconciliation. *Journal of Advanced Nursing*, **27**: 1242–9.

Coates, V. E. and Gormley, E. (1997) Learning the practice of nursing: views about preceptorship. *Nurse Education Today*, **17**: 91–8.

Colaizzi, P. (1978) Psychological research as a phenomenologist views it. In *Existential Phenomenological Alternatives for Psychology*, ed. R. Valle and M. Kings (New York: Oxford University Press); cited in by I. Holloway and S. Wheeler (1998) *Qualitative Research for Nurses* (Oxford: Blackwell Publishing).

Corben, V. (1999) Misusing phenomenology in nursing research: identifying the issues. *Nurse Researcher*, **6** (3): 52–66.

Cotty, M. (1996) Tradition and culture in Heidegger's being and time. *Nursing Inquiry*, **4** (2): 88–98.

Daloz, L. A. (1987) *Effective Teaching and Mentoring* (San Francisco, CA: Jossey-Bass); cited by N. Northcott (2000) Mentorship in nursing. *Nursing Management*, **7** (3): 30–2.

Darling, L. A. W. (1984) What do nurses want in a mentor? *Journal of Nursing Administration*, **3** (2).

Darling, L. A. W. (1985) What to do about toxic mentors. *Journal of Nursing Administration*, May: 43–4.

DoH (1999) *Making a Difference: Strengthening the Nursing, Midwifery and Health Visitor Contribution to Health and Healthcare* (London: Department of Health).

DoH (2000) *The NHS Plan. A Plan for Investment: A Plan for Reform* (London: Department of Health).

DoH (2003) *Agenda for Change: Proposed Agreement* (London: Department of Health).

Dolan, G. (2003) Assessing student nurse clinical competency: will we ever get it right? *Journal of Clinical Nursing*, **12** (1): 132–44.

Donovan, J. (1990) The concept and role of mentor. *Nurse Education Today*, **10** (4): 294–8.

Dreyfuss, H. (1987) Husserl, Heidegger and modern existentialism. In *The Great Philosophers: An Introduction to Western Philosophy*, ed. B. Magee (London: BBC Books) cited by A. J. Walters (1995) The phenomenological movement: implications for nursing research. *Journal of Advanced Nursing*, **22**: 791–9.

Duffy, K. (2004) *Failing Students*. www.nmc-uk.org

Dunn, S. and Hansford, B. (1997) Undergraduate nursing students' perceptions of their clinical learning environment. *Journal of Advanced Nursing*, **25** (6): 1299–1306.

Earnshaw, G. J. (1995) Mentorship: the students' views. *Nurse Education Today*, **15**: 274–9.

ENB (2000) Practice and Assessment: An evaluation of the assessment of practice at diploma, degree and post-graduate level in pre- and post-registration nursing and midwifery education. *Research Highlights* No. 43 (London: ENB).

ENB and DoH (2001a) *Preparation of Mentors and Teachers* (London: ENB/DoH).

ENB and DoH (2001b) *Placements in Focus* (London: ENB/DoH).

Ewan, C. and White, R. (1996) *Teaching Nursing – A Self-Instructional Handbook*, 2nd edn (London: Chapman and Hall); cited by A. Morton-Cooper and A. Palmer (2000) *Mentoring, Preceptorship and Clinical Supervision: A Guide to Professional Roles in Clinical Practice* (Cambridge, MA: Blackwell Publishing).

Farrell, G. A. (1997) Aggression in clinical settings: nurses' views. *Journal of Advanced Nursing*, **25**: 501–8.

Fields, H. (1994) Coaching and Mentoring. *Nursing Standard*, **8** (30): 106–12.

Freshwater, D. (2000) Cross-currents: against cultural narration in nursing. *Journal of Advanced Nursing*, **32** (2): 481–6.

Gilloran, A. (1995) Gender differences in care delivery and supervisory relationship: the case of psycho-geriatric nursing. *Journal of Advanced Nursing*, **21** (4): 652–8.

Gordon, M. F. and Grundy, M. (1997) From apprenticeship to academia: an adult branch programme. *Nurse Education Today*, **17**: 162–7.

Gray, M. and Smith, L. N. (1999) The professional socialization of diploma of higher education in nursing students (Project 2000): a longitudinal qualitative study. *Journal of Advanced Nursing*, **29** (3): 639–47.

Gray, M. A. and Smith, L. N. (2000) The qualities of an effective mentor from the student nurse's perspective: findings from a longitudinal qualitative study. *Journal of Advanced Nursing*, **32** (6): 1542–9.

Guba, E. and Lincoln, Y. (1989) *Fourth Generation Evaluation* (Newbury Park, CA: Sage Publications); cited by L. Whitehead (2004) Enhancing the quality of hermeneutic research: decision trail. *Journal of Advanced Nursing*, **45** (5): 512–18.

Hagerty, B. (1986) A second look at mentors. *Nursing Outlook*, **34** (1): 16–24; cited by M. Andrews and M. Wallis (1999) Mentorship in nursing: a literature review. *Journal of Advanced Nursing*, **29** (1): 201–7.

Hallett, C. (1995) Understanding the phenomenological approach to research. *Nurse Researcher*, **3** (2): 55–65.

Holloway, I. and Wheeler, S. (1998) *Qualitative Research for Nurses* (Oxford: Blackwell Science).

Jackson, D. and Mannix, J. (2001) Clinical nurse teachers: insights from students of nursing in their first semester of study. *Journal of Clinical Nursing*, **10** (2): 270–7.

Knapp, T. (1998) *Quantitative Nursing Research* (New York: Sage Publications).

Lloyd Jones, M., Walters, S. and Akehurst, R. (2001) The implications of contact with the mentor for pre-registration nursing and midwifery. *Journal of Advanced Nursing*, **35** (2): 151–60.

Lofmark, A. and Wikbald, K. (2001) Facilitating and obstructing factors for development of learning in clinical practice: a student perspective. *Journal of Advanced Nursing*, **34** (1): 43–50.

Lord, M. (2002) Making a difference: the implications for nurse education. *Nursing Times*, **98** (20): 38–40.

Mackenzie, J. (1997) 'A thorny problem for feminism': an analysis of the subjective work experiences of enrolled nurses. *Journal of Clinical Nursing*, **6** (5): 365–70.

Macleod Clark, J. (1998) Education for the future. *Nursing Management*, **5**.

Marriot, A. (1991) The support, supervision and instruction of nurse learners in clinical areas: a literature review. *Nurse Education Today*, **11**: 261–9.

Marrow, C. E. (1997) Primary nursing and student supervision: exemplars in practice. *Nurse Education Today*, **17**: 333–337.

Marrow, C. E. and Tatum, S. (1994) Student supervision: myth or reality? *Journal of Advanced Nursing*, **19**: 1247–55.

Merriam, S. (1983) Mentors and proteges: a critical review of the literature. *Adult Education Quarterly* 33: 161–73; cited by M. A. Gray and L. N. Smith (2000) The qualities of an effective mentor from the student nurse's perspective: findings from a longitudinal qualitative study. *Journal of Advanced Nursing*, **32** (6): 1542–9.

Morgan, R. (2002) Giving the student the confidence to take part. *Nursing Times*, **98** (35): 36–7.

Morle, K. M. F. (1990) Mentorship – is it a case of the emperor's new clothes or a rose by any other name? *Nurse Education Today*, **10**: 66–9.

Morton-Cooper, A. and Palmer, A. (2000) *Mentoring, Preceptorship and Clinical Supervision: A Guide to Professional Roles in Clinical Practice* (New York: Blackwell Sciences).

Muldoon, O. T. and Reilly, J. (2003) Career choice in nursing students: gendered constructs as psychological barriers. *Journal of Advanced Nursing*, **43** (1): 93–100.

Munhall, P. L. (2001) Ethical considerations in qualitative research. *Western Journal of Nursing Research*, **10** (2): 150–62.

Myrick, F. and Yonge, O. J. (2001) Creating a climate for critical thinking in the preceptorship experience. *Nurse Education Today*, **21**: 461–7.

Neary, M. (1999) Preparing assessors for continuous assessment. *Nursing Standard*, **13** (18): 41–7.

Neary, M. (2000a) Supporting students' learning and professional development through the process of continuous assessment and mentorship. *Nurse Education Today*, **20**: 463–74.

Neary, M. (2000b) Responsive assessment of clinical competence: part 1. *Nursing Standard*, **15** (9): 34–6.

Neary, M., Phillips, R. and Davies, B. (1996) The introduction of mentorship to Project 2000 in Wales. *Nursing Standard*, **10** (25): 37–9.

NMC (2003) *NMC Requirements for Mentors and Mentorship: NMC and QA Factsheet O/2003* (London: NMC).

NMC (2004) *Consultation on a Standard to Support Learning and Assessment in Practice* (London: NMC).

Nolan, C. A. (1998) Learning on clinical placement: the experience of six Australian student nurses. *Nurse Education Today*, **18**: 622–9.

Northcott, N. (2000) Mentorship in nursing. *Nursing Management*, **7** (3): 30–2.

Nunnally, J. C. and Bernstein, I. H. (1994) *Psychometric Theory*, 3rd edn (New York: McGraw-Hill); cited by T. Knapp (1998) *Quantitative Nursing Research* (New York: Sage Publications).

Phillips, R. M., Davies W. B. and Neary M. (1996a) The practitioner–teacher: a study in the introduction of mentors in the pre-registration nurse education programme in Wales: part 1. *Journal of Advanced Nursing*, **23** (5): 1037–44.

Phillips, R. M., Davies, W. B. and Neary, M. (1996b) The practitioner–teacher: a study in the introduction of mentors in the pre-registration nurse education programme in Wales: part 2. *Journal of Advanced Nursing*, **23** (5): 1080–8.

Polit, D. F. and Hungler, B. (1997) *Nursing Research: Methods, Appraisal and Utilization*, 4th edn (Philadelphia: Lippincott).

Polit, D. F. and Hungler, B. (1999) *Nursing Research: Principles and Methods*, 6th edn (Philadelphia: Lippincott).

RCN (2002) *Helping Students Get the Best from their Practice Placements: A Royal College of Nursing Toolkit* (London: Royal College of Nursing).

Reed, J. (1994) Phenomenology without phenomena: a discussion of the use of phenomenology to examine expertise in long-term care of elderly patients. *Journal of Advanced Nursing*, **19**: 336–41.

Robson, C. (1995) *Real World Research. A Resource for Social Scientists and Practitioner-Researchers* (Oxford: Blackwell Publishing).

Ryan, D. and Brewer, K. (1997) Mentorship and professional role development in undergraduate nursing education. *Nurse Educator*, **22** (6): 22–4.

Silverman, D. (1998) *Qualitative Research: Theory, Method and Practice* (London: Sage Publications).

Silverman, D. (2000) *Doing Qualitative Research: A Practical Handbook* (London: Sage Publications).

Spouse, J. (1996) The effective mentor: a model for student-centred learning in clinical practice. *Nursing Times Research*, **1** (2): 34–8.

Spouse, J. (1998) Learning to nurse through legitimate peripheral participation. *Nurse Education Today*, **18**: 345–51.

Spouse, J. (2001) Workplace learning: preregistration nursing student perspectives. *Nurse Education in Practice*, **1** (3): 149–56.

Stew, G. (1996) New meanings: a qualitative study of change in nursing education. *Journal of Advanced Nursing*, **23** (3): 587–93.

Stuart, C. C. (2003) *Assessment, Supervision and Support in Clinical Practice: A Guide for Nurses, Midwives and other Health Professionals* (London: Churchill Livingstone).

Suen, L. K. P. and Chow, F. L.W. (2001) Students' perceptions of the effectiveness of mentors in an undergraduate nursing programme in Hong Kong. *Journal of Advanced Nursing*, **36** (4): 505–11.

Tarling, M. and Crofts, L. (1998) *The Essential Researcher's Handbook: For Nurses and Health Care Professionals* (London: Bailliere Tindall).

UKCC (1986) *Project 2000: A New Preparation for Practice* (London: UKCC).

UKCC (1999) *Fitness for Practice: The UKCC Commission for Nursing and Midwifery Education* (London: UKCC).

University of Hull (2002) *Policy 8.2: Guidelines for Practice Placements: Assessment of Practice, Pre-registration*, Faculty of Health and Social Care, University of Hull, Hull.

Van der Zalm, J. and Bergum, V. (2000) Hermeneutic-phenomenology: providing living knowledge for nursing practice. *Journal of Advanced Nursing*, **31** (1): 211–18.

Waddell, K. (1995) Gender: nursing a gender. *Nursing Standard*, **9** (30): 62.

Walters, A. J. (1995) The phenomenological movement: implications for nursing research. *Journal of Advanced Nursing*, **22**: 791–9.

Watkins, M. (2000) Competency for nursing practice. *Journal of Clinical Nursing*, **9** (3): 338–46.

Watson, N. (1999) Mentoring today – the students' views: an investigative case study of pre-registration nursing students' experiences and perceptions of mentoring in one theory/practice module of the Common foundation programme on a Project 2000 course. *Journal of Advanced Nursing*, **29** (1): 254–62.

Watson, S. (2000) The support that mentors receive in the clinical setting. *Nurse Education Today*, **20**: 585–92.

Webb, C. (2002) Feminism, nursing and education. *Journal of Advanced Nursing*, **39** (2): 111–13.

Welsh, I. and Swann, C. (2002) *Partners in Learning: A Guide to Support and Assessment in Nurse Education* (Abingdon: Radcliffe Medical Press).

Wengraf, T. (2001) *Qualitative Research Interviewing* (London: Sage Publications).

While, A. (1996) Strengths in diversity. *Nursing Standard*, **10** (15): 51.

Whitehead, J. (2001) Newly qualified staff nurses' perceptions of the role transition. *British Journal of Nursing*, **8** (5): 330–9.

Whitehead, D. (2002) The academic writing experiences of a group of student nurses: a phenomenological study. *Journal of Advanced Nursing*, **38** (5): 498–506.

Whitehead, L. (2004) Enhancing the quality of hermeneutic research: decision trail. *Journal of Advanced Nursing*, **45** (5): 512–18.

Whiting, L. (2001) Analysis of phenomenological data: personal reflections on Giorgio's method. *Journal of Advanced Nursing*, **9** (2): 60–74.

Wilson-Barnett, J., Butterworth, T., White, E., Twinn, S., Davies, S. and Riley, L. (1995) Clinical support and the Project 2000 nursing student: factors influencing the process. *Journal of Advanced Nursing*, **21**: 1152–8.

Woodrow, P. (1994) Mentorship: perceptions and pitfalls for nursing practice. *Journal of Advanced Nursing*, **19**: 812–18.

Woodrow, P. (1999) Pulse oximetry: continuing professional development article 501. *Nursing Standard*, **13** (42): 42–6.

Index